Advances in Occupational Health and Safety Management

Advances in Occupational Health and Safety Management

Editor

Delfina Gabriela Garrido Ramos

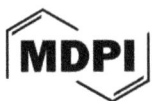

Basel • Beijing • Wuhan • Barcelona • Belgrade • Novi Sad • Cluj • Manchester

Editor
Delfina Gabriela Garrido Ramos
School of Engineering (ISEP)
Polytechnic of Porto
Porto, Portugal

Editorial Office
MDPI
St. Alban-Anlage 66
4052 Basel, Switzerland

This is a reprint of articles from the Special Issue published online in the open access journal *International Journal of Environmental Research and Public Health* (ISSN 1660-4601) (available at: https://www.mdpi.com/journal/ijerph/special_issues/OHSM).

For citation purposes, cite each article independently as indicated on the article page online and as indicated below:

Lastname, A.A.; Lastname, B.B. Article Title. *Journal Name* **Year**, *Volume Number*, Page Range.

ISBN 978-3-0365-9170-4 (Hbk)
ISBN 978-3-0365-9171-1 (PDF)
doi.org/10.3390/books978-3-0365-9171-1

© 2023 by the authors. Articles in this book are Open Access and distributed under the Creative Commons Attribution (CC BY) license. The book as a whole is distributed by MDPI under the terms and conditions of the Creative Commons Attribution-NonCommercial-NoDerivs (CC BY-NC-ND) license.

Contents

About the Editor vii

Preface ix

Delfina Ramos, Teresa Cotrim, Pedro Arezes, João Baptista, Matilde Rodrigues and João Leitão
Frontiers in Occupational Health and Safety Management
Reprinted from: *Int. J. Environ. Res. Public Health* **2022**, *19*, 10759, doi:10.3390/ijerph191710759 . 1

Ana Pimenta, Delfina Ramos, Gilberto Santos, Matilde A. Rodrigues and Manuel Doiro
Psychosocial Risks in Teachers from Portugal and England on the Way to Society 5.0
Reprinted from: *Int. J. Environ. Res. Public Health* **2023**, *20*, 6347, doi:10.3390/ijerph20146347 . . . 7

Delfina Ramos and Luis Almeida
Managing Nanomaterials in the Workplace by Using the Control Banding Approach †
Reprinted from: *Int. J. Environ. Res. Public Health* **2023**, *20*, 6011, doi:10.3390/ijerph20116011 . . . 19

Francisco Edison Sampaio, Manuel Joaquim Silva Oliveira, João Areosa and Emílio Facas
Prevalence of Comorbidity and Its Effects on Sickness-Absenteeism among Brazilian Legislative Civil Servants
Reprinted from: *Int. J. Environ. Res. Public Health* **2023**, *20*, 5036, doi:10.3390/ijerph20065036 . . . 29

Valentin Marian Antohi, Romeo Victor Ionescu, Monica Laura Zlati, Catalina Iticescu, Puiu Lucian Georgescu and Madalina Calmuc
Regional Regression Correlation Model of Microplastic Water Pollution Control Using Circular Economy Tools
Reprinted from: *Int. J. Environ. Res. Public Health* **2023**, *20*, 4014, doi:10.3390/ijerph20054014 . . . 41

Arie Arizandi Kurnianto, Gergely Fehér, Kevin Efrain Tololiu, Edza Aria Wikurendra, Zsolt Nemeskéri and István Ágoston
Analysis of the Return to Work Program for Disabled Workers during the Pandemic COVID-19 Using the Quality of Life and Work Ability Index: Cross-Sectional Study
Reprinted from: *Int. J. Environ. Res. Public Health* **2023**, *20*, 3094, doi:10.3390/ijerph20043094 . . . 65

Łukasz Jarosław Kozar and Adam Sulich
Green Jobs: Bibliometric Review
Reprinted from: *Int. J. Environ. Res. Public Health* **2023**, *20*, 2886, doi:10.3390/ijerph20042886 . . . 79

Marta Sousa, Pedro Arezes and Francisco Silva
Occupational Exposure to Incidental Nanomaterials in Metal Additive Manufacturing: An Innovative Approach for Risk Management
Reprinted from: *Int. J. Environ. Res. Public Health* **2023**, *20*, 2519, doi:10.3390/ijerph20032519 . . . 95

Farida Saleem and Muhammad Imran Malik
Safety Management and Safety Performance Nexus: Role of Safety Consciousness, Safety Climate, and Responsible Leadership
Reprinted from: *Int. J. Environ. Res. Public Health* **2022**, *19*, 13686, doi:10.3390/ijerph192013686 . 117

Dina Pereira, João Leitão and Ludovina Ramos
Burnout and Quality of Work Life among Municipal Workers: Do Motivating and Economic Factors Play a Mediating Role?
Reprinted from: *Int. J. Environ. Res. Public Health* **2022**, *19*, 13035, doi:10.3390/ijerph192013035 . 139

Xifeng Lu, Haijing Yu and Biaoan Shan
Relationship between Employee Mental Health and Job Performance: Mediation Role of Innovative Behavior and Work Engagement
Reprinted from: *Int. J. Environ. Res. Public Health* **2022**, *19*, 6599, doi:10.3390/ijerph19116599 . . . **157**

Suresh Sukumar, Shovan Saha, Winniecia Dkhar, Nitika C. Panakkal, Visakh Thrivikraman Nair, Tulasiram Bommasamudram, et al.
Knowledge of Medical Imaging Professionals on Healthcare-Associated Infections: A Systematic Review and Meta-Analysis
Reprinted from: *Int. J. Environ. Res. Public Health* **2023**, *20*, 4326, doi:10.3390/ijerph20054326 . . . **169**

About the Editor

Delfina Gabriela Garrido Ramos

Delfina Ramos holds a PhD in Industrial and Systems Engineering from the University of Minho. She also holds the title of Professor Honoris Causa at the University of Tourism and Management in Skopje, Macedonia. Additionally, she is an Invited Professor at the Institute of Engineering of Porto (ISEP). She conducts research as part of the Center ALGORITMI in the Industrial Engineering and Management (IEM) group, focusing on Ergonomics and Human Factors at the School of Engineering, University of Minho. She is also involved in research at the Associate Laboratory for Energy, Transports and Aerospace (LAETA-INEGI) at the University of Porto. Her research work centers around various areas including occupational health and safety, integrated management systems quality, environment and occupational health and safety, sustainability, project management, human factors and ergonomics, benchmarking, nanotechnologies, circular economy, and tourism. Delfina Ramos is an experienced auditor and consultant. She is a Certified Health and Safety High Technician and a senior member of the Professional Association of Engineers of Portugal. She also holds membership of the National Council of the College of Chemical and Biological Engineering for the 2022–2025 term. Moreover, she is a member of CT194 (Technical Commission for the Standardization of Nanotechnologies—SC4—Health, Safety, and Environment) at the Portuguese Quality Institute (IPQ). Delfina Ramos has earned specializations in Safety Engineering and Industrial Engineering and Management, both recognized by the Order of Engineers of Portugal.

Preface

In an increasingly interconnected world, partnerships between universities and corporations emerge as pivotal agents of change. Their collaborative efforts wield a profound impact on the global pursuit of the Sustainable Development Goals (SDGs). This book serves as a testament to the critical role they play in shaping our future, revealing significant market opportunities across diverse research domains.

The year 2021 marked a profound transformation in how we perceive and address safety and health in the workplace. On the occasion of the World Day for Safety and Health at Work, the International Labour Organization (ILO) issued a clarion call to nations worldwide. This call implored them to strengthen their occupational safety and health (OSH) systems, ensuring resilience to confront future health crises effectively. The solution, we are told, lies in substantial investments in OSH infrastructure, seamlessly integrated into comprehensive national emergency preparedness and response plans. The overarching objective is to safeguard the well-being of workers while fortifying the foundations of business continuity.

Within these pages, you will embark on a journey of exploration into the ever-evolving landscape of work environments. As economic challenges test our resolve, a resounding message echoes forth from the European Agency for Safety and Health at Work (EU-OSHA): the cost of inadequate occupational safety and health measures is not solely human but also financial. Furthermore, a multitude of case studies unveiled in this volume illustrate a direct correlation between proficient OSH management within organizations and the enhancement of overall performance and profitability.

This book, a collaborative endeavor of diverse contributors from around the globe, casts a wide net over the realms of Advances in Occupational Health and Safety Management and Risk Management. It aspires to provide a holistic view of these domains, shedding light on their multifaceted intricacies. It delves into topics as varied as the mechanics of occupational health and safety management systems, the art of risk assessment, the cultivation of resilient systems, the influence of psychosocial factors, the impact of human factors and ergonomics, the criticality of cost-benefit analysis, and the imperative for accident prevention.

But this book transcends the ordinary. It casts its gaze into the horizon of emerging risks with profound health and safety implications. It unravels the intricacies of navigating the circular economy, digitization, nanomaterials, green jobs, and telework, examining their potential effects on worker well-being. Furthermore, it navigates the uncharted waters of artificial intelligence in occupational health and safety management and delves into the implications of Industry 4.0 on the health and safety of the workforce.

As we embark on this collective odyssey through the pages that follow, let us remember that the pursuit of knowledge is a journey, not a destination. May the insights contained herein serve as beacons, guiding us toward a future where the principles of safety, health, and sustainability form the bedrock of our endeavors.

Let us delve deep, challenge conventions, and emerge armed with the wisdom and innovation needed to shape a world where every workplace is a haven of safety, every task is infused with purpose, and every individual's well-being is protected.

Delfina Gabriela Garrido Ramos
Editor

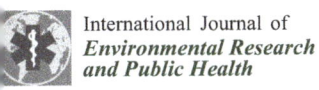

Editorial

Frontiers in Occupational Health and Safety Management

Delfina Ramos [1,2,3,*], Teresa Cotrim [4,5], Pedro Arezes [3], João Baptista [2,6,7], Matilde Rodrigues [3,8] and João Leitão [9,10,11]

1. School of Engineering, Polytechnic of Porto, ISEP, 4249-015 Porto, Portugal
2. INEGI—Instituto de Ciência e Inovação em Engenharia Mecânica e Engenharia Industrial, 4200-465 Porto, Portugal
3. Algoritmi Centre, School of Engineering, University of Minho, 4800-058 Guimarães, Portugal
4. Ergonomics Laboratory, Faculdade de Motricidade Humana, Universidade de Lisboa, 1499-002 Cruz Quebrada, Portugal
5. Research Centre for Architecture, Urbanism and Design (CIAUD), Faculdade de Arquitetura, Universidade de Lisboa, 1349-063 Lisboa, Portugal
6. Associated Laboratory for Energy, Transports and Aeronautics, LAETA (PROA), Faculty of Engineering, University of Porto, 4200-465 Porto, Portugal
7. Porto Biomechanics Laboratory, Faculty of Sport, University of Porto, 4200-450 Porto, Portugal
8. Research Centre on Environment and Health, Department of Environmental Health, School of Health, Polytechnic Institute of Porto, 4200-072 Porto, Portugal
9. NECE–Research Unit in Business Sciences, Faculty of Human and Social Sciences, University of Beira Interior (UBI), Estrada do Sineiro, 6200-001 Covilhã, Portugal
10. Centre for Management Studies of Instituto Superior Técnico (CEG-IST), University of Lisbon, 1649-004 Lisboa, Portugal
11. Instituto de Ciências Sociais (ICS), University of Lisbon, 1649-004 Lisboa, Portugal
* Correspondence: dgr@isep.ipp.pt

Overview

This Special Issue of the *International Journal of Environmental Research and Public Health* is devoted to the "Frontiers in Occupational Health and Safety Management". This issue intends to contribute to the knowledge in the field regarding the new challenges for Occupational Safety and Health (OSH) management. This concern is stated in the EU Strategic Framework on Health and Safety at Work for 2021–2027, which sets out the key actions needed to improve the health and safety of workers in the years to come. This new strategy focuses on three cross-cutting objectives, namely, anticipating and managing change in the context of green, digital, and demographic transitions; improving the prevention of work-related accidents and diseases and striving towards a Vision Zero approach to work-related deaths; and increasing the preparedness to respond to current and future health crises [1]. This strategy is expected to have a significant impact on the management of OSH at all levels, including companies from all sectors. It is also a basis for increasing the awareness and funding support for the improvement of the health and safety of workers. The European Agency for Safety and Health at Work (EU-OSHA) has an important role in implementing this strategy at the European level, but also in coordination with the numerous National Agencies.

The COVID-19 pandemic has had a profound impact on nearly every aspect of the world of work. The frontiers of OSH were pushed when outbreaks of SARS-CoV-2 were observed in workplaces, exposing workers, their families, and communities to the risk of infection. In addition to the risk of infection, workers in all sectors face additional hazards that have emerged due to new work practices and procedures adopted to mitigate the spread of the virus. Teleworking, for example, has led to ergonomic and psychosocial risks with some 65% of surveyed companies reporting that workers' morale has been difficult to sustain while working from home [2,3]. Additionally, self-reported symptoms of computer vision syndrome have increased in several settings [4]. The time spent by workers looking at the computer screen during the pandemic has increased due to the long working hours, thereby increasing eye and vision complaints. To face these problems, new guidance has emerged with respect to working safely during the COVID-19 pandemic, providing a set of guidelines to manage the risks that have been arising and to enable the effective and timely adaptation to changing situations (e.g., ISO/PAS 45005:2020 [5]).

The COVID-19 pandemic, by showing that organisations were not prepared to lead with this new risk, drew attention to emergency management, particularly for organizations in the field of public health. The International Labour Organization (ILO), on the World Day for Safety and Health at Work (28 April 2021), called on countries to implement resilient OSH systems for future health emergencies. This will require investments in OSH infrastructure and its integration into comprehensive national crisis emergency preparedness and response plans to protect the safety and health of workers and support business continuity. Thus, organizational resilience has been given a new boost [2].

Resilience can be defined as the process and outcome of successfully adapting to difficult or challenging life experiences, especially through mental, emotional, and behavioural flexibility and adjustment to external and internal demands. The concept of resilience has become very popular, especially in the 21st century. In the perspective of organisations, it becomes clear that they must be resilient to rapid technological, environmental, or other types of changes and install or remove controls quickly and efficiently. Therefore, dynamic decision making on risk controls will challenge the traditional strategies of OHS [6]. Risk management, also considered as uncertainty management, allows organisations to attempt to prepare for the unexpected by minimising risks and extra costs before they happen [7]. From the individual point of view, self-confidence is a good means to cope with the stresses of life and plays an important part in resilience. Becoming more confident in one's personal abilities, including the ability to respond to and deal with a crisis, is a great way to build resilience for the future. This concept has become increasingly important with the COVID-19 crisis and has also a certain connection with OSH.

The industry revolution has completely changed the way work is executed. At the same time that it brought solutions for OSH, it also brought new risks that need to be recognized and minimized. The frontiers in OSH changed again with the concept of Industry 4.0, which is now evolving towards Industry 5.0. The human factor becomes the central axis for the formation of smart cyber-physical socio-technical systems that are integrated into workplaces' physical and cultural host environments. New risks have emerged, leading to a potential transformation of OSH, and giving rise to a new model called OSH 5.0, in which innovation, digitalization, and cultural transformations constitute sources of value in work and in its development contexts, in parallel with the concept of Industry 5.0 [8]. Therefore, the frontiers of OSH are enlarged within this context.

There is a gradual transition to a circular economy, which is a key driver of the EU's goal of achieving carbon neutrality by 2050 while creating sustainable growth and jobs. The circular economy has significant policy and regulatory implications that will affect future jobs. It will also have consequences for workers' safety and health. There is, for instance, an impact on jobs in hazardous sectors related to maintenance and repair as well as disassembly and recycling, which can have a negative impact on working conditions [9]. The circular economy contributes to better and greater environmental sustainability and a better intervention at the social level [10]. The circular economy also leads to changes in organizational processes and/or redesigning tasks, which can have an impact on job content and satisfaction. The circular economy also influences the enlargement of the frontiers of OSH [9].

Technological advancement is often a double-edged sword in that it presents both risks and opportunities. The increasing use of artificial intelligence (AI) is continuously transforming jobs and work tasks. Although AI-based systems in the workplace offer many benefits, there is a growing debate on how they impact OSH. The automation (or semi-automation) of cognitive tasks in particular introduces concerns about workers' psychosocial wellbeing that must be addressed by policymakers. The recent EU-OSHA report on 'Artificial Intelligence and automation of cognitive tasks: Implications for occupational safety and health' identifies a number of key risks that should be addressed by policymakers through analysing labour law and data protection regulation. The most obvious concern is the threat of job loss, followed by feelings of precarity at work and poor mental health. As intelligent programs more efficiently process forms, applications, claims, legal documents, etc., it will no longer be necessary for humans to complete these 'mind-numbing' and alienating tasks [11].

The impact of artificial intelligence on the workplace might create opportunities but also new challenges for OSH, its management, and its regulation. Artificial intelligence has also facilitated the emergence of new forms of monitoring and managing workers based on the collection of large amounts of real-time data. These novel forms may provide an opportunity to improve OSH surveillance, reduce exposure to various risk factors, and provide early warnings of stress, health problems, and fatigue. However, they might also give rise to legal, regulatory, and ethical questions, as well as concerns for OSH [12]. Again, Artificial Intelligence broadens the frontiers of OSH.

Big data refers to data sets that contain greater variety, arriving in increasing volumes and with greater velocity, as they are too large or complex to be dealt with by traditional data-processing application software. According to Wang and Wang [13], big data has an important influence on safety management in various fields where its applications are becoming more prevalent. The analysis results of big data have become an important reference influencing safety-related decision making.

The implementation of integrated management systems allows organizations to achieve efficient results in reducing risks and increasing productivity, providing a better understanding of how management systems influence the OSH risk management in organizations, particularly in SMEs. The success of the integration of risk management in OSH depends on both technical and human aspects [14].

In the last decade, there has been a rapid emergence of nanotechnology into several consumer products, which has led to concerns regarding the potential risks for human health following consumer exposure. There is also a concern in terms of occupational safety and health, related to the exposure of workers involved in the manufacturing, processing, and handling of consumer goods containing nanomaterials. Exposure to engineered nanomaterials has been associated with several health effects including pulmonary inflammation, genotoxicity, carcinogenicity, and circulatory effects. Textiles are one of the most heavily traded commodities in the world. The textile industry is already an important user of nanotechnologies and there are a significant number of "nanotextiles" in the market, including many consumer skin-contact goods, which have been introduced by the incorporation of nanoparticles [15]. The risk for the workers and for the consumers is linked to the characteristic properties of nanomaterials that make them different from their macroscale counterparts and are determined by the physicochemical properties of the nanomaterial, the interactions with the materials, and the potential exposure levels. The growing concern about the possible negative effects of nanomaterials on humans and on the environment can lead to restrictions for consumer products incorporating nanoparticles. There are many studies about the penetration of nanoparticles into the skin, related, for instance, to sunscreens and cosmetics, which are often based on nanomaterials. In fact, only the smaller nanoparticles seem to be able to penetrate the undamaged skin, although if the skin is injured, larger nanoparticles can penetrate [15]. Nanotechnology is no doubt a concern and broadens the frontiers of OSH.

Industrial intelligence is a global trend. In developed countries, industrial intelligence has been developing under relatively mature economic and technology conditions, known as a tech-led pattern. In other words, industrial intelligence occurs naturally under the mature conditions of economic and technological conditions. In addition, one of the most critical conditions for industrial intelligence involves the skills of workers. Recent research argues that industrial intelligence creates better technology that reduces occupational injuries [16].

Recent research argues that robots could replace workers in dangerous work environments, for instance, in chemical and mining industries, with a strong impact on the reduction of occupational injuries [16,17]. However, according to Yang et al. [18], robot applications do not have a persistent impact on occupational injuries and can even increase the rate of occupational injuries in developing countries.

Concerning the more familiar occupational injuries, as outlined by Leitão et al. [19], there is still room for addressing the traditional motivators and hygiene factors associated with the promotion of the quality of working life (QWL), such as having an appropriate salary, having a safe work environment, and benefiting from occupational healthcare; thus, increased attention should be devoted to burnout factors, the so-called de-motivators, as a moderator of the relationship between QWL and the contribution to productivity at the organisational level. In this scope, the intelligent and learning algorithms and technologies could play a preventative role.

Implementing Industry 4.0 and interconnected robotization in industrial enterprises promotes occupational changes. It is essential to develop cooperation and collaboration between a robot and a human in a common robotized workplace so that robotization is safe and effective. A robotic device that works in collaboration with a human operator is called a cobot. Workplace robotization is particularly suitable for work environments that involve hazardous chemical substances that are carcinogenic and toxic to humans. Robotization also helps to improve workplace ergonomics and to avoid, for humans, very laborious and often repetitive work [17]. The automation of tasks with robots can remove workers from hazardous situations, and cobots can facilitate access to work for aging workers or those with disabilities [12]. The use of robots also presents a broadening of the frontiers of OSH.

Author Contributions: D.R., T.C., P.A., J.B., M.R. and J.L., conceived, wrote, and revised the manuscript. All authors have read and agreed to the published version of the manuscript.

Funding: This research received no external funding.

Acknowledgments: The authors wish to acknowledge the support of the *IJERPH* staff and the work of the anonymous reviewers.

Conflicts of Interest: All authors declare no conflict of interests.

References

1. European Commission (EC). EU Strategic Framework on Health and Safety at Work 2021–2027. In *Occupational Safety and Health in a Changing World of Work*; European Commission: Brussels, Belgium, 2021.
2. International Labour Organization (ILO). Safety and Health at Work. *Occupational Safety and Health Inspection*. 2022. Available online: https://www.ilo.org/global/topics/safety-and-health-at-work/areasofwork/occupational-safety-and-health-inspection/lang--en/index.htm (accessed on 11 May 2022).
3. International Labour Organization (ILO). *Anticipate, Prepare and Respond to Crises: Invest Now in Resilient OSH Systems*; International Labour Office: Geneva, Switzerland; ILO: Geneva, Switzerland, 2021; ISBN 9789220344460.
4. Li, R.; Yin, B.; Qian, Y.; Chen, D.; Li, X.; Zhu, H.; Liu, H. Prevalence of Self-Reported Symptoms of Computer Vision Syndrome and Associated Risk Factors among School Students in China during the COVID-19 Pandemic. *Ophthalmic Epidemiol.* **2021**, *29*, 363–373. [CrossRef] [PubMed]
5. ISO/PAS 45005; Occupational Health and Safety Management—General Guidelines for Safe Working during the COVID-19 Pandemic. ISO: Geneva, Switzerland, 2020.
6. European Agency for Safety and Health at Work (EU-OSHA). *The Development of Dynamic Risk Assessment and Its Implications for Occupational Safety and Health*; Discussion Paper; EU-OSHA: Bilbao, Spain, 2021. Available online: https://osha.europa.eu/en/publications/development-dynamic-risk-assessment-and-its-implications-occupational-safety-and-health (accessed on 11 May 2022).
7. Ramos, D.G.G.; Almeida, L. (Eds.) *Risk Management–An Overview*; Business Issues, Competition and Entrepreneurship; Nova Science Publishers: New York, NY, USA, 2021; ISBN 978-1-68507-177-6. [CrossRef]
8. Ávila-Gutiérrez, M.J.; Suarez-Fernandez de Miranda, S.; Aguayo-González, F. Occupational Safety and Health 5.0—A Model for Multilevel Strategic Deployment Aligned with the Sustainable Development Goals of Agenda 2030. *Sustainability* **2022**, *14*, 6741. [CrossRef]
9. European Agency for Safety and Health at Work (EU-OSHA). Circular Economy and Its Effects on OSH. 2022. Available online: https://osha.europa.eu/en/emerging-risks/circular-economy (accessed on 11 May 2022).

20. Ramos, D.; Fonseca, L.; Gonçalves, J.; Carvalho, R.; Carvalho, S.; Santos, G. Cost-Benefit Analysis of Implementing Circular Economy in a Portuguese Company: From a Case Study to a Model. *Qual. Innov. Prosper.* **2022**, *26*, 52–69. [CrossRef]
21. EU-OSHA. European Agency for Safety and Health at Work (EU-OSHA). Policy Brief. Cognitive Automation: Impact, Risks and Opportunities for Occupational Safety and Health. 2022. Available online: https://osha.europa.eu/en/publications/cognitive-automation-impact-risks-and-opportunities-occupational-safety-and-health (accessed on 11 May 2022).
22. EU-OSHA. European Agency for Safety and Health at Work (EU-OSHA). In *Impact of Artificial Intelligence on Occupational Safety and Health*; Policy Brief; EU-OSHAl: Bibao, Spain, 2021.
23. Wang, B.; Wang, Y. Big data in safety management: An overview. *Saf. Sci.* **2021**, *143*, 105414. [CrossRef]
24. Ramos, D.; Afonso, P.; Rodrigues, M.A. Integrated management systems as a key facilitator of occupational health and safety risk management: A case study in a medium sized waste management firm. *J. Clean. Prod.* **2020**, *262*, 121346. [CrossRef]
25. Almeida, L.; Ramos, D. Health and safety concerns of textiles with nanomaterials. *IOP Conf. Series: Mater. Sci. Eng.* **2017**, *254*, 102002. [CrossRef]
26. Sattari, F.; Macciotta, R.; Kurian, D.; Lefsrud, L. Application of Bayesian network and artificial intelligence to reduce accident/incident rates in oil & gas companies. *Saf. Sci.* **2021**, *133*, 104981.
27. Pauliková, A.; Gyurák Babeľová, Z.; Ubárová, M. Analysis of the Impact of Human–Cobot Collaborative Manufacturing Implementation on the Occupational Health and Safety and the Quality Requirements. *Int. J. Environ. Res. Public Health* **2021**, *18*, 1927. [CrossRef] [PubMed]
28. Yang, S.; Zhong, Y.; Feng, D.; Li RShao, X.F.; Liu, W. Robot application and occupational injuries: Are robots necessarily safer? *Saf. Sci.* **2022**, *147*, 105623. [CrossRef]
29. Leitão, J.; Pereira, D.; Gonçalves, Â. Quality of Work Life and Contribution to Productivity: Assessing the Moderator Effects of Burnout Syndrome. *Int. J. Environ. Res. Public Health* **2021**, *18*, 2425. [CrossRef] [PubMed]

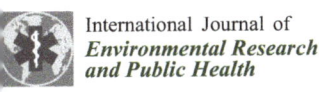 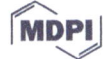

Article

Psychosocial Risks in Teachers from Portugal and England on the Way to Society 5.0

Ana Pimenta [1], Delfina Ramos [2,3,4,*], Gilberto Santos [1], Matilde A. Rodrigues [4,5] and Manuel Doiro [6]

1. Department of Industrial and Product Design, School of Design, Polytechnic Institute Cavado Ave, 4750-810 Barcelos, Portugal; gsantos@ipca.pt (G.S.)
2. School of Engineering, Polytechnic of Porto, ISEP, 4249-015 Porto, Portugal
3. Associate Laboratory for Energy, Transports and Aerospace (LAETA-INEGI), Rua Dr. Roberto Frias 400, 4200-465 Porto, Portugal
4. Algoritmi Research Centre/LASI, School of Engineering, University of Minho, 4800-058 Guimaraes, Portugal; mar@ess.ipp.pt
5. Center for Translational Health and Medical Biotechnology Research, School of Health of Polytechnic of Porto, 4200-072 Porto, Portugal
6. Department of Business Organization and Marketing, Vigo University, 36310 Vigo, Spain; mdoiro@uvigo.es
* Correspondence: dgr@isep.ipp.pt

Abstract: Being a teacher is one of the most demanding jobs, as a result of this responsibility, these workers face many psychosocial risks. This study aims to characterize and compare psychosocial factors in Portuguese and British teachers and discuss how new developments in technology, namely digital technology can improve education and, in particular, contribute to fewer issues related to mental health. The Copenhagen Psychosocial Questionnaire Medium Version (COPSOQ II) was applied to the teachers of six Portuguese schools (three public schools and three private schools), three British public schools and three private schools with an international British curriculum (Switzerland, Spain and Portugal). The results showed that cognitive, emotional, and quantitative demands, as well as work rhythm and work/family conflict, are the key psychosocial factors among these teachers. Differences were found between the teachers of both countries. Some models are proposed, through the proposals of Society 5.0, for their minimization and/or removal. Society 5.0 is the vision of a new human-centered society in the fifth stage launched by Japan in April 2016, and it is cited in our study with the hope that it will contribute to solving many problems of today's society.

Keywords: COPSOQ II; education; psychological risks; occupational health; Society 5.0

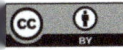

1. Introduction

Mental health problems are one of the most relevant disorders in occupational settings [1,2]. It is estimated that mental health problems are responsible for around 50% to 60% of all lost workdays [1]. In fact, many psychosocial risk factors often have a high impact on people's lives and lead to illnesses such as burnout, stress, anxiety, and depression [1,3]. One of the jobs in which there has been a significant increase in these problems is the teaching profession [2]. The mental health condition of teachers with different academic degrees continues to be a concern in different countries, as it can lead them to abandon the profession, as well as negatively influence students during the teaching-learning process [4]. Different risk factors have been contributing to this scenario, making it important to characterize them and implement appropriate measures to minimize psychosocial risks in the teaching profession.

It is undeniable that the world is changing rapidly due to the advancement of new technologies beyond the advancement of information technologies, leading us from the evolution of our society to the super-intelligent society called Society 5.0 [5]. This is a human-centered society that balances economic advancement with resolving social problems, and a system that integrates physical spaces and cyberspace [6,7]. Given this, the quality of life can be improved by applying Society 5.0 in education, especially for teachers in middle and secondary schools [6]. In Society 5.0, people expect social reform (innovation); with this, we will create a society that faces its future looking through its eyes, breaking the pattern that exists of being in stagnation. This will be a society where its members can show respect that will transcend generations, and all citizens can have an active and pleasant life [6].

In this study, we aim to characterize and compare psychosocial factors in Portuguese and British schoolteachers, identifying the main factors that affect teachers and providing possible solutions to minimize psychosocial risks according to the data evidence. These schools work mainly to ensure that students complete their secondary studies and do their assessments to join universities.

Through the comparison of the two countries' realities and curriculums, we wish to discuss findings in light of Society 5.0, by understanding how new developments in technology can help education to become better, with fewer issues related to mental health. It is the opinion of the authors of this work that Society 5.0 will contribute to the creation of a better future, which is based on the most advanced technologies, but which will have the human being at its center. It promises the creation of new value through innovation and the simultaneous promotion of economic development and effective solutions to social challenges. It will free individuals from the countless constraints to which they are subject today and will focus on imagination and creativity. It will be an intelligent society capable of achieving the sustainable development goals towards the ideal society [5,6].

2. Literature Review
2.1. Psychosocial Risks in Education Teachers

Teachers are the key elements of educational services, as they are responsible for the development of educational programs and education of students at different levels. In their daily work, they deal with different demands. Their duties include planning and preparing classes, providing additional support to students, applying teaching-learning methodologies that ensure student's participation and engagement, grading tests and documenting progress, assigning homework, providing individual support, attending several meetings with co-workers and students' parents, promoting extracurricular projects, and completing other administrative tasks. Usually, a good teacher becomes an example for several students and a source of inspiration and motivation. However, it is essential to ensure their workability, particularly regarding mental health.

Psychosocial risks are of particular concern for teachers, since they have been related to high turnover and high absenteeism, which when referring to teachers have a negative impact on the students' academic success [8,9]. A recent meta-analysis showed that burnout (exhaustion, depersonalization, and reduced accomplishment) and job satisfaction have an important role in teachers' intentions to leave the profession [4].

According to the literature, teachers are exposed to psychosocial risk factors that can jeopardize their mental health. Psychosocial risks stem from aspects of how work is organized, social factors at work and in the work environment, equipment, and hazardous tasks. In this workgroup, having to deal with challenging students is a common concern, as identified in the report ESENER in 2019 [10]. In fact, some studies have shown the importance of students' bad behavior on teachers' mental health [11,12]. However, other psychosocial risk factors are also relevant; particularly those related to demands and stressors that teachers experience daily beyond students' behaviors. Baeriswy et al. [11] emphasized conflicts with parents, workload, and prolonged working hours in emotional exhaustion in homeroom teachers. Time pressure and discipline problems were predictive of emotional exhaustion. Skaalvik and Skaalvik [13] verified that when teachers experience a feeling of value consonance, supervisory support, and positive relations with colleagues and parents, they report a feeling of belonging. Mijakoski et al. [14], through a literature review, identified different determinants of teacher exhaustion, including job satisfaction, work climate or pressure, teacher self-efficacy, neuroticism, perceived collective exhaustion, and classroom disruption.

Burnout is a highly prevalent phenomenon among teachers. For example, Bermejo-Toro et al. [15] showed that between 10 and 20% of teachers could suffer from high burnout levels and between 20 and 40% from moderate levels. Fernet et al. [16] stated burnout is predicted by changes in teachers' perceptions of the school environment, in particular demands (e.g., work overload, role conflict) and resources (e.g., teacher efficacy, support by colleagues), and motivational factors (autonomous motivation and self-efficacy).

2.2. Society 5.0 and Its Role in Teachers' Mental Health and Well-Being Improvement

Society 5.0 is the vision of a new human-centered society in the fifth stage launched by Japan in April 2016. It is cited in our study with the hope that it will contribute to solving many problems of today's society.

Society 5.0 is technology-based, focused on people, and encompasses a multitude of 'smart' applications. The important thing here is that this model puts people right at the heart of it. Originally coined by the Japanese government, Society 5.0 stands for an intelligent, fully networked, and sustainable society [17]. In Society 5.0, people expect a better society than the current one, that is, a society that faces its future where its members will be able to show intergenerational respect, and citizens will be able to live better [6]. To be able to reach this point, it will be necessary to start deep reforms in several areas, namely, enterprise reform, individual reforms, and social problem solving.

The purpose of this system will be to use information and communication technologies to help in the process of improving everyone's lives. As long as retirement ages are not extended without compromising the state of the economy, which stops when that happens, citizens have a good level of health, allowing them to enjoy their last years without constraints, for example, such as musculoskeletal injuries [18].

It is also the objective of Society 5.0 that all citizens have a quality of life. So, that their profession does not lead them to have health problems, whether physical, psychological, or mental during their career.

According to Salgues [5], keywords for Society 5.0 include: (i) adaptability, (ii) agility, (iii) mobility, and (iv) reactivity. These are linked to the fact that mutations, changes, and evolutions are constantly observed in our daily lives, reflected in our structure, knowledge, and skills. Adaptability, agility, and reactivity are crucial and require the implementation of the Industry 4.0 model, which implies the use of additive techniques that increase the consumption of a few resources for producing the goods. However, mobility has effects on means of transport and in our homes, and we see that we are increasingly in a more mobile and interconnected age. In this new society, Society 5.0 translates to a "new world", in which exchange is the most important factor. There will be the concept of the primacy of issues involving economic exchanges and the primacy of ideas. In western democracies, what prevailed for years has been the transaction of goods, and its performance of the means of transport led to globalization, but the primacy of ideas is what will take precedence. For example, China in 1992 developed its soft power of primacy of ideas, and consequently today we see all of its economic development. France is also an example of this, in another field designated as cultural exceptions. This leads us to the concept that the export of ideas and knowledge has become a source of wealth in a period in which the export of goods is in decline and the demand for services is increasing [19]. In developed countries, namely in the United States of America, a high percentage of young law graduates encounter great difficulties in professional insertion. This happens with the help of AI (artificial intelligence). The internet of things and cybernetics, in some cases, offer legal advice in just seconds both for simple and more complex legal cases with an accuracy level of 90% (above 70% of human accuracy). As a result, it is expected that in the coming years, this profession will see a reduction in staff: 90% fewer lawyers and only those who are specialized will survive. It is expected, according to Salgues [5], that as early as 2030, the computer will be able to compete with human intelligence. It is easy to see, even nowadays, that our mobile phones already have image recognition software, which can be used for many functions: for example, looking for people, which is dethroning professional physiognomists.

Social acceptance, however, is a prerequisite to creating Society 5.0. Many fear change—or are skeptical about technological progress—and this must be addressed. There's a growing fear that AI-powered automation will lead to mass redundancies, and some commentators have said that up to 800 million jobs will go by 2030. This can be a terrible reality, which we are approaching. Hence, the education system must be geared towards the new Society 5.0—both in terms of research and teaching. Universities and schools have a duty to adapt their educational programs for digital natives, particularly when it comes to preparing for tomorrow's job market [17]. The implementation of appropriate measures for a new way of teaching, in which teachers are the main players, is an absolute necessity.

3. Materials and Methods

3.1. Study Design

This is a cross-sectional study, whose aim is the characterization of psychosocial factors among teachers from European public and private schools, using the Portuguese and British curriculum. The research questions that guided the study were based on schools that work primarily to ensure that students finish their secondary studies and take their assessments to enter universities, as described in the introduction. The difference between public schools in England and private international schools' curriculum is that there is more coursework to cover, which will lead teachers in private international schools to have more pressure while teaching the British syllabus.

There are similarities between these schools' countries. Public school teachers only do their contact time with their pupils and have free periods to cope with all work required from the job. Apart from their contact time with students, private school teachers have to cover lessons to replace their peers, exam invigilation, and a more extended shift day than public school teachers. Consequently, they have an increased workload after they leave school. The research questions that guided the study were: What are the main psychosocial risk factors that affect all teachers?; What are the main differences between the psychosocial factors among Portuguese teachers and British teachers?; What are the main differences between the psychosocial factors among private and public schools? The schools that participated in the study were chosen firstly because they met the criteria established for the study and also because the Heads were interested to know how their teachers were feeling at that time and wanted to assess the psychological state of their teachers due to an increase in sick leaves.

3.2. Instruments

The Portuguese middle version of COPSOQ II [20] was used to assess the psychosocial factors among all the teachers using the Portuguese curriculum. The questionnaire was applied in international schools. Teachers could be of different nationalities and they had knowledge of the British curriculum.

Psychosocial risk analysis was performed using questionnaires on the Google Forms platform to ensure data confidentiality. In response to the questionnaires, respondents responded privately. These answers were not disclosed to the hierarchical superiors of the educational establishment.

National and international public and private schools participated in the study, namely:

- 3 Portuguese public schools with a Portuguese curriculum (North Region, Lisbon, and South Region);
- 3 private schools with Portuguese curriculum (North Region, Lisbon, and South Region);
- 3 public schools in the City of London with a British curriculum;
- 3 private schools with an international British curriculum (Switzerland, Spain, and Portugal).

The selected schools are essentially dedicated to preparing students for the completion of secondary education and conducting exams for access to university education. These schools began their activities in different decades, but they all have the objective of promoting the academic success of their students in common. Emphasis was given to the number of students admitted to universities. It was decided that only teachers from the 3rd cycle and secondary education (teachers with students aged between 13 and 18 years old) would be studied at the school. This choice was based on the fact the tasks performed by this group of workers are exposed to greater psychosocial risks as they deal with a group of students with an average of 25 students during school periods.

The questionnaire was applied online, following a previous contact given the informed consent by the teachers. *The Copenhagen Psychosocial Questionnaire II* (COPSOQ II) was sent via email to be completed, which could be done on computers on the school premises or at home. These results were stored in the Google forms database.

The items of COPSOQ II are measured using a five-point Likert scale, and the results of the scales can be presented from one to five points or transformed using the cutting points of 2.33 and 3.66 in order to obtain a traffic light graphic [20].

The variables measured on a Likert scale were analyzed through the presented categories, while the quantitative variables were analyzed from the measured values, such as the average obtained for each question (for questions on a scale of 1 to 5, a value greater than 3 is greater than the midpoint of the scale), the standard deviation associated with each question representing the absolute dispersion of responses, the coefficient of variation illustrating the relative dispersion of responses, the minimum and maximum values observed for the answers given to the various questions. An internal consistency analysis was also carried out, allowing the study of the properties of measurement scales and the questions that integrate them. Cronbach's Alpha is the most used model in the social sciences for checking scales' internal consistency and validity, measuring how a set of variables represent a given dimension. An internal consistency coefficient value measured by Cronbach's Alpha greater than 0.80 is considered adequate, and an internal consistency coefficient between 0.60 and 0.80 is considered acceptable. Statistical tests used in this study serve to ascertain whether the differences observed in the sample are statistically significant, that is, whether the conclusions of the sample can be inferred for the population. The value of 5% is a reference value used in Social Sciences to test hypotheses; it means that we establish the inference with an error probability of less than 5%. As the sample size is in these conditions, it will not be necessary to verify the assumption and parametric tests can be applied. As the groups under study can be considered significant, the parametric Student's *t*-test is used to analyze a quantitative variable in both classes of a dichotomous qualitative variable to verify the significance of the differences between the means observed for both the groups of the dichotomous variable. The t-test poses the following hypotheses:

- **H1.** *There is no difference in means between the groups of the dichotomous variable.*
- **H2.** *There is a difference in means between the groups of the dichotomous variable.*

When the test value of the t-test is greater than 5%, the null hypothesis is accepted. That is, there are no differences between the two groups. The null hypothesis is rejected when the test value is less than 5%. Therefore, there are differences between the two groups. The use of the chi-square test is addressed; in the face of two nominal variables or a nominal and an ordinal variable, the appropriate test to verify the relationship between each pair of variables is the chi-square, in which we have the hypotheses:

- **H3.** *The two variables are independent, that is, there is no relationship between the categories of one variable and the categories of the other.*
- **H4.** *The two variables present a relationship between themselves, that is, there is a relationship between the categories of one variable and the categories of the other.*

The null hypothesis is rejected when the test value is less than 5% (0.05), concluding that the two variables are related. When the test value is greater than the 5% reference value, we cannot reject the null hypothesis that the two variables are independent; it is concluded that they are unrelated.

3.3. Participants

The sample encompassed 340 teachers from public (N = 170) and private schools (N = 170), following the Portuguese (N = 170) and British (N = 170) curriculum (Table 1). These teachers belong to European schools located in different countries: six Portuguese schools following the Portuguese curriculum, three of them private and the remaining three public; three British public schools located in London, following the British curriculum; and three international private schools following the British curriculum, and located in Switzerland, Spain, and Portugal.

Table 1. Sample characterization.

	Portuguese Curriculum		British Curriculum	
	Public School	Private School	Public School	Private School
Number of teachers	85	85	85	85
Gender	F M	F M	F M	F M
	74 11	74 11	80 5	84 1
Total	170		170	
		340		

We also collected the data about the age group of each teach for each specific school (Table 2). The schools chosen for the project were chosen because the students had similar backgrounds, high expectations, and engagement to work at school. So, if students do not differ so much, the teachers will face similar pressures that will introduce the same psychosocial risks. Also, regarding the differences between British and Portuguese curricula, the international schools deliver both syllabi (British and the local curriculum), and the differences between the syllabus created some problems between colleagues (teachers) arguing about who works more or has the most demanding syllabus. It was this behavior between peers (that could lead to psychosocial risks) that led to the present study.

Table 2. Sample characterization in terms of age.

		Age			
		<30 Years	30 < Years < 40	40 < Years < 50	>50 Years
Portugal—Public	N	0	29	39	17
	% no Grupo	0.0%	34.1%	45.9%	20.0%
Portugal Private	N	10	44	25	6
	% no Grupo	11.8%	51.8%	29.4%	7.1%
International Public	N	24	33	21	7
	% no Grupo	28.2%	38.8%	24.7%	8.2%
International Private	N	22	32	14	17
	% no Grupo	25.9%	37.6%	16.5%	20.0%

4. Results

The global assessment of the psychosocial factors among the sample of all teachers of this study showed the presence of several risk factors, mainly related to the dimension work demands, but also present in the dimensions of interpersonal relations and work-individual interface. Also concerning are the results obtained through the health and well-being scales.

According to the respondents, the main risk factors, showed in red label in Figure 1 (from right to left), are those presenting the higher percentages of respondents, which were: 89.7% for cognitive demands; 80.6% for emotional demands; 76.5% for pace of work; 72.9% for quantitative demands; 70.6% for work/family conflicts; and 65% for labor conflicts. Among the health and well-being scales, exhaustion (or burnout), showed the higher percentage of unfavorable results (68.8%), which means a big risk.

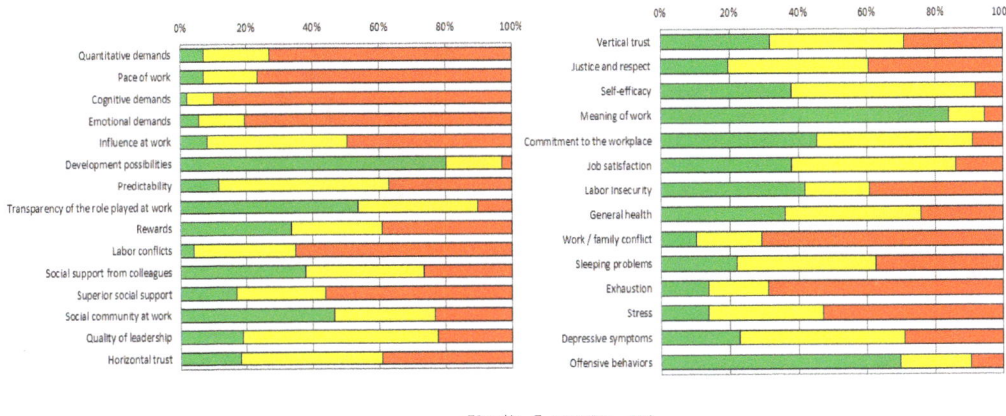

Figure 1. Description of COPSOQ II scales by a traffic light graphic among all teachers.

There are issues that help to minimize the risk, of which we highlight: meaning of work, development possibilities, transparency of the role-played at work, and social community at work, among others.

As this study was carried out for Portuguese teachers and foreign teachers, we wanted to know if the health risks for Portuguese teachers were different from those of international teachers. Also, it is important to note that Portuguese schools (public or private) have a massive bureaucratic workload that puts more pressure on teachers' shoulders, and they believe that this factor makes their life difficult.

For this analysis, we used descriptive statistics and T-tests to check if they are the same or if the risks are different.

The horizontal axis of Figure 2 represents the means of all responses obtained for each case. An asterisk* has been added to the most significant results. Thus, by analyzing Figure 2, it is possible to confirm that significant statistical differences exist between these groups on some study scales while others are not significant. Therefore, for these results and looking only to those that exist, on statistical difference, we can state that for teachers in Portugal, when we compare with teachers from other countries, the main risks are, among others, emotional demands, cognitive demands, work/family conflict, labor conflicts, and exhaustion, that is, burnout. In comparison, the risks that involve more teachers in the international system are, among others: development possibilities, meaning of work, pace of work, social community at work.

It is possible to confirm that work conditions are varied, which can create tensions and different perspectives for teachers.

As this study was carried out for public and private schools, we wanted to know if the risks of public education teachers are different from those private education teachers.

It is necessary to be aware that when we speak about public schools, these are schools that have public funding from the local authorities. It's called public because the taxpayer pays for it. When referencing private schools, which are paid for by the students' parents or careers, the school provides the British curriculum if it is called private international. The factors: pace of work, quantitative demands, labor conflicts, horizontal trust, work/labor conflicts and exhaustion (or burnout), are more prevalent for teachers in private schools. The horizontal axis of Figure 3 represents the means of all responses obtained for each case. An asterisk * has been added to the most significant results. Thus, as it is shown in Figure 3, the differences observed are not statistically significant. In the sample, according to Figure 3, the factors cognitive demands, emotional demands, development possibilities, social community at work, quality of leadership, general health, sleeping problems, stress, and depressive symptoms are more prevalent for public school teachers.

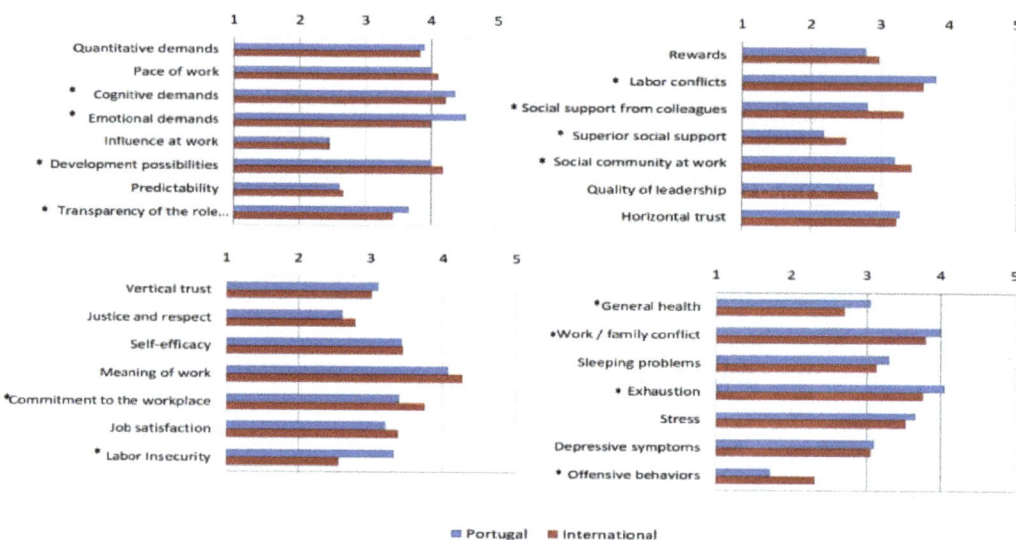

Figure 2. Statistical differences between groups in different countries. *: The ones with the * sign are the statistically significant.

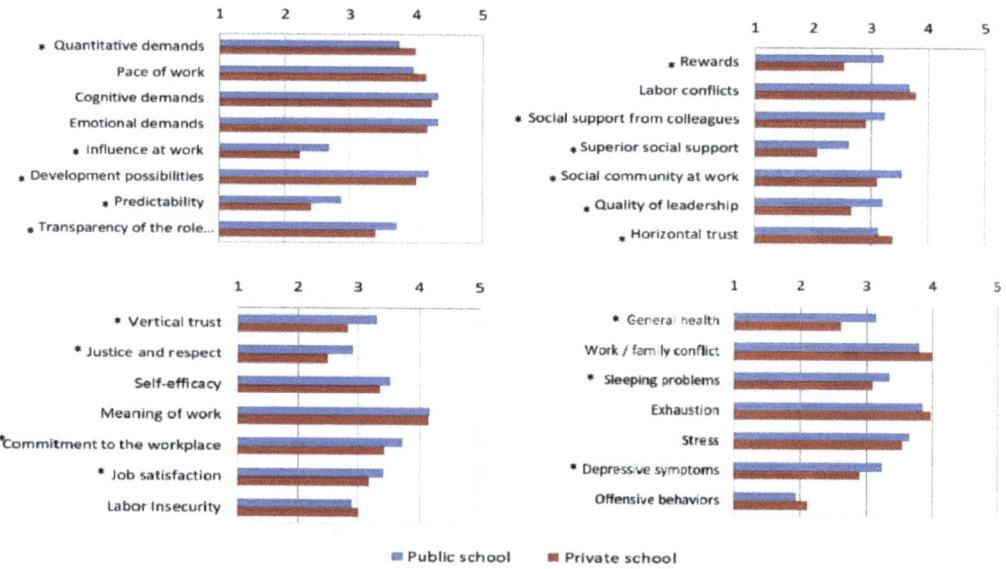

Figure 3. Statistical differences between public and private schools. *: The ones with the * sign are the statistically significant.

The factor labor insecurity is more prevalent for teachers in private education. The factor "meaning of work" does not differ between the two groups.

Not all the differences observed are statistically significant. The ones with the * sign are the statistically significant. When we analyze the results given by Portuguese teachers, we can verify the risks do not differ much among all samples. When we analyze the differences between private and international public education, we find that from the statistical analysis, we can say that the proof value is less than 5% for Work/family conflict and Predictability.

From the obtained results, it is possible to verify that teachers are exposed to the same risks, but they can change in order. Still, they are the same, and the first seven are in decreasing order cognitive demands, emotional demands, pace at work, quantitative demands, work/family conflict, exhaustion (or burnout), and labor conflicts. However, countries have different bureaucracies and syllabuses in their education system, so the risks will be different.

When checking the risks regarding public or private management at school, it is possible to see that exhaustion (or burnout), and work/family conflict are present in all of them and are important factors. However, the Portuguese teachers have other associated risks, and they are different due to the organization and requirements of the school. Teachers that work with the British syllabus do not have statistically significant differences; only the general health and rewards level are very different.

5. Discussion

Many authors, from the most varied countries, have published studies on exhaustion work of teachers, which is teacher burnout. For instance, Li et al. [21] conducted a study in China designed to examine how achievement goals, burnout, and school context relate to beginning teachers' turnover intention in China. The results showed that mastery goals and performance-avoidance goals were related to teachers' turnover intention because of burnout. They made a study to examine how achievement goals, burnout, and the school context relate to teachers beginning to work to turnover their intentions due to reasons that lead them to burnout, such as mastery goals, performance-avoidance goals, time, pressure and discipline problems.

Saloviita and Pakarinen [22] conducted a study on Finnish teachers. This study documented several associations between teacher burnout and background variables. This work is in line with the work presented here as it confirms the existence of burnout in teachers.

Prasojo et al. [23] comducted research on Indonesian education. The dataset presents a relationship for possible predictors of burnout. The study developed by these researchers suggests that emotional exhaustion (characterized by emotional and quantitative demands in this study), depersonalisation (in labour conflicts), and reduced personal accomplishment are the three components that lead people to develop burnout.

Hassan and Ibourk [24] conducted a study to test burnout and job satisfaction among Moroccan elementary school teachers. The results of the study confirmed the two-dimensionality of the burnout measurement scale.

Brown and Biddle [25] did a study in the USA in which the participants were teachers. The results showed that the professional protection factor of working in a positive school climate showed a negative indirect effect specifically on burnout.

From all the studies mentioned here, which also includes our study, we can demonstrate that teacher burnout is a serious problem at an international level. We know that the risks really exist, and we have to learn to minimize them [26,27].

Digital transition can have an important role in teachers' mental health by reducing their workload. If the work becomes more accessible and more efficient, prolonging working hours, a relevant risk factor of emotional exhaustion, is avoided, and the teachers have more time to develop more timely health-promoting actions [11]. Despite recent changes in schools using online platforms, it is not expected to look to AI as a digital transition; however, it must be seen as a tool for teachers to decrease their workload. With the evolution towards Society 5.0, teachers must be able to get a better quality of life. It's also a fact that using artificial intelligence, big data, and the internet of things does not only have benefits, and we are at the start of this transition, so this means that the systems are not as accurate as they should be and will also process tasks in a stringent line. So, although everything requires some teacher supervision, this will also lead to more workload depending on the subjects. Also, because there will be development of the system and leaving the traditional methods used in schools, this can lead to a more complex overall system that some teachers will not be able to follow and will leave some teachers behind (creating more psychosocial risks).

By the results obtained during our study, and other studies referenced, their mental health is affecting their quality of life. It is not difficult to explain that psychosocial risks like the pace of work, quantitative demands required from leadership, and work/family conflicts generated by the workload and labor conflicts with students and colleagues will significantly impact teachers' mental health. This affects peace of mind and, in some cases, the interaction with pupils, colleagues and family can be quite demanding and challenging to manage. We cannot forget that people of all ages use sarcasm and irony, so they want to undermine others in a way that their language and actions cannot target them.

These risks are a relay that brings distress to their lives, but no one may notice it. However, they can be noticed by work colleagues, leadership, and also family members. All can see changes in their attitudes, such as error-making decisions and feelings of guilt and anxiety. Also, their physiological health shows signs like tiredness and different problems in their musculoskeletal system, which can lead to mistakes or accidents.

With the help of artificial intelligence and internet of things, perhaps it will be possible to reduce in a significant way the risks regarding quantitative demands and the pace of work that will lead to a decrease in work/family conflict. Therefore, Big Data allied to artificial intelligence can reduce the amount of work by providing regular updates to teachers. It will also help by having access to worksheets and assessments, assisting the teachers in knowing what each student's weaknesses are to provide accurate feedback or resources that will help him to thrive. Of course, there is a need for an online platform that needs to be updated continuously and should have different languages.

Allowing teachers worldwide to be able to connect and work together will create support from colleagues even if at that school they do not have that support. It is also possible to develop new platforms with a lot more resources that can help teachers reach the goals required by their managers. One of the biggest causes of stress for teachers is marking assessments, especially when they have to mark exams that are important to provide access to universities. Due to different perspectives, different training, and because the teams that support the examiner markers sometimes do not provide an answer in useful time, this can produce unfairness when grading. Therefore, we can request cybernetics help to perform the correction of assessments. With this, we will be ensuring uniformity for all students using the same rules for everyone, and of course accelerating the process to make sure that results and feedback will be provided to students a lot faster. If we can decrease the workload for a teacher, they will able to do better work, providing a better balance in life with work and family. This, in turn, will lead to a decrease in stress eliminating depression symptoms, insomnia and exhaustion, or burnout. These work improvements will help them value their job, and not affect them in the way as it is does today. A double effect will be created: an increase in satisfaction for the teacher who will be a more effective teacher and will make sure that students will have better preparation for their future. On the other hand, it will be possible to decrease the amount of money spent every year in health care for these professionals minimizing the financial impact for governments.

6. Limitations and Future Research

As limitations of this work, we can consider the low number of schools and countries involved. As future research, we propose expanding the number of schools and countries, because as we see in this work, the psychosocial risks of teachers is a common problem in many countries.

7. Conclusions

It is possible to conclude that the risks teachers face are the same in any education system. Furthermore, those risks are cognitive demands, emotional demands, the pace of work, quantitative demands, work/family conflicts, exhaustion (or burnout), and labor conflicts. However, regarding countries/syllabus, those risks are for certain, different. Thus, we can conclude that the working conditions that cause these feelings of discontent or tension are different in different countries. Therefore, in Portugal, differences between the public and private system of education are statistically different, impacting teachers' lives.

There are, however, some limitations to this study; several teachers from the private schools were not comfortable answering this questionnaire. Another aspect that influenced the results is the massive difference in how the teachers in Portugal get their jobs because they might have to distance themselves from relatives when moving country, increasing the risk of psychosocial risks. It was also necessary to complement this study with other analysis, like TISES (*Teacher Interpersonal Self-efficacy Scale*) and MBI-ES (*Maslach Burnout Inventory*™), to show more critical factors and their real impact.

It is necessary to help teachers to resolve problems like burnout and work/family conflict; with these problems dealt with, they will be able to develop a better life, which will lead to fewer emotional, psychological, and physical issues. Measures need to be taken to improve the life of these professionals. In conclusion, Society 5.0, with the help of robotics, Big Data, and artificial intelligence can be the chance to help teachers recover their mental wellness. However, it is imperative to start to think of them as vital to reduce the psychosocial risks to improve the quality of life for teachers.

Author Contributions: Conceptualization, A.P.; methodology, D.R. and M.D.; validation, D.R. and M.A.R.; formal analysis, A.P.; investigation, D.R. and G.S.; data curation, A.P.; writing—original draft preparation, A.P.; writing—review and editing, A.P., D.R., G.S., M.A.R. and M.D.; visualization, M.D.; supervision, D.R. and G.S.; All authors have read and agreed to the published version of the manuscript.

Funding: This research received no external funding.

Institutional Review Board Statement: According to the Portuguese legislation, this study carried out in the field of Occupational Health and Safety does not require a pre-approval of an Ethical Committee.

Informed Consent Statement: Informed consent was obtained from all subjects involved in the study.

Acknowledgments: The authors wish to acknowledge the support of the IJERPH staff and the work of the anonymous reviewers. All author shave consented to the acknowledgement.

Conflicts of Interest: All authors declare no conflict of interest.

References

1. EU-OSHA. *Psychosocial Risks in Europe Prevalence and Strategies for Prevention*; Publications Office of the European Union: Luxembourg, 2014.
2. Eurofound. *Sixth European Working Conditions Survey—Overview Report (2017 Update)*; Publications Office of the European Union: Luxembourg, 2016.
3. Leka, S.; Jain, A.; World Health Organization. *Health Impact of Psychosocial Hazards at Work: An Overview*; World Health Organization: Geneva, Switzerland, 2010.
4. Madigan, D.J.; Kim, L.E. Towards an understanding of teacher attrition: A meta-analysis of burnout, job satisfaction, and teachers' intentions to quit. *Teach. Teach. Educ.* **2021**, *105*, 103425. [CrossRef]
5. Salgues, B. *Society 5.0: Industry of the Future, Technologies, Methods and Tools*, 1st ed.; John Wiley & Sons: Hoboken, NJ, USA, 2018; Volume 1.
6. Harayama, Y.; Fukuyama, M. Society 5.0: Aiming for a New Human-Centered Society—Hitachi Global, July/August, 1–6. *Hitachi Rev.* **2017**, *66*, 554–555.
7. Cabinet Office, Goverment of Japan. Science and Technology, Policy, Council for Science, Technology and Innovations—Society 5.0. 2017. Available online: https://www8.cao.go.jp/cstp/english/society5_0/index.html (accessed on 15 November 2019).
8. Schonfeld, I.S. Stress in 1st-Year Women Teachers: The Context of Social Support and Coping. *Genet. Soc. Gen. Psychol. Monogr.* **2001**, *127*, 133–168. [PubMed]
9. Sorensen, L.C.; Ladd, H.F. The hidden costs of teacher turnover. *AERA Open* **2020**, *6*, 2332858420905812. [CrossRef]
10. ESENER. Third European Survey of Enterprises on New and Emerging Risks: Overview Report How European Workplaces Manage Safety and Health. 2019. Available online: https://osha.europa.eu/en/publications/esener-2019-overview-report-how-european-workplaces-manage-safety-and-health (accessed on 3 January 2023).
11. Baeriswyl, S.; Bratoljic, C.; Krause, A. How homeroom teachers cope with high demands: Effect of prolonging working hours on emotional exhaustion. *J. Sch. Psychol.* **2021**, *85*, 125–139. [CrossRef] [PubMed]

12. Simões, F.; Calheiros, M.M. A matter of teaching and relationships: Determinants of teaching style, interpersonal resources and teacher burnout. *Soc. Psychol. Educ.* **2019**, *22*, 991–1013. [CrossRef]
13. Skaalvik, E.M.; Skaalvik, S. Teacher job satisfaction and motivation to leave the teaching profession: Relations with school context, feeling of belonging, and emotional exhaustion. *Teach. Teach. Educ.* **2011**, *27*, 1029–1038. [CrossRef]
14. Mijakoski, D.; Cheptea, D.; Marca, S.C.; Shoman, Y.; Caglayan, C.; Bugge, M.D.; Gnesi, M.; Godderis, L.; Kiran, S.; McElvenny, D.M.; et al. Determinants of Burnout among Teachers: A Systematic Review of Longitudinal Studies. *Int. J. Environ. Res. Public Health* **2022**, *19*, 5776. [CrossRef] [PubMed]
15. Fernet, C.; Guay, F.; Senécal, C.; Austin, S. Predicting intraindividual changes in teacher burn-out: The role of perceived school environment and motivational factors. *Teach. Teach. Educ.* **2012**, *28*, 514–525. [CrossRef]
16. Bermejo-Toro, L.; Prieto-Ursúa, M.; Hernández, V. Towards a model of teacher well-being: Personal and job resources involved in teacher burnout and engagement. *Educ. Psychol. Int. J. Exp. Educ. Psychol.* **2015**, *36*, 481–501. [CrossRef]
17. Grunwitz, K. The future is Society 5.0. *Comput. Fraud. Secur.* **2019**, *8*, 20. [CrossRef]
18. Keidanren (Japan Business Federation). Toward Realization of the New Economy and Society—Reform of the Economy and Society by the Deepening of "Society 5.0". 2016. Available online: http://www.keidanren.or.jp/en/policy/2016/029_outline.pdf (accessed on 12 November 2019).
19. Santos, G.; Afonseca, J.; Murmura, F.; Félix, M.J.; Lopes, N. Critical success factors in the management of ideas as an essential component of innovation and business excellence. *Int. J. Qual. Serv. Sci.* **2018**, *3*, 214–232. [CrossRef]
20. Fernandes da Silva, C.; Amaral, V.; Pereira, A.; Bem-haja, P.; Pereira, A.; Rodrigues, V. *Copenhagen Psychosocial Questionnaire, COPSOQ II*; Universidade de Aveiro: Aveiro, Portugal, 2012.
21. Li, R.; Liu, H.; Chen, Y.; Yao, M. Why teachers want to leave? The roles of achievement goals, burnout and perceived school context. *Learn. Individ. Differ.* **2021**, *89*, 102032. [CrossRef]
22. Saloviita, T.; Pakarinen, E. Teacher burnout explained: Teacher-, student-, and organisation-level variables. *Teach. Teach. Educ.* **2021**, *97*, 103221. [CrossRef]
23. Prasojo, L.D.; Habibi, A.; Yaakob, M.F.M.; Pratama, R.; Yusof, M.R.; Mukminin, A.; Suyanto; Hanum, F. Dataset relating to the relationship between teacher self-concept and teacher efficacy as the predictors of burnout: A survey in Indonesian education. *Data Brief* **2020**, *30*, 105448. [CrossRef]
24. Hassan, O.; Ibourk, A. Burnout, self-efficacy and job satisfaction among primary schools teachers in Morocco. *Soc. Sci. Humanit. Open* **2021**, *4*, 100148.
25. Brown, S.P.; Biddle, C. Testing a teacher costs to caring resilience model to identify burnout mediators. *Teach. Teach. Educ.* **2023**, *127*, 104078. [CrossRef]
26. Rebelo, M.F.; Silva, R.; Santos, G. The integration of standardized management systems: Managing business risk. *Int. J. Qual. Reliab. Manag.* **2017**, *34*, 395–405. [CrossRef]
27. Vilhena, E.; Ramos, D.; Veloso Neto, H.; Vilaça, C. Psychosocial Working Climate in a Portuguese Metallurgical Industry. *Stud. Syst. Decis. Control.* **2022**, *406*, 521–531.

Disclaimer/Publisher's Note: The statements, opinions and data contained in all publications are solely those of the individual author(s) and contributor(s) and not of MDPI and/or the editor(s). MDPI and/or the editor(s) disclaim responsibility for any injury to people or property resulting from any ideas, methods, instructions or products referred to in the content.

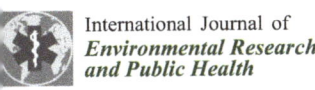

Article

Managing Nanomaterials in the Workplace by Using the Control Banding Approach [†]

Delfina Ramos [1,2,3,*] and Luis Almeida [4]

1. ISEP—School of Engineering, Polytechnic of Porto, 4249-015 Porto, Portugal
2. Associate Laboratory for Energy, Transports and Aerospace (LAETA-INEGI), Rua Dr. Roberto Frias 400, 4200-465 Porto, Portugal
3. Algoritmi Research Centre/LASI, School of Engineering, University of Minho, 4800-058 Guimarães, Portugal
4. Department of Textile Engineering, University of Minho, 4800-058 Guimarães, Portugal
* Correspondence: dgr@isep.ipp.pt
† This paper is an extended version of our paper published in Ramos, D., Almeida, L., Gomes M. Application of Control Banding to Workplace Exposure to Nanomaterials in the Textile Industry. In: Arezes P. et al. (eds) Occupational and Environmental Safety and Health. Studies in Systems, Decision and Control, vol 202. Springer, Cham. Pages 105–113, https://doi.org/10.1007/978-3-030-14730-3_12.

Abstract: Nanomaterials offer new technical and commercial opportunities. However, they may also pose risks to consumers and the environment and raise concerns about occupational health and safety. An overview of the standardization in the area of nanomaterials is presented. Focus is given to the standard ISO/TS 12901-2:2014, which describes the use of a control banding approach for controlling the risks associated with occupational exposures to nano-objects and their aggregates and agglomerates greater than 100 nm. The article also presents a case study on a textile finishing company that implements two chemical finishes containing nanomaterials. A risk analysis was conducted to assess the hazards associated with workers handling nanomaterials. Control banding was applied, and measures such as appropriate ventilation and use of protective equipment are proposed to mitigate risks. In some cases, additional measures, such as a closed booth and smoke extractor, are required. The safety data sheets are a primary source of information on how to handle and care for products containing nanomaterials, but the information provided is still limited in terms of the specific hazards and risks posed by nanomaterials.

Keywords: nanomaterials; occupational health and safety; risk management; control banding; standardization; textiles

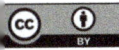

1. Introduction

1.1. Nanomaterials

Nanomaterials are incredibly small particles, as tiny as 10,000 times smaller than a human hair. To be considered as "nano", they must have at least one dimension that is less than 100 nanometers. They can be found in various everyday products, such as food, cosmetics, textiles, electronics, etc. [1,2].

Nanomaterials have unique characteristics that make them very valuable. This is due not only to their miniature size but also factors such as shape and surface area. In reality, the properties of nanomaterials may differ significantly from those of the same materials at larger scales [1,2].

Due to these distinctions in properties, nanomaterials bring new and exciting possibilities to different industries and areas, such as engineering, information technology, medicine, and pharmaceuticals. However, the same characteristics that give nanomaterials their special properties can also lead to potential impacts on human health and the environment [1–4].

Nanomaterials can be found naturally, such as in volcano emissions, or as a result of human activities, such as diesel exhaust fumes or tobacco smoke. Of particular interest are manufactured nanomaterials designed specifically for a certain use, which are already being incorporated into a vast array of products and applications.

Some nanomaterials have been used for many years, such as synthetic amorphous silica in concrete and food products, while others are more recent discoveries, such as nano-titanium dioxide, used as a UV blocking agent in paints and sunscreens; nano-silver, used as an anti-microbial in textiles and medical applications; or carbon nanotubes, which are used for their mechanical strength, light weight, heat dissipation properties, and electrical conductivity in fields such as electronics, energy storage, spacecraft and vehicle structures, and sports equipment. The market for nanomaterials is rapidly growing and new generations of nanomaterials are being developed at a fast pace. Note that despite the numerous advantages of nanomaterials, there is still a significant amount of knowledge missing regarding their potential health risks [1,4].

In fact, there are significant concerns regarding the health effects of nanomaterials [4]. The Scientific Committee on Emerging and Newly Identified Health Risks (SCENIHR) found that there are proven health hazards associated with a number of manufactured nanomaterials. Not all nanomaterials necessarily have a toxic effect, however, and a case-by-case approach is necessary while ongoing research continues [2].

The most significant effects of nanomaterials have been observed in the lungs, including inflammation, tissue damage, fibrosis, and the generation of tumors. The cardiovascular system may also be affected. Some types of carbon nanotubes have been shown to have effects similar to asbestos. Nanomaterials have been found to reach other organs and tissues, such as the liver, kidneys, heart, brain, skeleton, and soft tissues. The small size and large surface area of particulate nanomaterials in powder form can pose a risk of explosion, while their coarser materials may not [2,5].

Workers can be exposed to nanomaterials in various work environments where nanomaterials are used, handled, or processed, which can cause them to become airborne and potentially inhaled or come into contact with the skin. This type of exposure is most common during the production stage, but workers throughout the supply chain may also come into contact with nanomaterials without realizing it [4]. This raises concerns about the lack of measures in place to prevent exposure, making it crucial to educate workers about the potential risks. The European Agency for Safety and Health at Work (EU-OSHA) has published several resources on risk awareness and communication related to nanomaterials in the workplace [1].

1.2. Legislation and Standardization

It is important to emphasize that, in 2014, the European Commission published a recommendation regarding the definition of nanomaterials, which has recently been revised (Commission Recommendation of 10 June 2022):

> "Nanomaterial means a natural, incidental or manufactured material consisting of solid particles that are present, either on their own or as identifiable constituent particles in aggregates or agglomerates, and where 50 % or more of these particles in the number-based size distribution fulfil at least one of the following conditions: (a) one or more external dimensions of the particle are in the size range 1 nm to 100 nm; (b) the particle has an elongated shape, such as a rod, fiber or tube, where two external dimensions are smaller than 1 nm and the other dimension is larger than 100 nm; and (c) the particle has a plate-like shape, where one external dimension is smaller than 1 nm and the other dimensions are larger than 100 nm" [2].

Within the European Union, there is legislation in place to protect workers from the potential risks associated with nanomaterials, even though the legislation does not explicitly mention these materials. The Framework Directive 89/391/EEC, the Chemical Agent Directive 98/24/EC, and the Carcinogen and Mutagen Directive 2004/37/EC, as well as the regulations on chemicals such as Registration, Evaluation, Authorization and Restriction of Chemicals (REACH) and Classification, Labelling and Packaging (CLP), are particularly relevant in this context. This means that employers must assess and manage the risks of nanomaterials in the workplace.

If the use and generation of nanomaterials cannot be eliminated or substituted by less hazardous materials and processes, the exposure of workers must be minimized through preventive measures following a hierarchy of control that prioritizes elimination, substitution, engineering controls, administrative controls, and personal protective equipment in that order. Although many uncertainties still exist, there is a high level of concern about the safety and health hazards of nanomaterials. Therefore, employers and workers must take a precautionary approach to risk management and the selection of prevention measures [1,4].

Standard documents are essential to support the effective implementation of legislation. Standards cover terminology, test methods, material specifications, management systems, and other relevant areas. The authors of this text recently published a review of standards related to the occupational risk and safety of nanotechnologies [6]. A summary and update of this review is presented below.

At the international level, ISO has been developing a large set of standards related to nanotechnology, especially within ISO Technical Committee 229, created in 2005. Working group three deals specifically with health, safety, and environmental aspects of nanotechnologies.

At the European level, the Technical Committee CEN TC 352, created in 2006, is engaged in standardization in the field of nanotechnologies. The standards that have already been published or are under preparation include those that deal with science-based health, safety, and environmental practices.

The European Commission has recognized the importance of standards in supporting legislation and has issued a mandate to the European standardization bodies to develop testing methods and tools for characterizing, understanding the behavior of, and assessing the exposure to nanomaterials. This exposure assessment takes into account the health and safety of workers, as well as the protection of the consumers and of the environment [5].

The coordination of this mandate falls under CEN/TC 352, but multiple CEN and ISO technical committees are involved in its execution. Several European standards have already been published under this mandate, and others are currently being developed. Many of these standards are related to occupational health and safety.

Up to now (April 2023), 32 European standards have been published, including 26 EN/ISO documents developed in conjunction with ISO/TC229. Nine new standards are being prepared. The updated list can be consulted at https://standards.cen.eu/, accessed on 15 April 2023.

Related to ISO/TC229, up to now (February 2023), 102 standard documents have already been published and 32 are under development covering health and safety aspects. The following documents are especially relevant:

- ISO/TR 12885:2018—Nanotechnologies—Health and safety practices in occupational settings;
- ISO/TS 12901-1:2012—Nanotechnologies—Occupational risk management applied to engineered nanomaterials—Part 1: Principles and approaches;
- ISO/TS 12901-2:2014—Nanotechnologies—Occupational risk management applied to engineered nanomaterials—Part 2: Use of the control banding approach;
- ISO/TR 13121:2011—Nanotechnologies—Nanomaterial risk evaluation;
- ISO/TR 13329:2012—Nanomaterials—Preparation of material safety data sheet (MSDS).

In 2006, the Organization for Economic Co-operation and Development (OECD) established the Working Party on Manufactured Nanomaterials (WPMN) as a subsidiary body of the OECD Chemicals Committee. This program is focused on examining the implications of manufactured nanomaterials for human health and the environment. Since its inception, the WPMN has published more than 100 documents under the "Safety of Manufactured Nanomaterials" series, some of which are related to standards. A complete list of all freely downloadable documents can be found at: http://www.oecd.org/env/

ehs/nanosafety/publications-series-safety-manufactured-nanomaterials.htm, accessed on 15 April 2023 [6].

At the European level, it is also important to mention the Malta Initiative, which was launched during the Maltese EU Council Presidency in 2017. Although this is a self-organized group without any legally binding status, it involves 18 European countries, several Directorates-General of the European Commission, the European Chemicals Agency (ECHA), authorities, research institutions, NGOs, universities, and industry representatives. The goal of this initiative is to make legislation enforceable, particularly in the chemicals sector. To achieve this, it is necessary to ensure that essential test, measurement, and verification procedures are available. The work of the Malta Initiative is focused on amending the OECD Test Guidelines in the area of nanomaterials to ensure that the REACH Regulation is duly adapted to fully cover materials at the nanoscale [6].

1.3. Control Banding Approach Applied to Engineered Nanomaterials

The control banding approach has been widely recommended for the selection of exposure controls for engineered nanomaterials. This approach is particularly useful for controlling workplace exposure to potentially hazardous agents with unknown or uncertain toxicological properties and where quantitative exposure estimations are lacking [6–9].

Already in 2009, the National Institute for Occupational Safety and Health NIOSH) published an extensive review about control banding [4]. There are several control banding tools available, such as NanoSafer, Stoffenmanager-Nano, NanoTool, Precautionary Matrix, ANSES, etc., which can lead to different results [8,9]. In the present study, the ISO Technical Specification ISO/TS 12901-2:2014 was chosen as it is an internationally recognized method.

The control banding process, as defined in ISO/TS 12901-2:2014, involves several elements, including information gathering, assignment of nano-objects to a hazard band based on a comprehensive evaluation of all available data, description of potential exposure characteristics based on workplace scenarios, definition of recommended work environments and handling practices by applying control banding methods, and evaluation of the control strategy or risk banding. Factors such as toxicity, in vivo biopersistence, the ability of particles to reach and be deposited in various regions of the respiratory tract, and their potential to elicit biological responses are considered when assigning a hazard band to each material. Actual exposure measurement data and the potential for dust generation during processes are also taken into account when defining exposure scenarios at the workplace.

A new registration system for nanomaterials has been introduced under REACH Regulation, which took effect in January 2020 (Commission Regulation (EU) 2018/1881 of 3 December 2018). It is recommended that chemical suppliers incorporating nanomaterials provide more information on hazards and risk mitigation measures in safety data sheets based on the guidelines provided in ISO/TR 13329:2012. This information is necessary for the implementation of the control banding approach [10].

More recently, the new Commission Regulation (EU) 2020/878 was introduced on 18 June 2020, which amends Annex II to REACH, providing requirements for compiling safety data sheets used to provide safety information on hazardous chemical substances and mixtures in the EU. This regulation, which came into full force in January 2023, provides more detailed requirements to be included in the safety data sheets of chemicals that include nanoforms.

1.4. Use of Nanotechnology in Textiles

Nanotechnology is frequently used in textile products to provide specific functionalities, such as incorporating nanoparticles into textile materials. The common effects include antibacterial effects (using, for instance, nanosilver), ultraviolet protection (using nano-titanium oxide), and self-cleaning through the nanostructuring of the surface. The durability of nanoparticles in textiles depends not only on their attachment to the fabric but also on the impact of the fabric's lifecycle, which can cause damage to the textile material or the bond between the nanoparticle and fibers due to abrasion, mechanical stress, UV radiation, body fluids, water, detergents, and temperature changes [11–13].

Nanoparticles can interact with the human body through inhalation, ingestion, and skin contact, with skin contact being the most relevant pathway for textiles. As part of the European Commission's mandate, CEN/TC248 (Textile and Textile Products) has developed a specific test method for skin exposure to nanomaterials. The technical report CEN/TR 17222:2019 titled "Textile products and nanotechnologies—Guidance on tests to simulate nanoparticle release—Skin exposure" has been published [14]. This method is based on existing textile standard test methods, which include the extraction of nanomaterials using artificial perspiration solutions under physical stress (a method adapted by Goetz et al. [15]) and measuring the release to the air from the textile due to mechanical action [11,12].

2. Materials and Methods

2.1. Control Banding: ISO/TS 12901-2:2014

The control banding approach was originally developed by the pharmaceutical industry to safely handle new chemicals with limited or no toxicity data. This practical method can also be utilized to manage the risk of exposure to possibly hazardous agents in the workplace that have unknown or uncertain toxicological properties, such as nanomaterials, where quantitative exposure estimations are not available.

Developing a control banding approach for nanomaterials presents a significant challenge, as it is necessary to determine which parameters and criteria are relevant to assign a nano-object to a control band and which operational strategies to implement. Producers or importers are responsible for identifying whether their product contains nanomaterials and must provide relevant information in safety data sheets, labels, etc., in accordance with existing regulations. By utilizing this information, companies and employees can recognize potential hazards and implement appropriate controls [4,6,11,12,16].

ISO/TS 12901-2:2014 mentioned above is a Technical Specification developed by the ISO that presents a guide to the use of control banding in managing occupational risks associated with engineered nanomaterials. Given the level of uncertainty in assessing potential work-related health risks from nano-objects, including aggregates and agglomerates larger than 100 nm, control banding is a valuable tool for risk assessment and management of nanomaterials. The control banding process outlined in this standard includes several elements, which are well-summarized in the infographic presented in the standard and briefly described below.

First, information must be gathered, and if there are limited or no data available, "reasonable worst-case assumptions" should be used along with management practices appropriate for those options. Then, hazard banding is used to assign a hazard band to nano-objects based on a comprehensive evaluation of available data, taking into account parameters such as toxicity, in vivo biopersistence, and respiratory tract deposition. Exposure banding is used to assign an exposure scenario to an exposure band, taking into account the physical form and amount of the nano-object, dust generation potential, and actual exposure measurement data. Next, control banding is implemented proactively or retroactively to define recommended work environments and handling practices based on hazard banding and fundamental factors mitigating anticipated exposure potential. Finally, periodic and as-needed reviews are conducted to ensure that the information, evaluations, decisions, and actions from the previous steps are kept up to date [4,7,11,12].

ISO/TS 12901-2:2014 describes five hazard bands, as summarized in Table 1 [7].

Table 1. Hazard bands.

Category	Hazard
HB A	No significant risk to health
HB B	Slight hazard—slightly toxic
HB C	Moderate hazard
HB D	Serious hazard
HB E	Severe hazard

Details of the allocation of the different hazard bands can be found in Table 1 in the standard.

In terms of exposure banding, the standard proposes four levels from EB 1 to EB 4 corresponding to increased levels of exposure to nanomaterials. In the case of production processes where nanomaterials are handled in liquid form, exposure banding using the levels EB1 or EB2 is normally suggested. When nano-objects are in suspension in a liquid, the choice depends on the amount of liquid and number of nano-objects involved, as well as the potential for aerosol generation [12].

Table 2 presents the control measures proposed in the standard.

Table 2. Specific control measures for risk mitigation bands.

Level of Risk	Control Measure
CB 1	Natural or mechanical general ventilation
CB 2	Local ventilation: extractor hood, slot hood, arm hood, table hood, etc.
CB 3	Enclosed ventilation: ventilated booth, fume hood, closed reactor with regular opening
CB 4	Full containment: glove box/bags, continuously closed systems
CB 5	Full containment and review by a specialist: seek expert advice

Control banding can be determined by combining the hazard bands and the potential exposure band. The corresponding matrix included in ISO/TS 12901-2:2014 is presented in Table 3 [7].

Table 3. Control band matrix as a result of hazard and exposure potential bands.

Hazard Band	Exposure Band			
	EB 1	EB 2	EB 3	EB 4
HB A	CB 1	CB 1	CB 1	CB 2
HB B	CB 1	CB 1	CB 2	CB 3
HB C	CB 2	CB 3	CB 3	CB 4
HB D	CB 3	CB 4	CB 4	CB 5
HB E	CB 4	CB 5	CB 5	CB 5

2.2. Case Study

In a case study conducted by Ramos et al. [11], the methodology of control banding was applied in a Portuguese textile finishing company specialized in producing knitted fabrics. The study focused on the use of nanomaterials in two chemical finishes—namely, mosquito repellent and antibacterial finish—which were applied to specific customers' textile products. The risk analysis was mainly focused on four workers who were involved in preparing the finishing baths and operating the stenter frame for knitted fabric finishing [4,7,11,12].

The safety data sheets for the two chemicals, in accordance with the CLP regulation (Regulation EC No 1272/2008), present the hazard statements (H) and precautionary statements (P) shown in Tables 4 and 5.

Table 4. Product A (mosquito repellent).

Product A (Mosquito Repellent)	
Hazard Statements (H)	**Precautionary Statements (P)**
H319—causes serious eye irritation	P233—keep container tightly closed P261—avoid breathing dust/fume/gas/mist/vapors/spray P305 + P351 + P338—if in eyes, rinse cautiously with water for several minutes; remove contact lenses, if present and easy to do; continue rinsing P305 + P351 + P338—if in eyes, rinse cautiously with water for several minutes; remove contact lenses, if present and easy to do; continue rinsing P403 + P233—store in a well-ventilated place, keep container tightly closed P501—dispose of contents/container according to local/regional/national/international legislation

Table 5. Product B (antibacterial finish).

Product B (Antibacterial Finish)	
Hazard Statements (H)	**Precautionary Statements (P)**
H302—harmful if swallowed H318—causes serious eye damageH332—harmful if inhaled	P233—keep container tightly closed P261—avoid breathing dust/fume/gas/mist/vapors/spray P280—wear protective gloves/protective clothing/eye protection/face protection P273—avoid release to the environment
H410—very toxic to aquatic life with long-lasting effects	P301 + P312—if swallowed, call a poison center or doctor/physician if you feel unwell P305 + P351 + P338—if in eyes, rinse cautiously with water for several minutes, remove contact lenses, if present and easy to do, continue rinsing P501—dispose of contents/container to approved incineration unit

The two chemicals, delivered in cans in an aqueous suspension, are applied to cotton knitted fabrics through padding and heat setting in a stenter frame. It should be noted that neither the product information nor the safety data sheets explicitly mention that these chemicals contain nanomaterials, although this information is indirectly provided by the suppliers. In one case, the information just states that the remaining composition of the product is kept secret by the company.

The risk analysis primarily focused on the four workers involved in the preparation of the finishing baths, starting in the chemical warehouse, and in the operation of the stenter frame. The workers' tasks included opening the cans, weighing the required amount for each batch, transporting the chemicals to the production process, transferring the chemicals to the stenter frame (via automatic dispenser), mixing and preparing the chemicals (with the addition of water), and, finally, developing the finishing process in the stenter.

3. Results and Discussion

The hazard band HB B was selected for product A (mosquito repellent) due to the potential for serious eye irritation. Exposure band EB 2 was chosen because it is in a suspension form and used in quantities greater than 1 L, with low potential for aerosol formation. During production, the exposure of workers to nanomaterials is low, resulting in the selection of EB 1. The control band CB 1, which includes natural or mechanical general ventilation, was chosen in accordance with Table 2.

The company has already implemented all of the measures recommended in this study, ISO/TS 12901-2: 2014, and the product safety data sheet for product A. Workers wear protective glasses, 0.7 mm thick butyl rubber gloves, protective clothing, and a respiratory mask when vapors are released. The results of the control banding process for the different tasks performed by workers handling product A are shown in Table 6.

Table 6. Selection of control bands for product A (mosquito repellent).

Task	Hazard Band	Exposure Band	Control Band
Opening of the packaging and weighing of the chemicals	HB B	EB 2	CB 1
Transportation and trans-shipment	HB B	EB 2	CB 1
Preparation and start	HB B	EB 2	CB 1
Production	HB B	EB 1	CB 1

Product A has potential to cause serious eye irritation, so hazard band HB B was chosen for all tasks performed by the workers. Exposure Band EB2 was selected for all tasks except the production phase, as the chemical is in a suspension form with low potential for aerosol formation but is used in quantities greater than 1 L. For the production phase, EB 1 was selected due to the low exposure of workers to the chemicals. In accordance with Table 3, the corresponding control band CB 1 was chosen, needing only natural or mechanical general ventilation [12].

The company has already implemented all suggested measures for product A, including personal protective equipment (PPE), such as protective glasses, gloves, clothing, and respiratory masks.

Table 7 presents the results of the control banding process applied to the different tasks performed by the workers involved in handling product B.

Table 7. Selection of control bands for product B (antibacterial finish).

Task	Hazard Band	Exposure Band	Control Band
Opening of the packaging and weighing of the chemicals	HB C	EB 2	CB 3
Transportation and trans-shipment	HB C	EB 2	CB 3
Preparation and start	HB C	EB 2	CB 3
Production (stenter)	HB C	EB 1	CB 2

Product B has potential to cause serious eye damage and other health issues. Therefore, the hazard band HB C was selected for all tasks performed by the workers. Exposure band EB 2 was selected since this chemical is in a suspension form with low potential for aerosol formation but is used in quantities greater than 1 L. However, in the case of the production phase, where worker exposure to nanomaterials is low, EB 1 was chosen. In accordance with Table 3, the corresponding control band for product B is CB 3 for all tasks except for the production process, where CB 2 is suggested. CB3 involves the need for enclosed ventilation (a ventilated booth, fume hood, closed reactor with regular opening) whereas, for the production process, local ventilation is sufficient, such as an extractor hood, slot hood, arm hood, table hood, etc.

The company has implemented measures recommended by the product safety data sheet and ISO/TS 12901-2:2014. Workers wear protective glasses, nitrile rubber gloves, protective clothing, and respiratory protection when vapors are released. Further measures requiring more investment will be implemented at a later stage [12].

4. Conclusions

The control banding approach was used to suggest risk mitigation measures based on work station analysis and supplier information concerning the chemicals used.

Although there are, in most cases, still no legal occupational exposure limits, it is recommended that the company conduct exposure measurements for chemicals with nanoscale materials at the workplace as these limits can come up in the future.

The lack of information on specific nanomaterials and corresponding risks in safety data sheets is a major issue. To address this, it is suggested that suppliers include more detailed hazard and risk information in safety data sheets based on ISO/TR 13329:2012 recommendations [10].

Note that, since January 2023, within the European Union, it is required to include information concerning the nanoforms present in chemicals.

It is also recommended to measure occupational exposure to engineered nanomaterials; for instance, using the method used by Iavicoli et al. [17].

The use of other control banding tools is also suggested for future work, allowing a comparison of the results obtained.

It is worth noting that ISO/TS 12901-2 is currently under revision, so updating the present study in the future is also recommended.

Author Contributions: Conceptualization, D.R. and L.A.; methodology, D.R. and L.A.; investigation, D.R. and L.A.; resources, D.R. and L.A.; data curation, D.R.; writing—original draft preparation, D.R. and L.A.; writing—review and editing, D.R. and L.A. All authors have read and agreed to the published version of the manuscript.

Funding: This research received no external funding.

Institutional Review Board Statement: Not applicable.

Informed Consent Statement: Informed consent was obtained from all subjects involved in the study.

Data Availability Statement: Not applicable.

Conflicts of Interest: The authors declare no conflict of interest.

References

1. EU-OSHA. European Agency for Safety and Health at Work (EU-OSHA). *Managing Nanomaterials in the Workplace.* 2022. Available online: https://osha.europa.eu/en/emerging-risks/nanomaterials (accessed on 15 April 2023).
2. European Commission; Official Journal of the European Union. Commission Recommendation of 10 June 2022 (2022/C 229/01). Definition of Nanomaterial. 2022. Available online: https://ec.europa.eu/environment/chemicals/nanotech/faq/definition_en.htm (accessed on 15 April 2023).
3. Ramos, D.; Cotrim, T.; Arezes, P.; Baptista, J.; Rodrigues, M.; Leitão, J. Frontiers in Occupational Health and Safety Management. *Int. J. Environ. Res. Public Health* **2022**, *19*, 10459. [CrossRef] [PubMed]
4. Lentz, T.; Niemeier, R.; Geraci, C.L. *Qualitative Risk Characterization and Management of Occupational Hazards: Control Banding (CB): A Literature Review and Critical Analysis*; The National Institute for Occupational Safety and Health (NIOSH): Washington, DC, USA, 2009. [CrossRef]
5. Almeida, L.; Ramos, D. Particle Technology and Textiles Review of Applications. In De Gruyter STEM; Cornier, J., De Gruyter, F.P., Eds., Berlin, Germany; Chapter VII—Governance/Legislation/EU Legal Framework-REACH.; Occupational Health Aspects (EU); De Gruyter, Berlin, Germany, 2022. Available online: https://www.degruyter.com/document/isbn/9783110670776/html (accessed on 15 April 2023).
6. Ramos, D.; Almeida, L. Overview of Standards Related to the Occupational Risk and Safety of Nanotechnologies. *Standards* **2022**, *2*, 7. [CrossRef]
7. *ISO/TS 12901-2: 2014*; Nanotechnologies—Occupational Risk Management Applied to Engineered Nanomaterials—Part 2: Use of the Control Banding Approach. International Organization for Standardization: Geneva, Switzerland, 2014.
8. Eastlake, A.; Zumwalde, R.; Geraci, C. Can Control Banding be Useful for the Safe Handling of Nanomaterials? A Systematic Review. *J. Nanoparticle Res.* **2016**, *18*, 169. [CrossRef] [PubMed]

9. Jiménez, A.S.; Varet, J.; Poland, C.; Fern, G.J.; Hankin, S.M.; van Tongeren, M. A comparison of control banding tools for nanomaterials. *J. Occup. Environ. Hyg.* **2016**, *13*, 936–949. [CrossRef] [PubMed]
10. ISO/TR 13329:2012; Nanomaterials—Preparation of material safety data sheet (MSDS). International Organization for Standardization: Geneva, Switzerland, 2012.
11. Almeida, L.; Ramos, D. Health and safety concerns of textiles with nanomaterials. *IOP Conf. Series Mater. Sci. Eng.* **2017**, *254*, 102002. [CrossRef]
12. Ramos, D.; Almeida, L.; Gomes, M. Application of Control Banding to Workplace Exposure to Nanomaterials in the Textile Industry. In *Occupational and Environmental Safety and Health*; Studies in Systems, Decision and Control; Arezes, P., Baptista, J., Barroso, M., Carneiro, P., Cordeiro, P., Costa, N., Melo, R., Miguel, A., Perestrelo, G., Eds.; Springer: Cham, Switzerland, 2019; Volume 202, pp. 105–113. [CrossRef]
13. Wong, Y.; Yuen, C.; Leung, M.; Ku, S.; Lam, H. Selected Applications of Nanotechnology in Textiles. *Autex Res. J.* **2006**, *6*, 1–10.
14. CEN/TR 17222:2019; Textile Products and Nanotechnologies—Guidance on Tests to Simulate Nanoparticle Release—Skin Exposure. CEN, European Committee for Standardization: Geneva, Switzerland, 2019.
15. von Goetz, N.; Lorenz, C.; Windler, L.; Nowack, B.; Heuberger, M.; Hungerbühler, K. Migration of Ag- and TiO_2-(Nano)particles from Textiles into Artificial Sweat under Physical Stress: Experiments and Exposure Modeling. *Environ. Sci. Technol.* **2013**, *47*, 9979–9987. [CrossRef] [PubMed]
16. Gomes, J.; Miranda, R.; Esteves, M.; Albuquerque, P.C. Risk Assessment of Welding Operations and Processes in Terms of Ultrafine Particles Emissions. In *Risk Management: An Overview*; Ramos, D., Almeida, L., Eds.; Business Issues, Competition and Entrepreneurship, Nova Science Publishers: New York, NY, USA, 2021; Chapter 7; p. 157, ISBN 978-1-68507-177-6. [CrossRef]
17. Iavicoli, I.; Fontana, L.; Pingue, P.; Todea, A.M.; Asbach, C. Assessment of occupational exposure to engineered nanomaterials in research laboratories using personal monitors. *Sci. Total Environ.* **2018**, *627*, 689–702. [CrossRef]

Disclaimer/Publisher's Note: The statements, opinions and data contained in all publications are solely those of the individual author(s) and contributor(s) and not of MDPI and/or the editor(s). MDPI and/or the editor(s) disclaim responsibility for any injury to people or property resulting from any ideas, methods, instructions or products referred to in the content.

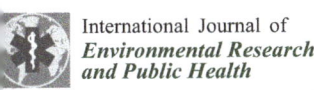

Article

Prevalence of Comorbidity and Its Effects on Sickness-Absenteeism among Brazilian Legislative Civil Servants

Francisco Edison Sampaio [1,*], Manuel Joaquim Silva Oliveira [1], João Areosa [2] and Emílio Facas [3]

1 Faculty of Engineering, University of Porto (FEUP), 4200-465 Porto, Portugal
2 Higher School of Business Sciences, Polytechnic Institute of Setubal, 2914-503 Setubal, Portugal
3 Department of Social and Work Psychology, University of Brasilia (UNB), Brasília 70910-900, Brazil
* Correspondence: sampaio.eng.trab@gmail.com; Tel.: +55-62-98562-1011

Abstract: Studies have shown there is an association of chronic diseases with working days lost, considering the impact of these pathologies on the levels of vulnerability of the individual's health, with an increased risk of work disability. This article is part of a more comprehensive investigation on the sickness absenteeism of civil servants of the legislative branch in Brazil, with the purpose of determining the comorbidity index (CI) of the individuals and its correlation with days of absence from work. Sickness absenteeism was counted from the data of 37,690 medical leaves, from 2016 to 2109, involving 4149 civil servants. The self-administered comorbidity questionnaire (SCQ) was used to estimate the CI, based on the diseases or chronic health problems declared by the participants. The average number of working days lost per servant per year was 8.73 days, totaling 144,902 days of absence. The majority of the servants (65.5%) declared at least one chronic health condition. A significant association between the CI scores and working days lost was observed (r = 0.254, p-value < 0.01), thus showing that the CI may be an important predictor of sickness absenteeism. Chronic diseases or health problems are a characteristic of the general population, often affecting working capacity.

Keywords: chronic disease; comorbidity; multimorbidity; sickness absenteeism; comorbidity index; civil servant

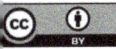

1. Introduction

Work absenteeism is a global phenomenon that affects public and private organizations with detrimental effects on employers, employees, government, and society. Globally, annual statistics indicate the occurrence of about 374 million non-fatal work accidents, which cause at least four days of absence from work. In addition, over 2.7 million worker deaths from occupational accidents or illnesses have been reported [1]. In Europe, sickness absenteeism averaged 11.5 days per worker per year from 1970 to 2019 [2]. In Brazil, a total of 2,934,155 occupational accidents were recorded from 2015 to 2019, of which 34% caused at least 16 days away from work. Of these accidents or occupational diseases, 85,603 occurrences involved Brazilian civil servants from the executive, legislative, and judiciary branches [3]. Moreover, the International Labor Organization (ILO) has reported negative economic effects at around 3.94% of the Gross Domestic Product worldwide each year due to work absenteeism [1].

Several studies on sickness absenteeism in the public service have reported some pathological predictors of work absences, including mental health problems, musculoskeletal disorders, trauma to different parts of the body, and respiratory system diseases, among others [4–7]. In this context, individuals with comorbidity may present a higher degree of absence from work due to the level of human vulnerability. In Australia, individuals with comorbidity reported greater symptom severity, poorer work performance, and a greater number of working days lost when compared to individuals with more favorable health conditions [8].

1.1. Work Absenteeism and Sickness Absenteeism

Work absenteeism is the absence or non-attendance of the worker at work, regardless of the reason and legality [9]. As reported by De Oliveira (2016, p. 14) [10], absenteeism can be understood as a phenomenon of multifactorial etiology, characterized by an unplanned absence from the workplace. In addition, absenteeism is understood as absences due to personal health problems, leading to medical leaves [4]. According to the ILO, absenteeism is the absence from work due to a worker's incapacity for the working tasks, caused by illness or an accident injury, or risk of transmission of some disease, excluding non-attendance at work resulting from pregnancy and imprisonment [11]. Sickness absenteeism is a phenomenon that affects private and public organizations since all work exercises can expose the worker to dangers inherent to the environment and general working conditions, regardless of the type of work. As reported by Rodrigues et al., (2013, p. 138) [5], absenteeism is a worldwide phenomenon of multidimensional character, resulting from non-specific complaints and declared illnesses, and its occurrence and evolution are influenced by socio-demographic, behavioral, and occupational factors, among others.

1.2. Comorbidity

The term comorbidity does not reflect a conceptual consensus or convergence regarding its application in health care, with distinct approaches from several authors and health institutions. However, there is no disagreement about the association of this health condition with incapacity to work, and therefore absenteeism from work. Briefly, comorbidity has been described as the coexistence of two or more diseases in a patient, taking as reference an index disease, while multicomorbidity comprises an equivalent condition regarding the presence of diseases or chronic health problems in the same individual, without considering a medical condition as reference or dominant [7,8]. When dealing with the conceptualization of comorbidity, Valderas et al., (2009) [12] recognize that although there is no agreement on the subject, comorbidity is most often defined according to a specific index condition (main or reference disease). In this regard, the author presents Feinstein's definition, which describes comorbidity as any additional different entity that has existed or may occur during the clinical course of a patient with an index disease under study. On the other hand, the author brings the concept of multimorbidity as the "co-occurrence" of multiple chronic or acute diseases and medical conditions in the same individual, with no reference to an index condition. As the proponents of the term multimorbidity prefer to focus on primary care, the term index disease is often not applied. Valderas et al., (2009) [12] refer to the morbidity burden, defined as the total burden of physiological dysfunction, or diseases with some impact on the physiological reserve of an individual. In turn, the term patient complexity can be defined as an interaction between the socioeconomic, cultural, environmental, and behavioral characteristics and the health conditions of the individuals, which can exert an influence on the morbidity burden. Figure 1 shows a graphic representation of these concepts.

According to the authors, comorbidity and multimorbidity are associated with adverse health outcomes. Eventually, the emphasis on an index disease may be important in specialized care. On the other hand, when primary care is the interest, the burden of multimorbidity becomes the focus, thus the patient should be treated as a whole, without privileging any specific medical condition [13]. Depending on the perspective of analysis, the differentiation between multimorbidity and comorbidity can be unreal since the same individual can be considered in both situations [13]. The conceptual relevance of comorbidity and multimorbidity is due to the impact of the approach on healthcare systems dealing with patients with multiple chronic conditions, which leads to a direction in research. In this regard, the term "comorbidity" was first proposed in 1970 by Feinstein to describe any pathology or health problem additional to an index disease. However, since 1976, the term "multimorbidity" has been used more frequently by researchers to designate the same thing as morbidity [14]. Due to a growing ambiguity in the adoption of the two terms, in 1996 Van den Akker et al. suggested keeping Feinstein's original concept for comorbidity, while multimorbidity was defined as the occurrence of multiple chronic or acute diseases and medical conditions in the same individual [14].

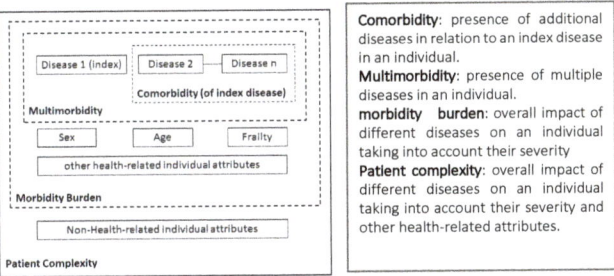

Figure 1. Comorbidity constructs, adapted from (Valderas et al., 2009 [12]).

Due to their representativeness in individual health, comorbidity and multicomorbidity should be considered highly relevant variables in studies aimed to estimate absenteeism due to illness in organizations, whether private or public. This article is part of a larger investigation on sickness absenteeism of civil servants that work in the Legislative Houses (Federal Senate, House of Representatives, and Legislative Assembly of the State of Goias—ALEGO) in Brazil, which aims to evaluate the prevalence of diseases or chronic health problems of the participants, as well as the effects of this medical condition on the number of working days lost by these servants.

2. Materials and Methods

2.1. Experimental Design

The present study consists of an observational, cross-sectional, and analytical quantitative approach to sickness absenteeism of civil servants working in the legislative branch in Brazil. The research was developed with the approval of the Ethics Committee of the Federal University of Goias, under register number 3.962.630 on 9 April 2020.

2.2. Participants

The counting of sick leave involved a total of 4149 servants who were absent from work for health reasons between January 2016 and December 2019. To evaluate the individual health condition determined through the comorbidity index, 447 electronic questionnaires answered voluntarily by the participants were validated, which meets the sample sizing requirements for a sampling error ≤ 0.5 and confidence level = 95%.

2.3. Measurements and Data Collection

The medical leaves with the reasons for absence and the respective working days lost by the servants, as well as the sociodemographic and occupational information, were made available by the organizations participating in the research, in a spreadsheet developed especially for this purpose. The health condition of the servants was evaluated using the self-administered comorbidity questionnaire (SCQ), developed, and validated by Sangha et al., (2003) [15]. All absent servants who agreed to participate in the study answered the SCQ in electronic format, under the condition of anonymity, which allowed for estimating the CI of the participants. This instrument allows the evaluation of the comorbidity condition from individual responses about the presence of diseases/chronic health problems, necessary medical treatments, and limitations imposed by medical conditions in the execution of activities. According to the SCQ, the higher the incidence of chronic diseases, combined with the need for medical treatment and restrictions in performing activities, the more serious the state of health. People with high CIs may have a higher level of personal health vulnerability, leading to a greater likelihood of work absences, especially when their health status is ignored in the workplace. Concerning the SCQ score, an individual can score a maximum of 3 points for each medical condition, consisting of 1 point for the presence of the active health problem, 1 point for the existence of medical treatment, and an additional point in case of functional limitation. The questionnaire presents 13 health problems and 3 additional possibilities, totaling a maximum score of 48 points or 39 points when the open items or closed items are used, respectively. Comorbidity was expressed as an index (CI) with a value between 0.00 (no morbidity) and 1.00 (maximum score on the questionnaire), obtained by the ratio between the score achieved by each individual and the maximum possible score.

2.4. Statistical Analysis

The counting and preliminary treatment of the sick leave data as well as the CI calculation were performed using Microsoft Office's Excel software, version 2302. The statistical analysis of absolute and relative frequencies and measures of position and dispersion and the correlation between variables were performed using IBM® SPSS Statistics (Statistical Package for the Social Sciences, Inc., Chicago, IL, USA)

3. Results

3.1. Sociodemographic and Occupation Characteristics

The servants that responded to the comorbidity survey (n = 447) were predominantly male (52.7%), married/stable union (69.1%), and a mean age above 46 years. Table 1 shows the sociodemographic details of the participants.

Table 1. Sociodemographic and occupation characteristics of the participants.

Variables		ALEGO	House of Deputies	Federal Senate	All LH
		n (%)	n (%)	n (%)	n (%)
Gender	Male	11 (61.1)	117 (48.4)	104 (57.8)	232 (52.7)
	Female	7 (38.9)	125 (51.6)	76 (42.2)	208 (47.3)
Marital status	Single/widowed	2 (11.1)	37 (15.3)	53 (29.5)	92 (20.9)
	Married/stable union	12 (66.7)	187 (77.3)	105 (58.3)	304 (69.1)
	Separated	4 (22.2)	18 (7.4)	22 (12.2)	44 (10.0)
Education	Elementary school	1 (5.6)	0 (0.0)	1 (0.6)	2 (0.4)
	High school	2 (11.1)	6 (2.5)	4 (2.2)	12 (2.7)
	College	7 (38.9)	29 (12.0)	33 (18.3)	69 (15.7)
	Specialization	6 (33.3)	141 (58.3)	110 (61.1)	257 (58.4)
	Master	2 (11.1)	44 (18.2)	26 (14.5)	72 (16.4)
	PhD	0 (0.0)	22 (9.0)	6 (3.3)	28 (6.4)
Age	M(SD) [1]	43.1 (10.0)	46.6 (7.6)	45.5 (9.1)	46.3 (9.4)
Working hours	M(SD) [1]	6.4 (0.6)	8 (0.0)	7.6 (0.6)	7.8 (0.5)
Length of service (Seniority)	M(SD) [1]	12.4 (12.4)	14.5 (8.3)	14.2 (9.7)	15.8 (10.5)

[1] Mean (Standard deviation).

3.2. Global Sickness Absenteeism Data

The work absences of civil servants from the three Legislative Houses (LH) were counted by the number of medical leaves (ML) granted and working days lost, which was taken as the parameter to portray absenteeism due to illness. In the study period (2016 to 2019), LHs issued a total of 37,690 ML, involving 4149 servants, which resulted in 144,902 working days lost. Table 2 presents a summary of these absences.

Table 2. Sickness absenteeism in the 3 Legislative Houses, from 2016 to 2019.

All Houses	Absences (Days)	Percentage (%)	Number of Absent Servants	Percentage (%)	Mean (d/s/yr)
ALEGO	4272	2.9	107	2.6	9.98
House of Deputies	103,981	71.8	2567	61.9	10.13
Federal Senate	36,649	25.3	1475	35.6	6.21
Total	144,902	100	4149	100	8.73

As shown in Table 2, The number of working days lost is quite different among the three LHs, probably due to the number of servants in these Legislative Houses and the criteria used by these organizations to measure absenteeism. The House of Deputies and the Federal Senate issue ML for absences starting from 1 day of absence due to health problems, while ALEGO recorded only absences of more than 3 days. The other cases of non-attendance at work, less than 4 days, were managed by the immediate superior. It is worth mentioning the annual average of working days lost per server (d/s/yr), as shown in the last column of Table 2, as it represents the real average of sickness absenteeism. In this sense, ALEGO and the House of Deputies had a very similar performance, around 10 d/s/yr, while the Federal Senate positioned well above these figures, with an average absence of 6.2 d/s/yr. It should be noted that, except for very few cases, ALEGO did not compute absences of 1 to 3 days in its general absenteeism register, which may have affected its average work absences. On the other hand, the much more favorable situation of the Federal Senate may be associated with a more adequate general working condition, among other factors.

3.3. Individual Health Condition (Comorbidities)

The individual health status of the servants regarding the presence of active or chronic health problems was evaluated using an electronic questionnaire (self-administered comorbidity questionnaire—SCQ), which allows the calculation of the CI. This index allows for estimating the situation of individuals regarding the existence or absence of permanent or long-term morbidities. An individual who declares no pathology or health problem has a CI score of 0.00. An individual with a pathology or chronic health problem without the need for medical treatment or restrictions in the performance of any type of activity receives a CI score of 0.02. Table 3 shows the CI scores determined in the three LHs.

A total of 154 servants (34.5%) declared no chronic health problems. In contrast, most respondents (65.5%) reported at least one chronic problem/illness. The highest frequency score (CI = 0.04) was registered in 77 cases and may correspond to the presence of two comorbidities or only one morbidity combined with the need for medical treatment, or difficulties to perform activities. The most serious situation, CI = 0.44, was declared by only one servant and corresponds to a health condition that can show a significant vulnerability. However, all cases with CI scores above 0.20 deserve more attention because it implies the presence of at least 4 pathologies/health problems combined with medical treatment and difficulties to perform activities.

Table 4 presents the distribution of individuals according to the number of diseases or health problems. Among those who declared a diagnosis of chronic diseases (293 individuals), 44.4% reported a single occurrence, while the remaining individuals, 55.6%, reported having two or more comorbidities.

Table 3. Comorbidity index (CI) for all LHs.

CI	Frequency	Percentage (%)	Cumulative Percentage (%)
0.00	154	34.5	34.5
0.02	29	6.5	40.9
0.04	77	17.2	58.2
0.06	41	9.2	67.3
0.08	33	7.4	74.7
0.10	16	3.6	78.3
0.13	30	6.7	85.0
0.15	18	4.0	89.0
0.17	11	2.5	91.5
0.19	12	2.7	94.2
0.21	6	1.3	95.5
0.23	2	0.4	96.0
0.25	8	1.8	97.8
0.27	2	0.4	98.2
0.29	1	0.2	98.4
0.31	3	0.7	99.1
0.33	2	0.4	99.6
0.35	1	0.2	99.8
0.44	1	0.2	100.0
Total	447	100.0	

Table 4. Distribution of comorbidity events.

Number of Diseases or Health Problems	Individuals	Percentage	Cumulative Percentage
0	154	34.5	34.5
1	130	29.1	63.5
2	65	14.5	78.1
3	52	11.6	89.7
4	33	7.4	97.1
5	7	1.6	98.7
6	4	0.9	99.6
7	1	0.2	99.8
9	1	0.2	100.0
Total	447	100.0	

Among the items suggested in the SCQ and those included by the participants, 622 records of diseases were reported, 362 referring to those in the questionnaire, and 260 new items informed by the servants. Among the chronic health problems included in the questionnaire, back pain was the most frequent, with 126 records, followed by hypertension and depression, with 70 and 54 records, respectively. On the other hand, the pathologies/chronic health problems directly declared by the respondents as "Other Health Problems", in the categories of Problem-1, Problem-2, and Problem-3, resulted in 156, 74, and 30 records, respectively. Figure 2 presents a graph with the frequency of the diseases/health problems, in percentages, resulting from the CI estimation among the servants from all LHs. All diseases/health problems reported by the participants (differing from those in the questionnaire) are represented by the categories Other Health Problems 1, 2, and 3, considering the vast list of specific pathologies reported by the servants. Figure 3 shows an overview of self-reported chronic diseases, in the form of a word cloud, highlighting back pain, hypertension, depression, and other musculoskeletal disorders (Other-DME) with higher frequencies.

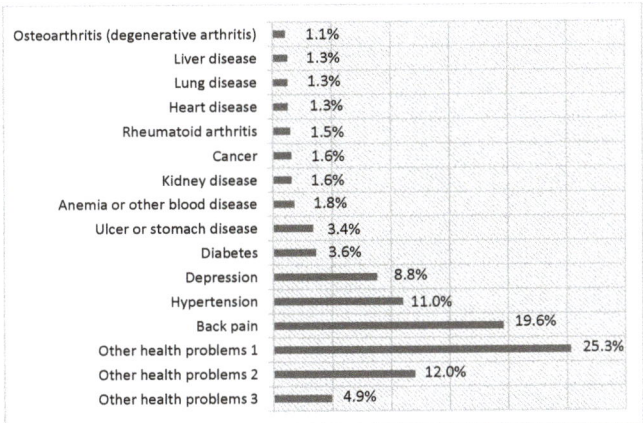

Figure 2. Frequency of chronic diseases/health problems.

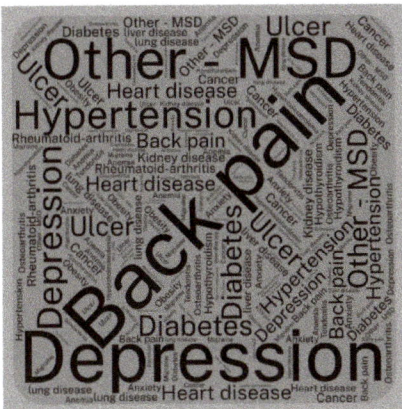

Figure 3. Chronic diseases/health problems among civil servants.

Other pathologies and health problems reported by the servants also proved to be very important in the estimation of the CI score. In order, the cases of diabetes, ulcers, anxiety, and hypothyroidism stand out. It is also worth noting the cases of cancer and kidney disease.

The CI score becomes more significant when it also reflects the need for the respective medical treatment, which denotes a condition that requires permanent control. Moreover, the health condition can evolve and become more serious when the comorbidity situation prevents or makes it difficult for individuals to perform work activities. Figures 4 and 5, respectively, show the percentage of servants with chronic diseases/health problems requiring medical treatment and those who have difficulties in performing work activities.

As shown in Figure 4, the vast majority of the civil servants with CI scores above zero (83%) received some type of treatment for their health situation. Moreover, 54% of these servants with comorbidities reported no difficulty performing any activity given their health condition. In contrast, 46% informed that the presence of chronic pathologies/health problems causes restrictions in performing activities.

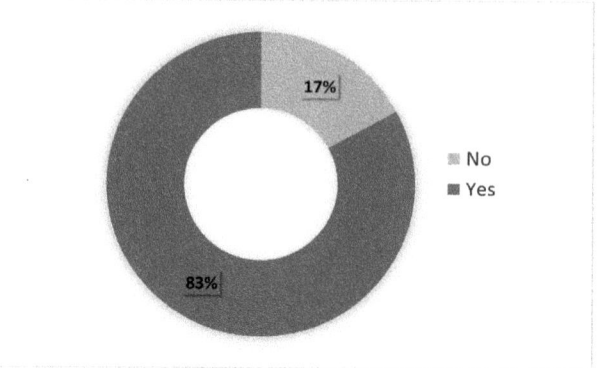

Figure 4. Individuals with CI > 0.00 with medical treatment.

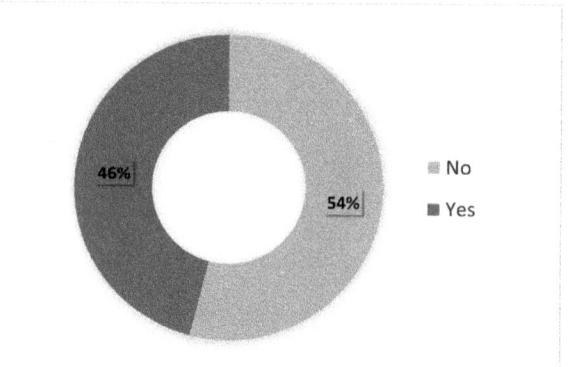

Figure 5. Individuals with CI > 0.00, with and without difficulties to perform activities.

The presence of chronic diseases or health problems can make individuals more vulnerable due to several factors, including a risk to personal health, and greater susceptibility of these individuals, due to daily exposures, to risk factors (at work or outside work), which can increase the degree of severity of the effects resulting from exposure.

3.4. Correlation between Comorbidity Index (CI), Working Days Lost, and Sociodemographic Variables

The association between the individual health status measured by the CI, and the absenteeism measured in working days lost, as well as the sociodemographic variables were analyzed through bivariate correlation. Higher CI scores indicate a level of increased vulnerability to individuals' health and may influence work absences. Table 5 shows the result of this analysis through Pearson's coefficient.

The CI scores were positively and significantly associated with the work absences of the servants at a 1% level (r = 0.254, p-value < 0.01), thus an increase in the level of vulnerability of the individual's health due to chronic diseases is associated with an increase in the working days lost. Moreover, the CI was positively and significantly associated with both the age of the servants at a 5% level (r = 0.116, p-value < 0.05) and the length of service (seniority) at a 1% level (r = 0.133, p-value < 0.01). Therefore, an increase in the age of the servants and their length of service is correlated with an increase in the CI score, which can lead to a longer time away from work. It should also be noted that age and seniority were statistically highly significant at a 1% level (r = 0.762, p-value < 0.01). Thus, the greater length of time on the job implies an increase in the servants' age, which represents a favorable situation for higher CI scores.

Table 5. Correlations between CI, working days lost, and sociodemographic variables.

Variables		Correlation				
		CI	Age	Seniority	Working Hours	Number of Working Days Lost
Age	(r)	0.116 *	1	-	-	-
	N	447	4149	-	-	-
Seniority	(r)	0.133 **	0.762 **	1	-	-
	N	447	4149	4149	-	-
Working hours	(r)	−0.046	−0.053 **	−0.045 **	1	-
	N	447	4149	4149	4149	-
Number of working days lost	(r)	0.254 **	0.107 **	0.117 **	0.032 *	1
	N	447	4149	4149	4149	4149

* The correlation is significant at the 0.05 level (2 extremities). ** The correlation is significant at the 0.01 level (2 extremities).

Sickness absenteeism, as already mentioned, is a multifactorial phenomenon; that is, it consists of a variable dependent on several other variables that act as predictors of work absences motivated by health problems. However, the CI proved to be a possible predictor of relative importance, considering the moderate correlation ($r = 0.254$) with the working days lost by the legislative servants from all LHs.

Regarding the prevalence of comorbidities according to the gender of the participants, no significant differences between genders were observed through the independent t-test ($t\ 445 = 0.039$; p-value = 0.969). There may be qualitative differences once male and female servants present differences in terms of the type of diseases or health problems.

4. Discussion

4.1. Sickness Absenteeism

The average annual rate of days of absence of civil servants of the three Legislative Houses in this study was 8.73 d/s/yr, which is relatively moderate when compared to other national and international cases of work absences in the public service due to health problems. The sickness absenteeism of civil servants of the City Halls of Goiania, between 2005 and 2010, and Coritiba, between 2010 and 2015, had an average of working days lost of 12.07 d/s/yr [4] and 23.04 d/s/yr, respectively [6]. Similar studies with civil servants in Canada and Australia indicated an average civil servant absence of 11.6 d/s/yr [5]. However, much lower values of days away from work in the public sector have been reported, as in the case of the UK countries that achieved an average annual working day loss of 4.4 d/s/yr in 2018.

The poorer results of sick leave in the legislative houses of the present study may be related to the less adverse general working conditions in the executive branch, mainly in the areas of education, health, and public security. These areas present frequent occurrences of absence from work due to health problems, considering the pathological potential of these sectors, due to direct contact with the public, high social demand for such services, or operational difficulties faced by educators and health and public safety professionals. Moreover, the legislative servants participating in this study perform only internal administrative activities of support to parliamentarians and have their own health service that provides care, including basic health promotion actions.

4.2. Comorbidity

The presence of chronic health diseases/conditions in the general population is a reality for millions of people. In Brazil, according to the National Health Survey, in 2019, 52% of the population aged 18 years or older reported having been diagnosed with at least one chronic disease, with hypertension standing out with 23.9% of individuals, and depression reaching 10.2% of the population [16]. This situation seems to be more comprehensive with the working population. The results of this study showed that most legislative staff (65.5%) reported at least one chronic disease or health problem, while the others (34.5%) reported no chronic pathology. Among the servants with chronic diseases or health problems, 44.4% reported a single occurrence, while 55.6% reported two or more comorbidities. A study conducted with more than 10,000 workers in the general population in Denmark found that 56.8% of the participants had one or more chronic diseases, which were associated with the risk of leaving for health treatment [17], corroborating the present research.

Back pain, hypertension, and depression were the pathologies with the highest frequency for all LHs, reaching 19.6, 11.0, and 8.8%, respectively, of all reported chronic diseases/problems, considering the category Other Health Problems 1, 2, and 3. Several studies corroborate the prevalence of these pathologies among workers and the general population, including civil servants. Serranheira et al., (2020) [18] investigated 735 workers from different occupational fields and reported that 69% of the respondents presented at least one episode of low back pain in 12 months, with the highest proportion of individuals presenting more than six episodes of low back pain per year among civil servants (31.8%). Research involving 4844 public service workers in Nigeria found a prevalence of 35% of cases of hypertension and 36.4% of prehypertension, with a slight predominance among male employees, while only 2% of employees diagnosed with hypertension were aware of their health condition [19]. Finally, a study evaluated the factors associated with temporary work incapacity among Brazilian university servants and found 30% of recurrent depressive disorders among 1753 cases of temporary incapacity for the 21 most prevalent diseases studied [20].

4.3. Comorbidity and Sickness Absenteeism

In general, sickness-related absenteeism is an outcome variable of several other variables within the work environment, in addition to external and individual factors. In this study, the main purpose was to assess the role of chronic diseases or problems in work absences.

The statistical analyses revealed that the CI that contemplates the presence of pathologies/chronic health conditions was highly significantly associated with the working days lost ($r = 0.254$, p-value = 0.01), therefore the number of days away from work increases with the increase in the CI score. This correlation was evidenced in other research involving civil servants. It is known that the chance of absenteeism among workers with chronic diseases is 6.34 times higher when compared to those in the opposite situation. Moreover, there is a higher probability of the occurrence of negative critical incidents with these individuals at work [21]. The presence of chronic diseases associated with a low capacity (physical and mental) for work is correlated with a high risk of long-term absence in the general working population [17]. A study on the association between comorbidities and general labor force participation of Australian workers with back pain showed that an individual with these conditions and heart disease was ten times more likely to be out of the labor force. Absenteeism was also associated with long-term work incapacity among workers with episodes of comorbid depressive disorders or anxiety [22]. Finally, multicomorbidity is common among young adult workers and is related to absenteeism as well as presenteeism at work [23].

In this study, a significant and positive correlation between the CI scores and age and length of service (seniority) was observed, i.e., the level of vulnerability of individual health of legislative workers to diseases and chronic health problems increases with increasing age and length of service. This finding demands attention since in some countries the multimorbidity rates for the population over 65 years of age are estimated at 80–90%, which may represent a greater susceptibility of older workers to the onset of diseases, leading to a greater occurrence of work disability or permanent disability to work.

The results showed no significant differences between men and women regarding the CI scores for the total number of participants, regardless of age or activity. This result may vary when some specific criteria are considered, including education, age, or specific pathology, among others. However, there is usually a prevalence of chronic diseases in the group of women in the general population. Regarding the population aged 18 years or older in Brazil in 2019, hypertension was more prevalent among women (26.4%) when compared to men (21.1%). Likewise, regarding diagnoses of depression, women showed a prevalence of 14.7% when compared to 5.1% among men [16]. More specific population extracts, such as the legislative staff participating in this research, do not necessarily reproduce the general profile of the population in terms of comorbidities.

5. Conclusions

The main purpose of this study was to evaluate the chronic health condition among civil servants that work in the legislative houses in Brazil, through the comorbidity index, as well as its effects on sickness-related absenteeism, expressed in working days lost.

The statistical analyses revealed that the vast majority of the participants had at least one chronic disease or health problem. In turn, the comorbidity index showed that at least 8 out of 10 of these individuals use medication or other medical treatment, and no less than four individuals reported difficulties or restrictions in performing some activity due to their health condition. Thus, it is reasonable to conclude that the population under study presents a profile strongly characterized by the presence of chronic health conditions, which affect the personal health of these individuals, imposing the need for some kind of medical monitoring and the risk of losing working capacity.

Regarding the effects of the chronic health condition on work absences assessed by the comorbidity index, it was evident that the individual health condition was strongly associated with the working days lost by the civil servants with diseases or chronic problems. Therefore, the presence of diseases or chronic health problems had important effects on the work absenteeism of this group of civil servants. As already discussed, absenteeism is a phenomenon of multifactorial etiology and may be associated with internal and external factors to work. However, individual characteristics such as the socio-demographic profile and individual health conditions act to mitigate or aggravate absences from work activities.

Studies aimed at detailing the prevalence of chronic health problems of workers and the impact of this medical condition on the reduction of working capacity can help in understanding sickness-related absenteeism, providing a more adequate and humanized management of work, with possible positive effects on people's health and productivity.

Author Contributions: Writing—review & editing, F.E.S.; Supervision, M.J.S.O., J.A. and E.F. All authors have read and agreed to the published version of the manuscript.

Funding: This research has not received any external funding.

Institutional Review Board Statement: This study was developed with the approval of the Ethics Committee of the Universidade Federal de Goiás, Brazil, under registration number 3.962.630 on 9 April 2020.

Informed Consent Statement: Informed consent was obtained from all subjects involved in the study.

Data Availability Statement: The data and information in this article can be found in the doctoral thesis: bsenteísmo-doença de servidores públicos do poder legislativo no Brasil, available from 6 December 2023, in the respository of the University of Porto, Portugal, at the request of the author who decided to publish a book, based on his research. access link: https://repositorio-aberto.up.pt/handle/10216/147784.

Conflicts of Interest: The authors declare no conflict of interest.

References

1. ILO (International Labour Organization). Safety and Health at Work. 2021. Available online: https://www.ilo.org/global/topics/safety-and-health-at-work/lang--en/index.htm (accessed on 6 August 2021).
2. European Health Information Gateway. Absenteeism from Work Due to Illness, Days per Employee per Year. 2021. Available online: https://gateway.euro.who.int/en/indicators/hfa_411-2700-absenteeism-from-work-due-to-illness-days-per-employee-per-year/ (accessed on 6 August 2021).
3. BRASIL, Secretaria da Previdência. Dados Estatísticos—Saúde e Segurança do Trabalhador. 2019. Available online: https://www.gov.br/previdencia/pt-br/assuntos/previdencia-social/saude-e-seguranca-do-trabalhador/dados-de-acidentes-do-trabalho (accessed on 7 July 2021).
4. Leão, A.L.D.M.; Barbosa-Branco, A.; Neto, E.R.; Ribeiro, C.A.N.; Turchi, M.D. Absenteísmo-doença no serviço público municipal de Goiânia. *Rev. Bras. Epidemiol.* **2015**, *18*, 262–277. [CrossRef] [PubMed]
5. Rodrigues, C.D.S.; De Freitas, R.M.; Assunção, A.; Bassi, I.B.; De Medeiros, A.M. Absenteísmo-doença segundo autorrelato de servidores públicos municipais em Belo Horizonte. *Rev. Bras. Estud. Popul.* **2013**, *30*, 135–154. [CrossRef]
6. Daniel, E.; Koerich CR, C.; Lang, A. The absenteeism profile among municipal public servants of the city of Curitiba, from 2010 to 2015 I O perfil do absenteísmo dos servidores da prefeitura municipal de Curitiba, de 2010 a 2015. *Rev. Bras. Med. Trab.* **2017**, *15*, 142–149. [CrossRef]
7. McGrandle, J.; Ohemeng, F.L.K. The conundrum of absenteeism in the Canadian public service: A wicked problem perspective. *Can. Public Adm.* **2017**, *60*, 215–240. [CrossRef]
8. Deady, M.; Collins, D.A.J.; A Johnston, D.; Glozier, N.; A Calvo, R.; Christensen, H.; Harvey, S.B. The impact of depression, anxiety and comorbidity on occupational outcomes. *Occup. Med.* **2021**, *72*, 17–24. [CrossRef] [PubMed]
9. Sampaio, E.; Baptista, J.S. Absenteeism of Public Workers—Short Review. In *Occupational and Environmental Safety and Health*; Springer International Publishing: Cham, Switzerland, 2019; pp. 345–353. [CrossRef]
10. de Oliveira, P.L. *Impacto das Características e Condições de Trabalho no Absentismo em Assistentes Operacionais de Escolas e Jardins de Infância*; Universidade Fernando Pessoa: Porto, Portugal, 2016.
11. Santi, D.B.; Barbieri, A.R.; Cheade, M.D.F.M. Absenteísmo-doença no serviço público brasileiro: Uma revisão integrativa da literatura. *Rev. Bras. De Med. Do Trab.* **2018**, *16*, 71–81. [CrossRef]
12. Valderas, J.M.; Starfield, B.; Sibbald, B.; Salisbury, C.; Roland, M. Defining Comorbidity: Implications for Understanding Health and Health Services. *Ann. Fam. Med.* **2009**, *7*, 357–363. [CrossRef] [PubMed]
13. Broeiro, P. Multimorbilidade e comorbilidade: Duas perspectivas da mesma realidade. *Rev. Port. Med. Geral E Fam.* **2015**, *31*, 150–160. [CrossRef]
14. Harrison, C.; Fortin, M.; Akker, M.V.D.; Mair, F.; Calderon-Larranaga, A.; Boland, F.; Wallace, E.; Jani, B.; Smith, S. Comorbidity versus multimorbidity: Why it matters. *J. Multimorb. Comorbidity* **2021**, *11*, 263355652199399. [CrossRef] [PubMed]
15. Sangha, O.; Stucki, P.D.m.G.; Liang, M.; Fossel, A.; Katz, J. The Self-Administered Comorbidity Questionnaire: A new method to assess comorbidity for clinical and health services research. *Arthritis Rheum.* **2003**, *49*, 156–163. [CrossRef] [PubMed]
16. Instituto Brasileiro de Geografia e Estatística. Pesquisa Nacional de Saúde; Rio de Janeiro. 2019. Available online: https://teca.ibge.gov.br/visualizacao/livros/liv91110.pdf (accessed on 6 August 2021).
17. Sundstrup, E.; Jakobsen, M.D.; Mortensen, O.S.; Andersen, L.L. Joint association of multimorbidity and work ability with risk of long-term sickness absence: A prospective cohort study with register follow-up. *Scand. J. Work Environ. Health* **2017**, *43*, 146–154. [CrossRef] [PubMed]
18. Serranheira, F.; Sousa-Uva, M.; Heranz, F.; Kovacs, F. Low Back Pain (LBP), work and absenteeism. *Work* **2020**, *65*, 463–469. [CrossRef] [PubMed]
19. Aladeneyi, I.; Adeneyi, O.V.; Owolabi, E.O.; Fawole, O.; Adeolu, M.; Goon, D.T.; Ajayi, A.I. Prevalence, awareness and correlates of hypertension among urban public workers in Ondo State, Nigeria. *Online J. Health Allied Sci.* **2017**, *16*, 1.
20. Dias, A.; Gómez-Salgado, J.; Bernardes, J.M.; Ruiz-Frutos, C. Factors affecting sick leave duration for non-work-related temporary disabilities in brazilian university public servants. *Int. J. Environ. Res. Public Health* **2018**, *15*, 2127. [CrossRef] [PubMed]
21. Fouad, A.M.; Waheed, A.; Gamal, A.; Amer, S.; Abdellah, R.F.; Shebl, F.M. Effect of Chronic Diseases on Work Productivity: A Propensity Score Analysis. *J. Occup. Environ. Med.* **2017**, *59*, 480–485. [CrossRef] [PubMed]
22. Hendriks, S.M.; Spijker, J.; Licht, C.M.; Hardeveld, F.; de Graaf, R.; Batelaan, N.M.; Penninx, B.W.; Beekman, A.T. Long-term work disability and absenteeism in anxiety and depressive disorders. *J. Affect. Disord.* **2015**, *178*, 121–130. [CrossRef] [PubMed]
23. Troelstra, S.A.; Straker, L.M.; Harris, M.; Brown, S.; van der Beek, A.J.; Coenen, P. Multimorbidity is common among young workers and related to increased work absenteeism and presenteeism: Results from the population-based raine study cohort. *Scand. J. Work. Environ. Health* **2020**, *46*, 218–227. [CrossRef] [PubMed]

Disclaimer/Publisher's Note: The statements, opinions and data contained in all publications are solely those of the individual author(s) and contributor(s) and not of MDPI and/or the editor(s). MDPI and/or the editor(s) disclaim responsibility for any injury to people or property resulting from any ideas, methods, instructions or products referred to in the content.

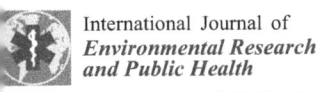

Article

Regional Regression Correlation Model of Microplastic Water Pollution Control Using Circular Economy Tools

Valentin Marian Antohi [1,2,*], Romeo Victor Ionescu [3], Monica Laura Zlati [1], Catalina Iticescu [4], Puiu Lucian Georgescu [4] and Madalina Calmuc [5]

1. Department of Business Administration, Dunarea de Jos University of Galati, 800001 Galati, Romania
2. Department of Finance, Accounting and Economic Theory, Transylvania University of Brasov, 500036 Brasov, Romania
3. Department of Administrative Sciences and Regional Studies, Dunarea de Jos University of Galati, 800201 Galati, Romania
4. Department of Chemistry, Physics and Environment, REXDAN Research Infrastructure, Dunarea de Jos University of Galati, 800008 Galati, Romania
5. REXDAN Research Infrastructure, Dunarea de Jos University of Galati, 800008 Galati, Romania
* Correspondence: valentin.antohi@ugal.ro

Abstract: Water pollution caused by microplastics represents an important challenge for the environment and people's health. The weak international regulations and standards in this domain support increased water pollution with microplastics. The literature is unsuccessful in establishing a common approach regarding this subject. The main objective of this research is to develop a new approach to necessary policies and ways of action to decrease water pollution caused by microplastics. In this context, we quantified the impact of European water pollution caused by microplastics in the circular economy. The main research methods used in the paper are meta-analysis, statistical analysis and an econometric approach. A new econometric model is developed in order to assist the decision makers in increasing efficiency of public policies regarding water pollution elimination. The main result of this study relies on combining, in an integrated way, the Organisation for Economic Co-operation and Development's (OECD) data on microplastic water pollution and identifying relevant policies to combat this type of pollution.

Keywords: microplastics; water pollution; water anti-pollution policies; circular economy

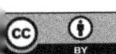

1. Introduction

The global economy, in its quest for economic efficiency during the period of extensive development (1970–2010), developed alternative materials based on polyethylene and polyurethane elastomer compounds. These compounds directly increase the marginal yield of production, but their impact on the environment and the health of the population has been neglected. In the case of water, microplastics are also found in sediments. The main characteristic of microplastics is their slow biodegradation, which leads to the formation of microplastic residues contaminating the environment and aquatic organisms. Poor aquatic wildlife health directly impacts human consumers in the food chain.

The presence of microplastics in the marine and freshwater aquatic environment has gradually increased and there is now a high rate of contamination of ecosystems and food chains, which are exposed to increasing amounts of new microplastics, hampering remediation efforts by the relevant entities.

Current research shows that the impact of microplastics on the environment, especially the aquatic environment, is devastating, leading to irreversible changes in the biodiversity of the aquatic macroenvironment and causing multiple diseases in the population.

In this context, our approach aims to demonstrate that anti-pollution policies, although heavily supported financially, are currently not very effective, particularly due to disparities in anti-pollution policies regarding types of plastic and at a regional level.

Regional disparities lead to the dissipation of efforts to combat pollution, and more effective pollution-control measures are needed.

In the case of microplastics, both consumption and production show a large regional disparity (see Figure 1).

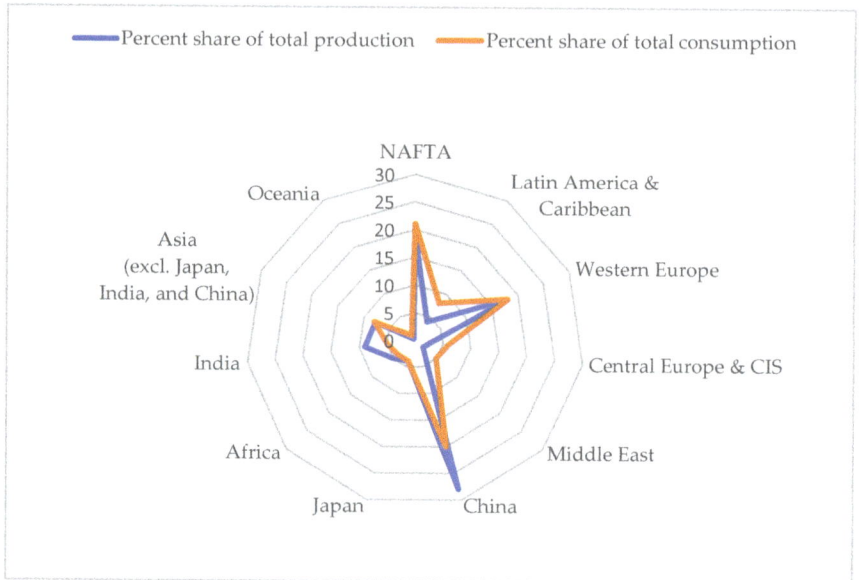

Figure 1. Regional disparities in microplastics consumption and production.

The authors have arrived at these disparity rates using statistics found in the United Nation's Environment Programme, "Mapping of Global Plastics Value chain and Plastics Loses to the Environment" [1].

We started our approach with the European Commission's implementation of the EU Plastic Strategy, which strongly emphasises the elimination of intentionally added microplastics in various products. This approach by the European Commission is supported by the European Chemicals Agency (ECHA). Unfortunately, there is no common concern in this area at the global level either, except for the relatively limited involvement of the OECD.

Returning to the EU27, some Member States have already banned by national legislation the intentional use of microplastics in consumer products. These bans cover a wide area, from food to cosmetics.

According to international statistics, 42,000 tonnes of microplastics end up in the environment every year in Europe [2]. The main sources of microplastic pollution in European waters are artificial turfs for sports fields and the wear and tear of larger pieces of plastic produced as commercial packaging waste.

In 2022, the European Commission launched a draft regulation on Registration, Evaluation, Authorisation and Restriction of Chemicals (REACH) regarding synthetic polymer microparticles [3], which came up for discussion among Member States at the end of 2022 and will be finalised in 2023.

The main directions are to set strict criteria for the release of non-degradable polymers, as the lower limit size of the particles has been eliminated.

In this case, one opposition came from the Committee for Socio-Economic Analysis (CASE) in December 2020, which supported imposing a lower limit of 1 nm for restricting microplastics.

In support of this scientific approach, we define the following research objectives:

O1. Determine the level of connection of microplastic water pollution to the regional microplastic limiting capacity;

O2. Determine the level of connection of water pollution with the level of implementation of the circular economy;

O3. Define a regional regression correlation model of microplastic water pollution control using circular economy tools;

O4. Define relevant public policy proposals to increase the effectiveness of actions to combat water pollution caused by microplastics.

The study continues with the Section 3, in which the model-building methodology is presented, followed by the Sections 4 and 5 in which the working hypotheses and policy proposals are demonstrated. The Section 6 is dedicated to conclusions.

2. Literature Review

The latest research in the field of microplastic water pollution presents significant, sometimes contradictory, aspects of pollution management, sources of pollution and its impact on the environment and human health.

An extremely unpleasant finding reveals that microplastics are widely found in aquatic environments. Authors such as Shi et al. [4] look for solutions regarding the efficient removal of microplastics from water and propose nano-Fe_3O_4 magnetic technology, which causes optimal magnetization of microplastics by surface adsorption. The next operation consists of magnet suction. The yield of this process varies between 62% and 87% in case of water pollution with polyethylene, polypropylene, polystyrene and polyethylene terephthalate, with dimensions of about 200–900 μm.

According to Wang et al. [5], cases of advanced microplastic-contaminated water, treatment technologies, exoelectrogen biofilm and associated microbial electrochemical processes occupy an important place. The analysis quantifies the impact of microplastics on the exoelectrogenic biofilm, with potential mechanisms revealed at the gene level. The authors believe that this approach can lay the methodological foundations for the future development of efficient water treatment technologies.

Since microplastics are present in both water resources and water supply systems (in pipes), some specialists, such as Chu et al. [6], focus on quantifying the presence of these microplastics throughout the distribution system. The analysis found that nylon and polyvinyl chloride were predominant in the water samples, but that the existence of efficient drinking water treatment plants and distribution systems prevented microplastics from entering the tap water. Furthermore, the authors note the necessary correlation between the stability of pipe scales and improved water quality and safety. Monitoring the presence of microplastics in water sources is also reviewed by Nicolai et al. [7], who use a new particle counter based on a real-time fluorescence emission analysis. The case study covers polyvinyl chloride and high-density polyethylene. The presence of microplastics in a drinking water treatment plant in Barcelona (Spain) is analyzed by Dronjak et al. [8]. The analysis focuses on microplastic particles in water with sizes between 20 μm and 5 mm. The authors use Fenton's reagent and hydrogen peroxide, as well as a zinc chloride solution. Visual identification was carried out with an optical and stereoscopic microscope, finally obtaining a microplastic removal yield of 98.3% from water, the main types of microplastics removed being polymers and synthetic cellulose, polyester, polyamide, polypropylene, polyethylene, polyurethane and polyacrylonitrile.

The conceptual approach to microplastic water pollution using reference materials is by Seghers et al. [9]. The authors support the use of a kit with microplastics immobilized in solid NaCl and a surfactant that they implemented for polyethylene terephthalate (PET) particles in water. Information on particle size distributions and shapes was obtained using laser diffraction, and the homogeneity of these particles was calculated using an ultra-microbalance.

Other authors, such as P. Wang et al. [10], propose the use of solar energy for the efficient removal of plastic particles from water. Basically, a bubble is created in a high-power density glass ball by focusing it in sunlight. It then collects the plastic particles into large clumps. The advantage of this method is that it does not use chemical or biological reagents or filters. Additionally, the costs of implementing the procedure are much lower than those of "classical" technologies.

An alarming finding is made by Karapanagioti and Kalavrouziotis [11], who state that "no microplastic removal treatment is currently used for drinking water". The authors analysed the presence of microplastics in waters from different regions of the world, such as Russia, India, Italy, Greece and Cyprus, finding a direct connection between microplastic concentrations in water and surrounding land uses. The studies involved direct sampling of water and soil as well as sampling organisms that interacted with microplastics, such as zooplankton or zebra mussels.

An alternative method of treating water pollution containing plastic is presented by Martin et al. [12] and consists of using iron oxide nanoparticles with hydrophobic coatings to magnetize waste plastic particles. The authors claim that this method allows for the complete removal of particles 2–5 mm in size, and almost 90% of nanoplastic particles 100 nm–1000 nm in size, using a simple 2-inch NdFeB permanent magnet.

The presence of microplastics in lake waters is reviewed by Viitala et al. [13], focusing on the Lake Saimaa sub-basin (Finland). The authors quantify the connection between the presence of the local wastewater treatment plant and the plastic concentration in different compartments of the receiving lake based on the collection of bottom sediment samples. These samples were analysed using pyrolysis-gas chromatography-mass spectrometry. The results showed the presence of higher concentrations of polyethylene (PE), polypropylene (PP) and polystyrene (PS) in the water near the wastewater treatment plant effluent discharge site compared to other sites.

Microplastic pollution is more pronounced in semi-enclosed seas to which many urban conurbations have access. Authors such as Trani et al. [14] have studied the case of the Mediterranean Sea since 2012, focusing on the Salento peninsula (Apulia, Italy). The analyses cover both surface waters and microplastics ingested by certain marine organisms. For this purpose, Neuston and Manta net monitoring were used and the level of microplastic contamination of different fish and mussel species was targeted. The results of the analysis show that microplastic water pollution is higher in the Adriatic Sea than in the Ionian Sea and that the concentration of microplastics at the sea surface and in the gastrointestinal tract of targeted species is higher. Another semi-enclosed sea is the Black Sea, whose plastic pollution is analysed by Strokal et al. [15] based on five scenarios modelled using a model assessing riverine inputs of pollutants to the sea (MARINA-Global) for 107 sub-basins. The authors state that European rivers flowing into the Black Sea discharge more than half of all microplastics and, as a result, make proposals for environmental policies capable of reducing pollution in the Black Sea to zero. Microplastic pollution of marine systems is the subject of an investigation by Yuan et al. [16] that reviews the current state of research in this area. The authors consider seafood consumption, lung inhalation and skin infiltration to be the main causes of human exposure to microplastics from the marine environment. The authors highlight the risks that microplastics in water pose on human health, referring to certain cancers and chronic and acute toxicity. The risks microplastics pose to human health are also addressed by Sarma et al. [17]. The authors conclude that urban wastewater flushing is the main source of microplastic water pollution. The impact of microplastics on human health through commercial fish, crustacean and bivalve species, is addressed by Sánchez-Guerrero-Hernández et al. [18], based on a case study of the main commercial fish species in Spain: the European anchovy and the European sardine. In order to determine the presence of microplastics in these fish, the authors used an alkaline organic oxidant (KOH-H_2O_2), which identified nylon as the main polymer found in both fish species. The impact of microplastics on health is the subject of a study by Kadac-Czapska et al. [19], who consider that the most common route of exposure is the gastrointestinal tract. In this context, microplastics (PET, PE, PP, PS, PVC, PA and PC) enter the human body through the consumption of fish, shellfish and water.

Technologies to remove microplastics from water are investigated by Gao et al. [20], who consider both technical processes and related costs. Furthermore, the authors refer to the practical efficiency of plastic removal technologies from water and their impact on the environment.

Microplastic pollutants < 5 mm in diameter from different countries and regions are reviewed by Yang et al. [21] in terms of abundance, morphology and polymer types in water and lake sediments. The authors conclude that the level of microplastic pollution depends on the level of local development and the economic structure of the areas analysed. The authors sound the alarm for an optimal microplastic pollution control system in lake systems.

The connection between microplastics (polyethylene and polyvinyl chloride), UV and bacteria (Gram-negative and Gram-positive) in water is presented by Manoli et al. [22]. The authors aim to quantify the effect of microplastics on UV disinfection performance in order to increase the efficiency of physical and chemical disinfection processes in different waters.

The increase in plastic production, the development of international trade in these products and plastic waste and the intensification of the use of plastics in the economy on the African continent are addressed by Deme et al. [23]. The authors study legislation supporting sustainable economic development in African countries and conclude that national policymakers' approaches are ineffective in this area. As a result, these authors support environmental policy decisions based on price, legislation and the implementation of the best practices in microplastics waste management.

An interesting analysis developed by Usman et al. [24] discusses plastic production, plastic waste management defects and human health. The analysis shows that the presence of microplastics in food and drinking water has long-term health effects on the population. The authors mention that "there is no regulation of plastic contamination of food and drinking water" and propose increased collaboration in this area at international and national levels. Microplastic water pollution can lead to rare forms of cancer, as shown in a study by Mocanu et al. [25]. This approach is also taken up in the research carried out by Nastase et al. [26].

Lofty et al. [27] critique the circular economy from the perspective of the use of sewage sludge generated by wastewater treatment plants in agriculture. The authors believe that there is a possibility that plastic successfully removed from sewage treatment plants and deposited in the soil may return to natural waters through runoff or seepage into groundwater. Based on official statistics provided by the European Commission and Eurostat, the authors state that the practice of spreading sludge on agricultural land can lead to the creation of an impressive global reservoir of plastic pollution. A contrary approach sees the circular economy as the key to a more sustainable use of plastic. The authors of this approach, Syberg et al. [28], consider that "explicit considerations of microplastics contamination are rarely taken into account in studies of the transition to a plastic circular economy". Furthermore, they state that there are situations and areas where recycling can lead to increased microplastic contamination. The circular economy from the perspective of microplastic water contamination is addressed by Syberg et al. [28], with the authors providing recommendations on how reducing microplastic contamination and transitioning to the circular economy can be interlinked in future research. Moreover, in the view of Cook et al. [29], the development of the circular economy must not have negative effects on human health and the environment. The authors use the scenario method to quantify the environmental impact of post-consumer plastic packaging resource recovery processes and recommend to developing countries the mechanical reprocessing of these plastics at the expense of chemical recycling procedures. In the framework of the circular economy, bioplastics represent a great challenge according to Rosenboom et al. [30] in the process of transforming them into high-quality materials. The authors stress the need for new regulations and financial incentives to support the sustainable recycling of these categories of bioplastics.

Perpetuation of plastic pollution along the food chain in the aquatic environment of the Vipacco River, northeastern Italy is studied by Bertoli et al. [31], who state that the main source of microplastic pollution in the aquatic environment is urban wastewater discharge. The effects of this pollution are quantified at the level of entire macrobenthic invertebrate communities and have results that are difficult to generalize. As a result, the authors stress the need for further studies. In this context, other authors, such as Mehinto et al. [32], propose a risk-management system for aquatic ecosystems. The authors establish four thresholds for plastic contamination of water based on studies in the literature, on the basis of which they define two mechanisms of effects: dietary dilution with thresholds ranging from ~0.5 to 35 particles/L and tissue translocation with thresholds ranging from ~60 to 4100 particles/L. Another model for risk assessment of marine water pollution with plastic is presented by Yuan et al. [33], who call for a screening strategy. This strategy allows the prioritisation of polymers of primary interest in marine waters: PUR, PVC, PAN, ABS, PMMA, SAN, TPU, UP, PET, PS and HDPE. The authors make recommendations to policy makers on how to better manage microplastics in marine waters. Microplastics are, according to Hossain et al. [34], one of the fastest-growing wastes in the world. The authors conduct an impressive meta-analysis of Australia's plastic waste management system in the context of the transition to the circular economy. The analysis shows that the most widespread forms of plastic in the environment are high-density polyethylene, polyethylene terephthalate and low-density polyethylene. In the case of microplastics, households generate the largest amount of PET and HDPE. The management of microplastic waste, including that found in water, is strongly influenced by the involvement of local and regional communities.

According to research by Campanale et al. [35], 50% of microplastic particles between 0.02 and 0.1 mm in size are transported by water runoff. The authors focus their research on temporary ponds, stormwater retention ponds and small streams, drawing attention to the extremely small number of studies (eight) conducted so far on the ecosystems and related to these water resources.

Other authors, such as Vuori and Ollikainen [36], point out that there are no standards regulating the amount of microplastics in wastewater. Their approach focuses on the cost-effectiveness of three types of wastewater treatment (activated sludge, rapid sand filtration and membrane bioreactor) and two sludge management technologies (anaerobic digestion and incineration), aiming to quantify the impact of microplastic pollution on the aquatic environment and aquatic ecosystems. The analysis concludes that the removal of microplastics from wastewater is technically feasible and economically profitable.

An interesting cause of increased water pollution caused microplastics is the impact of flooding on waste management facilities. According to Ponti et al. [37], these floods can release micropollutants into freshwater systems, impacting the marine environment, agricultural ecosystems and human health. Based on the existing situation in the UK, the authors propose a correlated analysis of the official waste statistics with rainfall and river flood extent maps. Furthermore, they believe that site-specific mitigation measures and containment systems capable of reducing the amount of flood-induced microplastics from waste management facilities are needed.

Risk management for aquatic ecosystems is considered by Mehinto et al. [32] to be closely related to pollution control measures that mitigate environmental emissions. The authors use four pollution risk thresholds, official statistical data, microplastic toxicity studies and a metanalysis in the field. Following this analysis, the authors make recommendations on the quantification of water pollution, including microplastics, and a more efficient identification of risk thresholds. Risk management of microplastic pollution of water sources is also addressed by Thornton Hampton et al. [38], who point out that there is no internationally unified approach to how microplastic concentrations should be reported. For this reason, the authors recommend that microplastic concentrations should be calculated at least by both mass and number.

An analysis of the degree of pollution of water sources caused by microplastics is carried out by Chakraborty et al. [39] and covers the period of 2015–2021. The authors use Raman spectroscopy and conclude that the most widespread microplastics in water sources are polystyrene (PS), polyethylene terephthalate (PET), polyethylene (PE) and polypropylene (PP). In addition to this, the authors define the main sources of microplastic water pollution as urban waste, fishing activities and industrial waste.

An interesting study carried out by Angelakis et al. [40] highlights, on the one hand, the historical evolution of water quality and, on the other hand, the current challenges for water quality management and protection. The authors believe that the analysis of the methods and solutions offered by the evolution of mankind in relation to the management of water sources is beneficial to look at for present and future solutions in this field.

The analysis of microplastic pollution in Italian marine waters is carried out by Sbrana et al. [41], in the context of European marine water protection legislation and its impact on marine ecosystems. The analysis reveals that the concentration of microplastics in the water decreases with distance away from the coast, except in areas where sea currents are very strong. Moreover, the concentration of plastic in surface waters is four times higher than in deep waters.

In the case of the Lis river basin (Portugal) and coastal area, microplastic pollution is analysed by Sá et al. [42], the authors using a sample of 105 companies in the area and comparing samples collected from surface water and sediment. The most common particles in the water analysed were polyethylene (37%), polyacrylate (18%) and polystyrene (18%), and in sediments, polyethylene terephthalate (29%) and polyacrylate (23%). The analysis concludes that factors contributing to the increase in microplastic water pollution are population growth, plastic production and environmental conditions conducive to the transmission of microplastic particles into water sources. A similar approach, carried out by Kittner et al. [43], considers microplastic pollution in the Danube River and aims to define a systematic pollution-monitoring strategy. Chemical analysis is performed using the thermal extraction desorption technique, gas chromatography/mass chromatography. Following the analysis of the collected samples, polyethylene, polystyrene and polypropylene were, alarmingly, found in abundance in the water.

The lack of standard protocols and technologies for removing microplastics from water through wastewater treatment plants is addressed by Sadia et al. [44], who review the efficiency of wastewater treatment plants and the possibility of converting microplastics into renewable energy sources. To this end, the authors developed a sustainable methodology for wastewater treatment.

Other authors such as Melchor-Martínez et al. [45] stress the need for sustainability of microplastic production under conditions of increasing economic efficiency. The authors conducted a meta-analysis of production methods, highlighting the environmental impact and mitigation of conventional and emerging plastics, as well as regulations in the field.

In terms of plastic recycling, according to Nikiema and Asiedu [46], only 9% of the 9 billion tonnes of plastic ever produced has so far been recycled. The authors reviewed microplastic removal technologies and their efficiency, starting with pollution sources and until microplastics reach the sea, covering stormwater, municipal wastewater treatment and drinking water. The final result provides a guide on implementable measures for the treatment and elimination of water pollution caused by microplastics.

A new technology for removing plastics from water sources is the use of superhydrophobic surfaces, which have a water contact angle of >150°. According to Rius-Ayra et al. [47], the increase in research related to this technology shows its importance. The authors believe that superhydrophobic materials allow the removal of five types of emerging pollutants, including microplastics.

The literature review is an argument in favour of the present scientific approach and highlights the need for a new approach in the field.

3. Materials and Methods

Since the intensification of global trade, interventions to limit environmental pollution caused by microplastics, especially in the aquatic environment, have become a priority for international environmental organisations. Several campaigns have been carried out to monitor pollution and inform stakeholders about its effects.

These issues have taken on a global dimension through OECD efforts to collect information on microplastic pollution. In our scientific research, we used OECD databases [48] for the period of 1990–2019 for the indicators presented in Table 1.

Table 1. Description of the indicators used in the analysis.

	Region	Symbol	Name	Unit of Measure	Databases (accessed on 3 January 2023)
1.	United States (US)				
2.	Canada (CAN)		plastic waste		https://stats.oecd.org/viewhtml.aspx?datasetcode=
3.	OECD America	PWCR	collected for		PLASTIC_WASTE_6&lang=en [49]
4.	OECD EU		recycling		
5.	OECD non-EU			tonnes (t) of	
6.	OECD Asia		plastic leakage to	plastics	https://stats.oecd.org/viewhtml.aspx?datasetcode=
7.	OECD Oceania	PLAE	aquatic		PLASTIC_LEAKAGE_5&lang=en [50]
8.	OECD Latin America (OECDLatAmerica)		environments		
9.	Other non-OECD EU (OthEU)				
10.	Other Eurasia (OthEurasia)	PUR	plastics use by		https://stats.oecd.org/viewhtml.aspx?datasetcode=
11.	Middle East North Africa (MENorthAfrica)		region		PLASTIC_USE_9&lang=en [51]
12.	Other Africa (OthAfrica)		plastic waste by		
13.	Non-OECD Asia (NonOEDASIA)	PWRELF	region and by		https://stats.oecd.org/viewhtml.aspx?datasetcode=
14.	China		end-of-life fate		PLASTIC_WASTE_5&lang=en [52]
15.	India				

Based on the collected data and literature review, we formulated the following research hypotheses:

H1. *At the global level, the policy to combat water pollution caused by microplastics is directly and proportionally oriented towards the reduction of regional pollution, with the awareness that this approach will have an effect of at least 98% in the total reduction in water pollution caused by microplastics. The hypothesis is a continuation of the results of the research by the authors Blanco et al., Chu et al., Dronjak et al., Karapanagioti and Kalavrouziotis, Nicolai et al., Seghers et al., Shi et al., P. Wang et al. and S. Wang et al. [4–11,53].*

H2. *Globally, plastic recycling mechanisms have been set up on the assumption that this will have a direct impact on reducing microplastic water pollution. The definition of this hypothesis was made in accordance with the results of the research undertaken by the authors Angelakis et al., Chakraborty et al., Kittner et al., Mehinto et al., Sá et al. and Thornton Hampton et al. [32,38–40,42,43].*

H3. *From the point of view of the coherence of water pollution reduction policies, there is an increasing trend in the dynamics towards the reduction in correlation errors of the indicators as the overall experience of the implementation of these policies increases. The construction of this hypothesis was based on research conducted by the authors Melchor-Martínez et al., Nikiema and Asiedu, Rius-Ayra et al. and Sadia et al. [44–47].*

H4. *At the EU level, against the background of intensified efforts to promote the circular economy, the disparities in terms of combating water pollution caused by microplastics are widening, especially for countries where the implementation of the circular economy is at an early stage. This hypothesis is also supported by research carried out by the authors Cook et al., Lofty et al., Rosenboom et al. and Syberg et al. [27–30].*

Using data reported by the OECD (Table 1), we performed a multiple regression correlation diagram for 15 regions in the world. It has as its pivot the dependent variable assimilated to the circular economy, i.e., the amount of plastic waste collected for recycling, which we treated in relation to the monitoring indicators of plastic waste produced at the regional level, end-of-life plastic waste and the impact of plastic pollution on the aquatic environment.

The system of regional equations for the variables in Table 1 is presented as follows:

$$\begin{cases} PWCR_{US} = 1.693 * PLAE_{US} + 0.043 * PUR_{US} + 0.068 * PWRELF_{US} - 0.742 \\ PWCR_{CAN} = 1.448 * PLAE_{CAN} - 0.086 * PUR_{CAN} + 0.143 * PWRELF_{CAN} - 0.111 \\ PWCR_{OECDAmerica} = 1.003 * PLAE_{OECDAmerica} - 0.173 * PUR_{OECDAmerica} + 0.236 * PWRELF_{OECDAmerica} + 0.14 \\ PWCR_{OECDEU} = 3.874 * PLAE_{OECDEU} - 0.158 * PUR_{OECDEU} + 0.2 * PWRELF_{OECDEU} - 1.7 \\ PWCR_{OECDNonEU} = -0.021 * PLAE_{OECDNonEU} - 0.272 * PUR_{OECDNonEU} + 0.509 * PWRELF_{OECDNonEU} - 0.299 \\ PWCR_{OECDASIA} = 0.094 * PLAE_{OECDASIA} - 0.275 * PUR_{OECDASIA} + 0.592 * PWRELF_{OECDASIA} + 0.115 \\ PWCR_{OECDOceania} = 21.215 * PLAE_{OECDOceania} - 0.009 * PUR_{OECDOceania} - 0.204 * PWRELF_{OECDOceania} + 0.003 \\ PWCR_{OECDLatAmerica} = 1.644 * PLAE_{OECDLatAmerica} + 0.084 * PUR_{OECDLatAmerica} - 0.175 * PWRELF_{OECDLatAmerica} - 0.083 \\ PWCR_{OthEU} = 11.154 * PLAE_{OthEU} - 0.014 * PUR_{OthEU} - 0.141 * PWRELF_{OthEU} + 0.045 \\ PWCR_{OthEurasia} = 4.762 * PLAE_{OthEurasia} + 0 * PUR_{OthEurasia} - 0.03 * PWRELF_{OthEurasia} - 0.025 \\ PWCR_{MENorthAfrica} = 1.096 * PLAE_{MENorthAfrica} - 0.029 * PUR_{MENorthAfrica} - 0.005 * PWRELF_{MENorthAfrica} + 0.065 \\ PWCR_{OthAfrica} = 0.611 * PLAE_{OthAfrica} + 0.073 * PUR_{OthAfrica} - 0.105 * PWRELF_{OthAfrica} - 0.06 \\ PWCR_{NonOECDASIA} = 1.06 * PLAE_{NonOECDASIA} - 0.037 * PUR_{NonOECDASIA} - 0.048 * PWRELF_{NonOECDASIA} + 0.156 \\ PWCR_{China} = 5.051 * PLAE_{China} + 0.05 * PUR_{China} - 0.158 * PWRELF_{China} - 0.525 \\ PWCR_{India} = 5.577 * PLAE_{India} + 0.035 * PUR_{India} - 0.226 * PWRELF_{India} - 0.029 \end{cases} \quad (1)$$

From the analysis of the system of equations constructed on the basis of the β coefficients of the 15 regional models, it is evident that the variable that best correlated with the outcome indicator of circular economy efficiency (dependent variable) is the indicator of monitoring the impact of plastic pollution on the aquatic environment. Thus, the impact of the circular economy results in long-term effects on the reduction of microplastic pollution, especially in China, India, Oceania and Europe (see Figure 2).

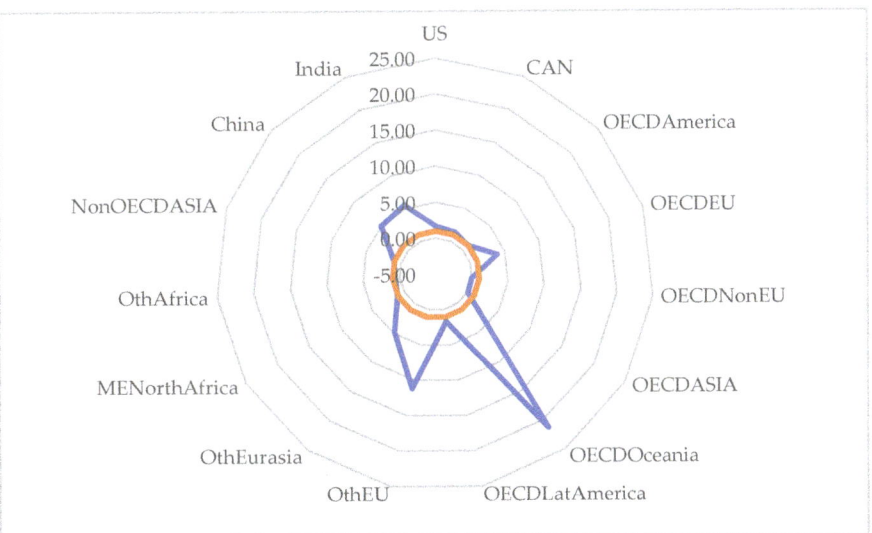

Figure 2. Correlation diagram of the effects of the implementation of the circular economy on the reduction of water pollution caused by microplastics (PWCR vs. PLAE).

The diagram shows that, at the level of the performing sample, the average correlation is 500%, i.e., the impact of reducing environmental plastic pollution generates a 5-fold reduction in the impact of microplastics on the aquatic environment in the circular economy, the maximum magnitude belonging to the Oceania region, where the impact is 21 times greater. At the European level, in OECD member countries, the impact is up to 3.8 times and up to 11 times in non-OECD member countries.

Non-EU countries show the lowest correlation between the two indicators, with an inversely proportional variation of 0.21%. This means that, in these countries, the impact of the circular economy is low and the strategies to reduce microplastic pollution are not in accordance with the global and European action guidelines.

After using a multiple regression correlation at the regional level (see Figure 3), it was observed that there is an inversely proportional relationship between plastic consumption and use in the regional circular economy of the USA, Canada, OECD America, OECD EU, OECD Non-EU, OECD Asia, OECD Oceania, Other EU, ME North Africa and non-OECD Asia. The average value of the inverse correlation is 10%. For the other regions analysed in the sample, the correlation is directly proportional, but reduced by a maximum of 8%, which shows that, in relation to the development objectives of clean industry, plastic consumption does not show significant changes. We consider this a major vulnerability of pollution policies, which, in this light, should focus additional efforts to improve public policies.

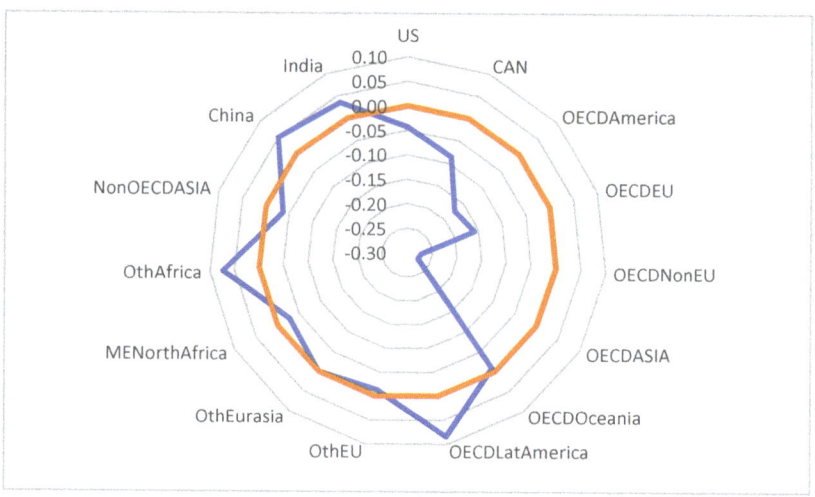

Figure 3. Correlation diagram of the effects of circular economy implementation on plastic use by region (PWCR vs. PUR).

Figure 4 shows a significant disparity in the correlation between the implementation of the circular economy and the reduction of the mass of end-of-life plastic waste, where developed regions of the world (USA, Canada, OECD America, OECD EU, OECD Non-EU, OECD Asia) have higher correlation rates. These regions have access to superior technologies to combat microplastic pollution according to its chemical properties with significant biological impact. The average correlation reaches 30%, with a maximum of 60% in the region of Asian OECD member states.

In the other regions analysed, the correlation is inversely proportional, which means that the policy to combat microplastic pollution does not meet the proposed goal, one explanation being the orientation of these regions towards commercial expansion and extensive economic growth.

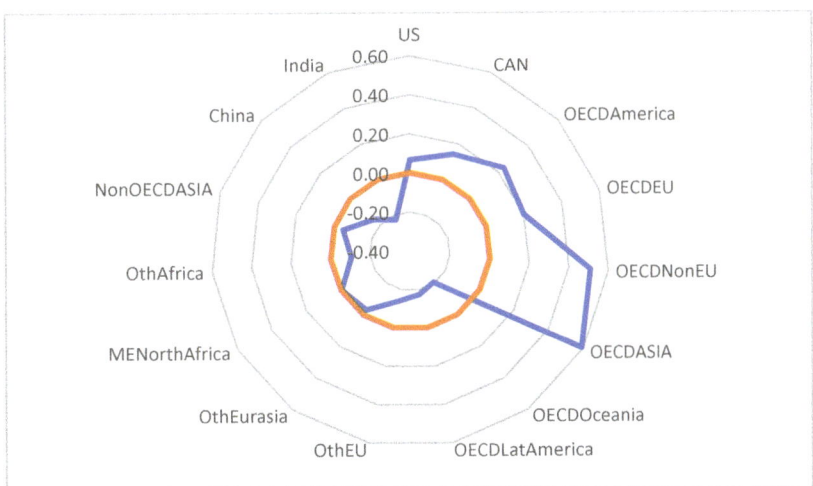

Figure 4. Correlation diagram of the effects of the implementation of the circular economy on end-of-life plastic waste (PWCR vs. PWRELF).

4. Results

Through the application of modelling techniques, the regional model was summarized, which generated statistically significant coefficients for all 15 regions studied, with the level of statistical significance exceeding 98% for these regions, with a standard maximum error estimate of 8% at the level of the sample studied, as shown in Table 2.

This validates hypothesis H1. At the global level, the policy to combat microplastic water pollution is directly and proportionally oriented towards the reduction of regional pollution, with the awareness that this approach will have an effect of at least 98% in the total reduction of microplastic water pollution.

Table 2 shows the distribution of the statistical F function values between the minimum value of 236.93 points and the maximum value of 5058.97 points, thus demonstrating a significant regional disparity of policies to combat microplastic water pollution. The maximum values are attributed to the regions: USA, OECD Latin America, Other Africa and non-OECD Asia. With respect to these regions, the analysis of the interval between 1990–2019 shows that the value of the circular economy's impact on microplastic water pollution reaches the maximum value at the correlation function.

At the opposite pole, the lowest values were recorded for the regions: OECD America, OECD Non-EU and OECD Asia. It should be mentioned that the level of Sig. coefficients assimilated to the F function is lower than the selected error representativeness threshold $\alpha = 0.05$, which allows for all 15 regions analyzed to reject the null hypothesis and maintain the alternative hypothesis. This allows the validation of the regional model to combat microplastic pollution. The ANOVA test is presented in Table 3.

The ANOVA statistical test for the regional models shows the statistical weight of the regression squares is allocated to the correlational function (98.5%), while the residual variable has an allocation of only 99.5%. This demonstrates that the model is valid and representative of the phenomenon studied, validating hypothesis H2. At the global level, plastic recycling mechanisms were created assuming that this approach will have a direct impact on reducing microplastic water pollution.

To prove hypothesis H3, we projected in Figure 5 the dynamic distributions of the evolution of the dependent variable in relation to its predicted values according to the regional PP-Plot distribution graph. From Figure 5, it follows that the error distribution of the dependent variable at the regional level has different error peaks ($\bar{y}$).

Figure 5 shows that, as experience increases and the current period approaches, the experience gained by policy makers in the field of pollution control helps straighten the trend curves, which proves hypothesis H3. From the point of view of coherence of water pollution abatement policies, there is an increasing trend to reduce the correlation errors of the indicators as the overall experience of implementing these policies increases.

Table 2. Model Summary.

Model	R	R Square	Adjusted R Square	Std. Error of the Estimate	Change Statistics					Durbin-Watson
					R Square Change	F Change	df1	df2	Sig. F Change	
1.	0.999 [a,b]	0.997	0.997	0.099143	0.997	2992.770	3	26	0.000	0.715
a. Predictors: (Constant), PWRELF$_{US}$, PUR$_{US}$, PLAE$_{US}$										
b. Dependent Variable: PWCR$_{US}$										
2.	0.998 [a,b]	0.997	0.997	0.013844	0.997	2857.987	3	26	0.000	0.831
a. Predictors: (Constant), PWRELF$_{CAN}$, PUR$_{CAN}$, PLAE$_{CAN}$										
b. Dependent Variable: PWCR$_{CAN}$										
3.	0.994 [a,b]	0.988	0.987	0.054194	0.988	727.162	3	26	0.000	0.456
a. Predictors: (Constant), PWRELF$_{OECDAmerica}$, PUR$_{OECDAmerica}$, PLAE$_{OECDAmerica}$										
b. Dependent Variable: PWCR$_{OECDAmerica}$										
4.	0.998 [a,b]	0.995	0.995	0.285726	0.995	1822.884	3	26	0.000	0.608
a. Predictors: (Constant), PWRELF$_{OECDEU}$, PUR$_{OECDEU}$, PLAE$_{OECDEU}$										
b. Dependent Variable: PWCR$_{OECDEU}$										
5.	0.991 [a,b]	0.982	0.980	0.099378	0.982	465.494	3	26	0.000	0.543
a. Predictors: (Constant), PWRELF$_{OECDNonEU}$, PUR$_{OECDNonEU}$, PLAE$_{OECDNonEU}$										
b. Dependent Variable: PWCR$_{OECDNonEU}$										
6.	0.982 [a,b]	0.965	0.961	0.156510	0.965	236.939	3	26	0.000	0.254
a. Predictors: (Constant), PWRELF$_{OECDASIA}$, PUR$_{OECDASIA}$, PLAE$_{OECDASIA}$										
b. Dependent Variable: PWCR$_{OECDASIA}$										
7.	0.998 [a,b]	0.997	0.997	0.003728	0.997	2865.476	3	26	0.000	1.108
a. Predictors: (Constant), PWRELF$_{OECDOceania}$, PUR$_{OECDOceania}$, PLAE$_{OECDOceania}$										
b. Dependent Variable: PWCR$_{OECDOceania}$										
8.	0.999 [a,b]	0.997	0.997	0.047812	0.997	3143.947	3	26	0.000	0.396
a. Predictors: (Constant), PWRELF$_{OECDLatAmerica}$, PLAE$_{OECDLatAmerica}$, PUR$_{OECDLatAmerica}$										
b. Dependent Variable: PWCR$_{OECDLatAmerica}$										
9.	0.998 [a,b]	0.996	0.996	0.004837	0.996	2360.164	3	26	0.000	0.491
a. Predictors: (Constant), PWRELF$_{OthEU}$, PUR$_{OthEU}$, PLAE$_{OthEU}$										
b. Dependent Variable: PWCR$_{OthEU}$										
10.	0.998 [a,b]	0.996	0.995	0.027975	0.996	1973.765	3	26	0.000	0.177
a. Predictors: (Constant), PWRELF$_{OthEurasia}$, PUR$_{OthEurasia}$, PLAE$_{OthEurasia}$										
b. Dependent Variable: PWCR$_{OthEurasia}$										
11.	0.998 [a,b]	0.996	0.995	0.027183	0.996	2052.844	3	26	0.000	0.454
a. Predictors: (Constant), PWRELF$_{MENorthAfrica}$, PUR$_{MENorthAfrica}$, PLAE$_{MENorthAfrica}$										
b. Dependent Variable: PWCR$_{MENorthAfrica}$										
12.	0.999 [a,b]	0.998	0.998	0.019682	0.998	4091.570	3	26	0.000	0.362
a. Predictors: (Constant), PWRELF$_{OthAfrica}$, PLAE$_{OthAfrica}$, PUR$_{OthAfrica}$										
b. Dependent Variable: PWCR$_{OthAfrica}$										
13.	0.999 [a,b]	0.998	0.998	0.047965	0.998	5058.977	3	26	0.000	1.023
a. Predictors: (Constant), PWRELF$_{NonOECDASIA}$, PUR$_{NonOECDASIA}$, PLAE$_{NonOECDASIA}$										
b. Dependent Variable: PWCR$_{NonOECDASIA}$										
14.	0.998 [a,b]	0.996	0.996	0.275743	0.996	2227.735	3	26	0.000	0.389
a. Predictors: (Constant), PWRELF$_{China}$, PLAE$_{China}$, PUR$_{China}$										
b. Dependent Variable: PWCR$_{China}$										
15.	0.998 [a,b]	0.996	0.995	0.074138	0.996	2115.586	3	26	0.000	0.294
a. Predictors: (Constant), PWRELF$_{India}$, PLAE$_{India}$, PUR$_{India}$										
b. Dependent Variable: PWCR$_{India}$										

In order to prove hypothesis H4, the authors analysed the results obtained by the proposed model (Equation (1)), finding that, at the level of the dependent variable assimilated to the circular economy, the correlation with the impact of water pollution caused by microplastics was strong, i.e., reducing the amount of plastic waste has the effect of reducing water pollution caused by microplastics by 3.8 times. It can be seen from equation 1 that the impact of the circular economy on the regional size of plastic consumption in the EU is inversely proportional, which can be presumed to have a causality with the high level of regional disparity in plastic consumption. In order to determine the level of regional disparity of plastic use in the EU, we accessed the Our World in Data database [54] for the year 2019 (the latest year for which official statistical data are available) and selected Member States for which we performed an algorithm to plot regional averages against the overall average for the following indicators: share of EU average mismanaged plastic waste (%); share of EU average mismanaged plastic waste to ocean (%) and share of EU average mismanaged plastic waste per capita (%) (see Table 4).

Table 3. ANOVA test.

	Model	Sum of Squares	df	Mean Square	F	Sig.
1.	Regression [a,b]	88.251	3	29.417	2992.770	0.000 [b]
	Residual	0.256	26	0.010		
	Total	88.507	29			

a. Dependent Variable: $PWCR_{US}$
b. Predictors: (Constant), $PWRELF_{US}$, PUR_{US}, $PLAE_{US}$

	Model	Sum of Squares	df	Mean Square	F	Sig.
2.	Regression [a,b]	1.643	3	0.548	2857.987	0.000 [b]
	Residual	0.005	26	0.000		
	Total	1.648	29			

a. Dependent Variable: $PWCR_{CAN}$
b. Predictors: (Constant), $PWRELF_{CAN}$, PUR_{CAN}, $PLAE_{CAN}$

	Model	Sum of Squares	df	Mean Square	F	Sig.
3.	Regression [a,b]	6.407	3.000	2.136	727.162	0.000 [b]
	Residual	0.076	26.000	0.003		
	Total	6.483	29.000			

a. Dependent Variable: $PWCR_{OECDAmerica}$
b. Predictors: (Constant), $PWRELF_{OECDAmerica}$, $PUR_{OECDAmerica}$, $PLAE_{OECDAmerica}$

	Model	Sum of Squares	df	Mean Square	F	Sig.
4.	Regression [a,b]	446.456	3.000	148.819	1822.884	0.000 [b]
	Residual	2.123	26.000	0.082		
	Total	448.578	29.000			

a. Dependent Variable: $PWCR_{OECDEU}$
b. Predictors: (Constant), $PWRELF_{OECDEU}$, PUR_{OECDEU}, $PLAE_{OECDEU}$

	Model	Sum of Squares	df	Mean Square	F	Sig.
5.	Regression [a,b]	13.792	3	4.597	465.494	0.000 [b]
	Residual	0.257	26	0.010		
	Total	14.048	29			

a. Dependent Variable: $PWCR_{OECDNonEU}$
b. Predictors: (Constant), $PWRELF_{OECDNonEU}$, $PUR_{OECDNonEU}$, $PLAE_{OECDNonEU}$

	Model	Sum of Squares	df	Mean Square	F	Sig.
6.	Regression [a,b]	17.412	3.000	5.804	236.939	0.000 [b]
	Residual	0.637	26.000	0.024		
	Total	18.049	29.000			

a. Dependent Variable: $PWCR_{OECDASIA}$
b. Predictors: (Constant), $PWRELF_{OECDASIA}$, $PUR_{OECDASIA}$, $PLAE_{OECDASIA}$

	Model	Sum of Squares	df	Mean Square	F	Sig.
7.	Regression [a,b]	0.119	3.000	0.040	2865.476	0.000 [b]
	Residual	0.000	26.000	0.000		
	Total	0.120	29.000			

a. Dependent Variable: $PWCR_{OECDOceania}$
b. Predictors: (Constant), $PWRELF_{OECDOceania}$, $PUR_{OECDOceania}$, $PLAE_{OECDOceania}$

	Model	Sum of Squares	df	Mean Square	F	Sig.
8.	Regression [a,b]	21.561	3	7.187	3143.947	0.000 [b]
	Residual	0.059	26	0.002		
	Total	21.621	29			

a. Dependent Variable: $PWCR_{OECDLatAmerica}$
b. Predictors: (Constant), $PWRELF_{OECDLatAmerica}$, $PLAE_{OECDLatAmerica}$, $PUR_{OECDLatAmerica}$

	Model	Sum of Squares	df	Mean Square	F	Sig.
9.	Regression [a,b]	0.166	3.000	0.055	2360.164	0.000 [b]
	Residual	0.001	26.000	0.000		
	Total	0.166	29.000			

a. Dependent Variable: $PWCR_{OthEU}$
b. Predictors: (Constant), $PWRELF_{OthEU}$, PUR_{OthEU}, $PLAE_{OthEU}$

	Model	Sum of Squares	df	Mean Square	F	Sig.
10.	Regression [a,b]	4.634	3.000	1.545	1973.765	0.000 [b]
	Residual	0.020	26.000	0.001		
	Total	4.654	29.000			

a. Dependent Variable: $PWCR_{OthEurasia}$
b. Predictors: (Constant), $PWRELF_{OthEurasia}$, $PUR_{OthEurasia}$, $PLAE_{OthEurasia}$

	Model	Sum of Squares	df	Mean Square	F	Sig.
11.	Regression [a,b]	4.551	3	1.517	2052.844	0.000 [b]
	Residual	0.019	26	0.001		
	Total	4.570	29			

a. Dependent Variable: $PWCR_{MENorthAfrica}$
b. Predictors: (Constant), $PWRELF_{MENorthAfrica}$, $PUR_{MENorthAfrica}$, $PLAE_{MENorthAfrica}$

	Model	Sum of Squares	df	Mean Square	F	Sig.
12.	Regression [a,b]	4.755	3.000	1.585	4091.570	0.000 [b]
	Residual	0.010	26.000	0.000		
	Total	4.765	29.000			

a. Dependent Variable: $PWCR_{OthAfrica}$
b. Predictors: (Constant), $PWRELF_{OthAfrica}$, $PLAE_{OthAfrica}$, $PUR_{OthAfrica}$

	Model	Sum of Squares	df	Mean Square	F	Sig.
13.	Regression [a,b]	34.916	3.000	11.639	5058.977	0.000 [b]
	Residual	0.060	26.000	0.002		
	Total	34.976	29.000			

a. Dependent Variable: $PWCR_{NonOECDASIA}$
b. Predictors: (Constant), $PWRELF_{NonOECDASIA}$, $PUR_{NonOECDASIA}$, $PLAE_{NonOECDASIA}$

Table 3. Cont.

	Model	Sum of Squares	df	Mean Square	F	Sig.
14.	Regression [a,b]	508.152	3	169.384	2227.735	0.000 [b]
	Residual	1.977	26	0.076		
	Total	510.129	29			

a. Dependent Variable: PWCR$_{China}$
b. Predictors: (Constant), PWRELF$_{China}$, PLAE$_{China}$, PUR$_{China}$

	Model	Sum of Squares	df	Mean Square	F	Sig.
15.	Regression [a,b]	34.885	3.000	11.628	2115.586	0.000 [b]
	Residual	0.143	26.000	0.005		
	Total	35.028	29.000			

a. Dependent Variable: PWCR$_{India}$
b. Predictors: (Constant), PWRELF$_{India}$, PLAE$_{India}$, PUR$_{India}$

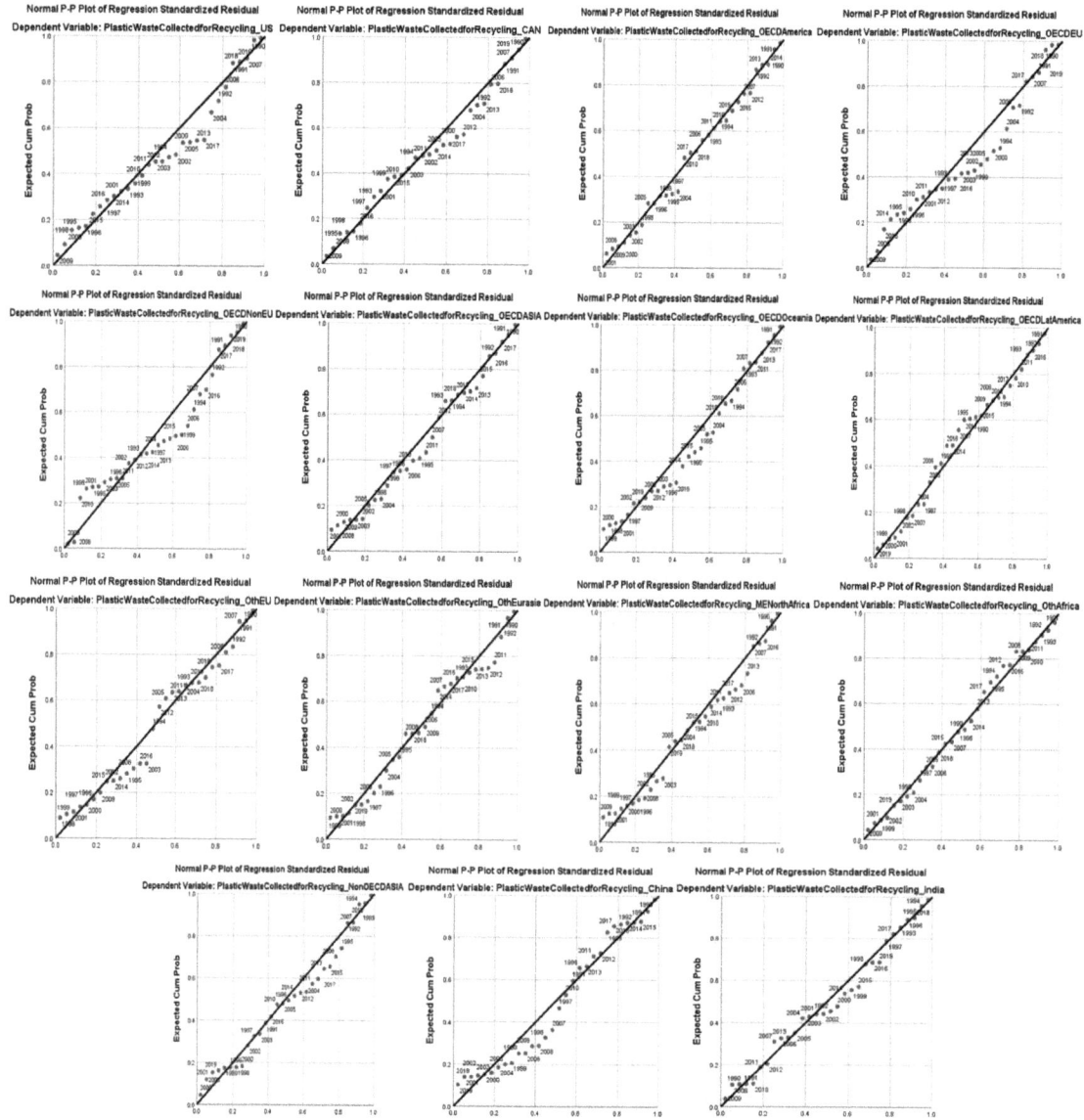

Figure 5. P-P Plot diagrams of regional distribution.

Table 4. Analysis of the degree of regional disparity on policies to combat plastic water pollution in the EU.

Country (2019)	Share of EU Average Mismanaged Plastic Waste (%)	Share of EU Average Mismanaged Plastic Waste to Ocean (%)	Share of EU Average Mismanaged Plastic Waste per Capita (%)	Std. Deviation
Belgium	19.70%	44.21%	27.41%	10.2%
Bulgaria	26.89%	15.00%	61.65%	19.8%
Croatia	151.36%	813.69%	588.16%	274.9%
Cyprus	7.22%	37.54%	96.66%	37.1%
Denmark	3.36%	23.39%	9.36%	8.4%
Estonia	5.18%	135.77%	62.65%	53.4%
Finland	22.61%	0.00%	65.60%	27.2%
France	239.68%	54.13%	59.06%	86.3%
Germany	437.21%	24.06%	84.01%	182.3%
Greece	38.87%	309.41%	59.57%	122.9%
Ireland	23.08%	0.00%	75.87%	31.8%
Italy	334.78%	102.57%	88.73%	112.9%
Latvia	8.24%	70.80%	69.34%	29.2%
Lithuania	8.95%	38.05%	52.02%	17.9%
Malta	2.23%	0.00%	81.50%	37.9%
Netherlands	131.42%	237.80%	123.36%	52.2%
Poland	121.86%	11.48%	51.62%	45.6%
Portugal	32.94%	111.50%	51.70%	33.5%
Romania	450.02%	61.98%	372.95%	167.7%
Slovakia	14.83%	0.00%	43.62%	18.1%
Slovenia	7.28%	79.38%	56.21%	30.1%
Spain	175.57%	75.43%	60.29%	51.2%
Sweden	36.71%	53.81%	58.70%	9.4%
Std deviation	136.0%	169.2%	123.7%	65.5%

The overall pollution disparity index calculated based on the standard deviation of the three regional data sets in Table 4 is 65%. Thus, there is a significant difference between policies to reduce plastic water pollution and policies to reduce plastic consumption per capita in the EU. At a regional level, the share of the EU average mismanaged plastic waste indicator has a disparity of 136%, close to the value of the disparity of the share of the EU average mismanaged plastic waste per capita indicator, which means that, in terms of communicating the effects on the environment, there is a successful communication effort in the EU, with 90% of European citizens aware of the consequences of pollution on the deterioration of environmental quality. This results from a comparison of regional disparities between the two indicators.

On the other hand, the Share of EU average mismanaged plastic waste to ocean indicator shows an increase in regional disparities, up to 169.2%, mainly due to the regional territorial configuration. The most advanced countries in implementing environmental policies in this area are Malta, Finland, Ireland and Slovakia. At the opposite end are Croatia, Greece, the Netherlands, Estonia and Portugal.

In the overall ranking for the three indicators, the highest levels of disparity were assessed for Croatia, Germany and Romania, with these countries showing the most fluctuating variations from the calculated EU average. These aspects demonstrate hypothesis H4. In the EU, as efforts to promote the circular economy intensify, the disparities in combating water pollution caused by microplastics are widening, especially for countries where the implementation of the circular economy is at an early stage.

5. Discussion

The research results allow the following aspects to be presented:

- In the US, the synergy between anti-pollution policies and the acceleration of the circular economy is marked by the period 2004–2013, which covers the global recession of 2007–2008, with a significant impact on the US economy;
- The period 2004–2012 was the impact period for Canada's economy, which takes on the effects of the US crisis;
- In OECD countries in the Americas, there was a reduction in errors relating to the projection of forecast values in relation to the trend line, the peaks being characterized by the period 1997–2004. This was against the backdrop of the terrorist attacks of 11 September 2001, followed by the stock market crisis and the effects of the war in Iraq in 2011–2003. These events redirected public policies towards security, minimising efforts for other policies such as pollution control;
- With 22 EU OECD member states, the distribution of errors is significant when compared to correct forecast rates and covers extended periods, namely 1992–1995, 2000–2004 and 2010–2014. In the first mentioned timeframe, major changes in the European economic policy occurred as a result of the fall of the communist regime in SE Europe. The second timeframe was assimilated to the EU enlargement efforts, which culminated in 2004 with the accession of 10 former communist states to the European bloc. The 2010–2014 timeframe represents the period of global recession triggered in 2007 in the US and rapidly propagated in the EU. This was a period that saw the bankruptcy of some renowned European institutions and the reshaping of European policies on financial risks and stock market trading risks. The phenomenon was boosted by the last two EU enlargements in 2007 and 2013;
- The distribution of errors was also transferred to the OECD Non-EU countries in the region, which, in the periods 1997–2000, 2005–2007 and 2010–2016, faced problems accessing the European single market and structural changes in trade due to EU regional reconfiguration;
- For Asian OECD member countries, the distribution of trend curves in relation to predicted values for the circular economy-like variable is superior, with more efficient correlations. The main disruptions the took place in 1995–2000 and 2011–2014. In the first period, the economies of these countries were heavily affected by the major financial crisis that began in Thailand involving the link between the Thai baht and the U.S. dollar. Indonesia, South Korea and Malaysia were involved in this crisis and their capital inflows were affected by more than $100 billion in the first year of the crisis. The effects of the Asian financial crisis spilled over into the economies of Russia and Brazil. The second period was a consequence of the global economic crisis that started in 2008;
- In Oceania's case, the values for the distribution of errors relative to the trend curve are flattened, the significant periods being 1990–1995 and 2012–2016;
- In the case of OECD Latin American countries, no significant error distributions were found, with the right-hand side of the forecast containing the likely values of the regression function;
- In the case of other non-OECD European countries, error distributions were found for the periods 1996–1999 (the fall of the communist regime and its consequences) and 2003–2014. These periods coincided with the reconfiguration of EU borders and the major global crisis of 2009;
- Non-OECD Eurasia shows the most significant errors distributed over the period 2011–2013, corresponding to the global crisis of the early 2010s;
- In the non-OECD African region, there are no significant distributions of errors to the right of the trend. The model is representative of this region;
- In non-OECD Asian countries, the period that witnessed function errors is clustered between 2012 and 2017 and was strongly influenced by the effects of the economic crisis in China in 201;

- At the level of the Chinese economy, there is a significant distribution of errors to the right of the trend for several periods, namely: 1990–1995, 1997–1999 and 2004–2009;

The Indian economy was characterized by significant error distribution in the periods of 1999–2000 and 2015–2019,

Based on the results of the analysis, we formulated the following proposals to improve public policies in the field of combating water pollution caused by microplastics (see Table 5).

Table 5. Proposals for improving public policies in the field of combating water pollution caused by microplastics.

Pollution Factor Plastics Polymer (Bioplastics–Dependent Variable)	Effectiveness of Implemented Control Measures	Public Policy Proposals	Graphical Distribution of Correlations with the Reference Pollutant Factor (Bioplastics) *
Marine coatings	Increased in relation to the reference pollutant factor bioplastics (superunit level of pollution reduction in the correlative assessment in relation to the dependent variable of value 4.255).	Introducing higher quality standards for paints used in the shipping industry in order to protect the environment and reduce water pollution caused by microplastics.	
Low-density polyethylene (LDPE) and Linear Low-Density Polyethylene (LLDPE)	Reduced in relation to the reference pollutant factor bioplastics (super-unit level of pollution reduction in the correlative assessment in relation to the dependent variable is close to 0, i.e., 0.043).	Realising an international agreement– on LDPE and LLDPE water pollution whereby plastic manufacturers declare the ingredients in their plastic products and their effects on health.	
High-density polyethylene (HDPE)	Reduced in relation to the reference pollutant factor bioplastics (super-unit level of pollution reduction in the correlative assessment in relation to the dependent variable is close to 0, i.e., 0.040).	Improving the management of HDPE waste to enable its recycling in terms acceptable to the circular economy.	

Table 5. Cont.

Pollution Factor Plastics Polymer (Bioplastics–Dependent Variable)	Effectiveness of Implemented Control Measures	Public Policy Proposals	Graphical Distribution of Correlations with the Reference Pollutant Factor (Bioplastics) *
Polypropylene (PP)	Reduced in relation to the reference pollutant factor bioplastics (sub-unit level of pollution re-reduction in the correlative assessment in relation to the dependent variable is close to 0, i.e., 0.032).	New public policies to control the production, consumption and use of PP in areas such as consumer packaging, plastic parts and textiles in the automotive industry.	
Polystyrene (PS)	Reduced in relation to the reference pollutant factor bioplastics (subunit level of pollution re-reduction in the correlative assessment in relation to the dependent variable is 0.112).	Realising new international agreements that reduce the production and use of PS in the construction, packaging, automotive, pharmaceutical and medical industries.	
Polyvinyl chloride (PVC)	Reduced in relation to the reference pollutant factor bioplastics (subunit level of pollution re-reduction in the correlative assessment in relation to the dependent variable is 0.046).	Implementation of new measures to improve the collection, treatment and proper disposal of PVC waste used in the construction, textile, electrical, cable and upholstery industries.	
Polyethylene terephthalate (PET)	Reduced in relation to the reference pollutant factor bioplastics (subunit level of pollution re-reduction in the correlative assessment in relation to the dependent variable is 0.089).	Adopting new measures to raise public awareness of the impact of PET on the environment and public health.	

Table 5. *Cont.*

Pollution Factor Plastics Polymer (Bioplastics–Dependent Variable)	Effectiveness of Implemented Control Measures	Public Policy Proposals	Graphical Distribution of Correlations with the Reference Pollutant Factor (Bioplastics) *
Polyurethane (PUR)	Reduced relative to the reference pollutant factor bioplastics (subunit level of pollution re-reduction in the correlative assessment relative to the dependent variable of 0.130).	New pollution mitigation policies for polyurethane elastomers used for furniture and vehicles as well as sound insulation materials.	
Fibres	Reduced relative to the reference pollutant factor bioplastics (subunit level of pollution re-reduction in the correlative assessment relative to the dependent variable of 0.037).	Adopting new policies to inform the public about the impact of fibres on the environment and public health.	
Road marking coatings	Increased in relation to the reference pollutant factor bioplastics (supra-unit level of pollution re-reduction in the correlative assessment in relation to the dependent variable of value 3.441).	Introduction into educational programmes at different levels of information on how to reduce pollution with road markings and pedestrian markings.	
Elastomers (tyres)	Reduced in relation to the reference pollutant factor bioplastics (subunit level of pollution re-reduction in the correlative assessment in relation to the dependent variable of 0.289).	Awareness of the problem of elastomer waste generation in the automotive industry which is significant and has a global environmental impact. Hence the need for sustainable recycling of this waste.	

* Arrived at by authors using official statistical data base [55].

The importance of this study lies in combining in an integrated way OECD data on microplastic water pollution and identifying relevant policies to combat this type of pollution.

6. Conclusions

The authors have achieved the objectives proposed in the research as defined in the introduction. The literature review allowed the development of research hypotheses, which were subsequently demonstrated in Sections 3 and 4 of the paper.

An interesting econometric model was built to study the connection between the factors contributing to the increase of microplastic water pollution. Following the implementation of this model at the OECD database level, proposals for improving public policies in the field of combating water pollution caused by microplastics were carried out.

The novelty of the econometric model and public policy proposals for decreasing water pollution caused by microplastics are the strengths of this scientific approach. The novelty of the approach lies in linking chemical elements with economic and social impacts at a regional level. The model is entirely unprecedented and is in no way an adaptation or update of an existing model. The public policy proposals in this area were also innovative.

This scientific work encountered difficulties, including the lack of official statistical information on water pollution caused by microplastics and the lack of a unified approach and common regulations at an international level.

The main limitation of this paper is the relatively small number of indicators used in the analysis. The authors propose to expand the number of indicators analysed and the statistical basis of observations through international collaboration, at least at the academic level, in a future scientific approach on the same topic.

Author Contributions: Conceptualization, V.M.A., R.V.I., M.L.Z., C.I., P.L.G. and M.C.; methodology, C.I., P.L.G., R.V.I., M.L.Z. and V.M.A.; validation, V.M.A., R.V.I., M.C. and M.L.Z.; formal analysis, C.I., M.C. and P.L.G.; investigation, C.I., R.V.I., P.L.G., M.C. and M.L.Z.; resources, C.I., P.L.G. and V.M.A.; data curation, V.M.A., C.I. and R.V.I.; writing—original draft preparation, R.V.I., V.M.A., M.L.Z., C.I., P.L.G. and M.C.; writing—review and editing, P.L.G.., M.L.Z., M.C. and C.I.; visualization, V.M.A. and C.I.; supervision, C.I. and R.V.I. All authors have read and agreed to the published version of the manuscript.

Funding: This research was funded by Fondo Proserpina S.R.L., grant number 2506/2022, "The Impact of Heavy Metals and Microplastics from Aquatic Organisms on Human Health".

Institutional Review Board Statement: Not applicable.

Informed Consent Statement: Not applicable.

Data Availability Statement: The data presented in this study are available on request from the corresponding author.

Acknowledgments: The technical support was provided by the Rexdan Research Infrastructure, the infrastructure created through the project An Integrated System for the Complex Environmental Research and Monitoring in the Danube River Area, REXDAN, SMIS code 127065, project co-financed by the European Regional Development Fund through the Competitiveness Operational Programme 2014–2020, contract no. 309/10.07.2020.

Conflicts of Interest: The authors declare no conflict of interest.

References

1. United Nations Environment Programme. Mapping of Global Plastics Value Chain and Plastics Losses to the Environment: With a Particular Focus on Marine Environment. Available online: https://wedocs.unep.org/20.500.11822/26745 (accessed on 3 January 2023).
2. European Chemicals Agency Microplastics. Available online: https://echa.europa.eu/ro/hot-topics/microplastics (accessed on 3 January 2023).

European Commission Comitology Register. Available online: https://ec.europa.eu/transparency/comitology-register/screen/documents/083921/1/consult?lang=en (accessed on 3 January 2023).

Shi, X.; Zhang, X.; Gao, W.; Zhang, Y.; He, D. Removal of Microplastics from Water by Magnetic Nano-Fe_3O_4. *Sci. Total Environ.* **2022**, *802*, 149838. [CrossRef] [PubMed]

Wang, S.; Xu, M.; Jin, B.; Wünsch, U.J.; Su, Y.; Zhang, Y. Electrochemical and Microbiological Response of Exoelectrogenic Biofilm to Polyethylene Microplastics in Water. *Water Res.* **2022**, *211*, 118046. [CrossRef] [PubMed]

Chu, X.; Zheng, B.; Li, Z.; Cai, C.; Peng, Z.; Zhao, P.; Tian, Y. Occurrence and Distribution of Microplastics in Water Supply Systems: In Water and Pipe Scales. *Sci. Total Environ.* **2022**, *803*, 150004. [CrossRef] [PubMed]

Nicolai, E.; Pizzoferrato, R.; Li, Y.; Frattegiani, S.; Nucara, A.; Costa, G. A New Optical Method for Quantitative Detection of Microplastics in Water Based on Real-Time Fluorescence Analysis. *Water* **2022**, *14*, 3235. [CrossRef]

Dronjak, L.; Exposito, N.; Rovira, J.; Florencio, K.; Emiliano, P.; Corzo, B.; Schuhmacher, M.; Valero, F.; Sierra, J. Screening of Microplastics in Water and Sludge Lines of a Drinking Water Treatment Plant in Catalonia, Spain. *Water Res.* **2022**, *225*, 119185. [CrossRef] [PubMed]

Seghers, J.; Stefaniak, E.A.; La Spina, R.; Cella, C.; Mehn, D.; Gilliland, D.; Held, A.; Jacobsson, U.; Emteborg, H. Preparation of a Reference Material for Microplastics in Water—Evaluation of Homogeneity. *Anal. Bioanal. Chem.* **2022**, *414*, 385–397. [CrossRef]

Wang, P.; Huang, Z.; Chen, S.; Jing, M.; Ge, Z.; Chen, J.; Yang, S.; Chen, J.; Fang, Y. Sustainable Removal of Nano/Microplastics in Water by Solar Energy. *Chem. Eng. J.* **2022**, *428*, 131196. [CrossRef]

Karapanagioti, H.K.; Kalavrouziotis, I.K. Microplastics in Water Bodies and in the Environment. *Water* **2022**, *14*, 1324. [CrossRef]

Martin, L.M.A.; Sheng, J.; Zimba, P.V.; Zhu, L.; Fadare, O.O.; Haley, C.; Wang, M.; Phillips, T.D.; Conkle, J.; Xu, W. Testing an Iron Oxide Nanoparticle-Based Method for Magnetic Separation of Nanoplastics and Microplastics from Water. *Nanomaterials* **2022**, *12*, 2348. [CrossRef]

Viitala, M.; Steinmetz, Z.; Sillanpää, M.; Mänttäri, M.; Sillanpää, M. Historical and Current Occurrence of Microplastics in Water and Sediment of a Finnish Lake Affected by WWTP Effluents. *Environ. Pollut.* **2022**, *314*, 120298. [CrossRef]

Trani, A.; Mezzapesa, G.; Piscitelli, L.; Mondelli, D.; Nardelli, L.; Belmonte, G.; Toso, A.; Piraino, S.; Panti, C.; Baini, M.; et al. Microplastics in Water Surface and in the Gastrointestinal Tract of Target Marine Organisms in Salento Coastal Seas (Italy, Southern Puglia). *Environ. Pollut.* **2023**, *316*, 120702. [CrossRef] [PubMed]

Strokal, V.; Kuiper, E.J.; Bak, M.P.; Vriend, P.; Wang, M.; van Wijnen, J.; Strokal, M. Future Microplastics in the Black Sea: River Exports and Reduction Options for Zero Pollution. *Mar. Pollut. Bull.* **2022**, *178*, 113633. [CrossRef]

Yuan, Z.; Nag, R.; Cummins, E. Human Health Concerns Regarding Microplastics in the Aquatic Environment—From Marine to Food Systems. *Sci. Total Environ.* **2022**, *823*, 153730. [CrossRef] [PubMed]

Sarma, H.; Hazarika, R.P.; Kumar, V.; Roy, A.; Pandit, S.; Prasad, R. Microplastics in Marine and Aquatic Habitats: Sources, Impact, and Sustainable Remediation Approaches. *Environ. Sustain.* **2022**, *5*, 39–49. [CrossRef]

Sánchez-Guerrero-Hernández, M.J.; González-Fernández, D.; Sendra, M.; Ramos, F.; Yeste, M.P.; González-Ortegón, E. Contamination from Microplastics and Other Anthropogenic Particles in the Digestive Tracts of the Commercial Species Engraulis Encrasicolus and Sardina Pilchardus. *Sci. Total Environ.* **2023**, *860*, 160451. [CrossRef] [PubMed]

Kadac-Czapska, K.; Knez, E.; Grembecka, M. Food and Human Safety: The Impact of Microplastics. *Crit. Rev. Food Sci. Nutr.* **2022**, 1–20. [CrossRef] [PubMed]

Gao, W.; Zhang, Y.; Mo, A.; Jiang, J.; Liang, Y.; Cao, X.; He, D. Removal of Microplastics in Water: Technology Progress and Green Strategies. *Green Anal. Chem.* **2022**, *3*, 100042. [CrossRef]

Yang, S.; Zhou, M.; Chen, X.; Hu, L.; Xu, Y.; Fu, W.; Li, C. A Comparative Review of Microplastics in Lake Systems from Different Countries and Regions. *Chemosphere* **2022**, *286*, 131806. [CrossRef]

Manoli, K.; Naziri, A.; Ttofi, I.; Michael, C.; Allan, I.J.; Fatta-Kassinos, D. Investigation of the Effect of Microplastics on the UV Inactivation of Antibiotic-Resistant Bacteria in Water. *Water Res.* **2022**, *222*, 118906. [CrossRef]

Deme, G.G.; Ewusi-Mensah, D.; Olagbaju, O.A.; Okeke, E.S.; Okoye, C.O.; Odii, E.C.; Ejeromedoghene, O.; Igun, E.; Onyekwere, J.O.; Oderinde, O.K.; et al. Macro Problems from Microplastics: Toward a Sustainable Policy Framework for Managing Microplastic Waste in Africa. *Sci. Total Environ.* **2022**, *804*, 150170. [CrossRef]

Usman, S.; Abdull Razis, A.F.; Shaari, K.; Azmai, M.N.; Saad, M.Z.; Mat Isa, N.; Nazarudin, M.F. The Burden of Microplastics Pollution and Contending Policies and Regulations. *Int. J. Environ. Res. Public Health* **2022**, *19*, 6773. [CrossRef] [PubMed]

Mocanu, H.; Mocanu, A.-I.; Moldovan, C.; Soare, I.; Postolache, P.A.; Nechifor, A. Rare and Unusual Benign Tumors of the Sinonasal Tract and Pharynx: Case Series and Literature Review. *Exp. Ther. Med.* **2022**, *23*, 334. [CrossRef] [PubMed]

Nastase, A.; Dima, S.O.; Lupo, A.; Laszlo, V.; Tagett, R.; Draghici, S.; Georgescu, M.E.; Nechifor, A.; Berbece, S.; Popescu, I.; et al. Molecular Markers for Long-Term Survival in Stage IIIA (N2) NSCLC Patients. *Cancer Genom. Proteom.* **2022**, *19*, 94–104. [CrossRef] [PubMed]

Lofty, J.; Muhawenimana, V.; Wilson, C.A.M.E.; Ouro, P. Microplastics Removal from a Primary Settler Tank in a Wastewater Treatment Plant and Estimations of Contamination onto European Agricultural Land via Sewage Sludge Recycling. *Environ. Pollut.* **2022**, *304*, 119198. [CrossRef]

28. Syberg, K.; Nielsen, M.B.; Oturai, N.B.; Clausen, L.P.W.; Ramos, T.M.; Hansen, S.F. Circular Economy and Reduction of Micro(Nano)Plastics Contamination. *J. Hazard. Mater. Adv.* **2022**, *5*, 100044. [CrossRef]
29. Cook, E.; Velis, C.A.; Cottom, J.W. Scaling up Resource Recovery of Plastics in the Emergent Circular Economy to Prevent Plastic Pollution: Assessment of Risks to Health and Safety in the Global South. *Waste Manag. Res.* **2022**, *40*, 1680–1707. [CrossRef]
30. Rosenboom, J.-G.; Langer, R.; Traverso, G. Bioplastics for a Circular Economy. *Nat. Rev. Mater.* **2022**, *7*, 117–137. [CrossRef]
31. Bertoli, M.; Pastorino, P.; Lesa, D.; Renzi, M.; Anselmi, S.; Prearo, M.; Pizzul, E. Microplastics Accumulation in Functional Feeding Guilds and Functional Habit Groups of Freshwater Macrobenthic Invertebrates: Novel Insights in a Riverine Ecosystem. *Sci. Total Environ.* **2022**, *804*, 150207. [CrossRef]
32. Mehinto, A.C.; Coffin, S.; Koelmans, A.A.; Brander, S.M.; Wagner, M.; Thornton Hampton, L.M.; Burton, A.G.; Miller, E.; Gouin, T.; Weisberg, S.B.; et al. Risk-Based Management Framework for Microplastics in Aquatic Ecosystems. *Microplastics Nanoplastics* **2022**, *2*, 17. [CrossRef]
33. Yuan, Z.; Nag, R.; Cummins, E. Ranking of Potential Hazards from Microplastics Polymers in the Marine Environment. *J. Hazard. Mater.* **2022**, *429*, 128399. [CrossRef]
34. Hossain, R.; Islam, M.T.; Ghose, A.; Sahajwalla, V. Full Circle: Challenges and Prospects for Plastic Waste Management in Australia to Achieve Circular Economy. *J. Clean. Prod.* **2022**, *368*, 133127. [CrossRef]
35. Campanale, C.; Galafassi, S.; Savino, I.; Massarelli, C.; Ancona, V.; Volta, P.; Uricchio, V.F. Microplastics Pollution in the Terrestrial Environments: Poorly Known Diffuse Sources and Implications for Plants. *Sci. Total Environ.* **2022**, *805*, 150431. [CrossRef]
36. Vuori, L.; Ollikainen, M. How to Remove Microplastics in Wastewater? A Cost-Effectiveness Analysis. *Ecol. Econ.* **2022**, *192*, 107246. [CrossRef]
37. Ponti, M.G.; Allen, D.; White, C.J.; Bertram, D.; Switzer, C. A Framework to Assess the Impact of Flooding on the Release of Microplastics from Waste Management Facilities. *J. Hazard. Mater. Adv.* **2022**, *7*, 100105. [CrossRef]
38. Thornton Hampton, L.M.; Brander, S.M.; Coffin, S.; Cole, M.; Hermabessiere, L.; Koelmans, A.A.; Rochman, C.M. Characterizing Microplastic Hazards: Which Concentration Metrics and Particle Characteristics Are Most Informative for Understanding Toxicity in Aquatic Organisms? *Microplastics Nanoplastics* **2022**, *2*, 20. [CrossRef]
39. Chakraborty, I.; Banik, S.; Biswas, R.; Yamamoto, T.; Noothalapati, H.; Mazumder, N. Raman Spectroscopy for Microplastic Detection in Water Sources: A Systematic Review. *Int. J. Environ. Sci. Technol.* **2022**. [CrossRef]
40. Angelakis, A.N.; Dercas, N.; Tzanakakis, V.A. Water Quality Focusing on the Hellenic World: From Ancient to Modern Times and the Future. *Water* **2022**, *14*, 1887. [CrossRef]
41. Sbrana, A.; Valente, T.; Bianchi, J.; Franceschini, S.; Piermarini, R.; Saccomandi, F.; de Lucia, A.G.; Camedda, A.; Matiddi, M.; Silvestri, C. From Inshore to Offshore: Distribution of Microplastics in Three Italian Seawaters. *Environ. Sci. Pollut. Res.* **2022**, *30*, 21277–21287. [CrossRef] [PubMed]
42. Sá, B.; Pais, J.; Antunes, J.; Pequeno, J.; Pires, A.; Sobral, P. Seasonal Abundance and Distribution Patterns of Microplastics in the Lis River, Portugal. *Sustainability* **2022**, *14*, 2255. [CrossRef]
43. Kittner, M.; Kerndorff, A.; Ricking, M.; Bednarz, M.; Obermaier, N.; Lukas, M.; Asenova, M.; Bordós, G.; Eisentraut, P.; Hohenblum, P.; et al. Microplastics in the Danube River Basin: A First Comprehensive Screening with a Harmonized Analytical Approach. *ACS ES&T Water* **2022**, *2*, 1174–1181. [CrossRef]
44. Sadia, M.; Mahmood, A.; Ibrahim, M.; Irshad, M.K.; Quddusi, A.H.A.; Bokhari, A.; Mubashir, M.; Chuah, L.F.; Show, P.L. Microplastics Pollution from Wastewater Treatment Plants: A Critical Review on Challenges, Detection, Sustainable Removal Techniques and Circular Economy. *Environ. Technol. Innov.* **2022**, *28*, 102946. [CrossRef]
45. Melchor-Martínez, E.M.; Macías-Garbett, R.; Alvarado-Ramírez, L.; Araújo, R.G.; Sosa-Hernández, J.E.; Ramírez-Gamboa, D.; Parra-Arroyo, L.; Alvarez, A.G.; Monteverde, R.P.; Cazares, K.A.; et al. Towards a Circular Economy of Plastics: An Evaluation of the Systematic Transition to a New Generation of Bioplastics. *Polymers* **2022**, *14*, 1203. [CrossRef] [PubMed]
46. Nikiema, J.; Asiedu, Z. A Review of the Cost and Effectiveness of Solutions to Address Plastic Pollution. *Environ. Sci. Pollut. Res.* **2022**, *29*, 24547–24573. [CrossRef] [PubMed]
47. Rius-Ayra, O.; Biserova-Tahchieva, A.; Llorca-Isern, N. Removal of Dyes, Oils, Alcohols, Heavy Metals and Microplastics from Water with Superhydrophobic Materials. *Chemosphere* **2023**, *311*, 137148. [CrossRef] [PubMed]
48. OECD. Stat Plastic Leakage from Mismanaged and Littered Waste. Available online: https://stats.oecd.org/viewhtml.aspx?datasetcode=PLASTIC_LEAKAGE_4&lang=en (accessed on 3 January 2023).
49. OECD. Stat Plastic Waste Collected for Recycling. Available online: https://stats.oecd.org/viewhtml.aspx?datasetcode=PLASTIC_WASTE_6&lang=en (accessed on 3 January 2023).
50. OECD. Stat Plastic Leakage to Aquatic Environments. Available online: https://stats.oecd.org/viewhtml.aspx?datasetcode=PLASTIC_LEAKAGE_5&lang=en (accessed on 3 January 2023).
51. OECD. Stat Plastics Use by Region. Available online: https://stats.oecd.org/viewhtml.aspx?datasetcode=PLASTIC_USE_9&lang=en (accessed on 3 January 2023).
52. OECD. Stat Plastic Waste by Region and End-of-Life Fat. Available online: https://stats.oecd.org/viewhtml.aspx?datasetcode=PLASTIC_WASTE_5&lang=en (accessed on 3 January 2023).
53. Blanco, H.; Leaver, J.; Dodds, P.E.; Dickinson, R.; García-Gusano, D.; Iribarren, D.; Lind, A.; Wang, C.; Danebergs, J.; Baumann, M. A Taxonomy of Models for Investigating Hydrogen Energy Systems. *Renew. Sustain. Energy Rev.* **2022**, *167*, 112698. [CrossRef]

54. Our World in Data Share of Global Mismanaged Plastic Waste. Available online: https://ourworldindata.org/grapher/share-of-global-mismanaged-plastic-waste?country=Asia~Africa~Europe~South+America~North+America~Oceania (accessed on 3 January 2023).
55. OECD. Stat Plastics Use by Polymer. Available online: https://stats.oecd.org/viewhtml.aspx?datasetcode=PLASTIC_USE_8&lang=en (accessed on 3 January 2023).

Disclaimer/Publisher's Note: The statements, opinions and data contained in all publications are solely those of the individual author(s) and contributor(s) and not of MDPI and/or the editor(s). MDPI and/or the editor(s) disclaim responsibility for any injury to people or property resulting from any ideas, methods, instructions or products referred to in the content.

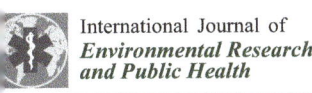

Article

Analysis of the Return to Work Program for Disabled Workers during the Pandemic COVID-19 Using the Quality of Life and Work Ability Index: Cross-Sectional Study

Arie Arizandi Kurnianto [1], Gergely Fehér [2,3,*], Kevin Efrain Tololiu [4], Edza Aria Wikurendra [5,6], Zsolt Nemeskéri [7] and István Ágoston [1]

1. Doctoral School of Health Sciences, University of Pécs, 7621 Pécs, Hungary
2. Center for Occupational Medicine, Medical School, University of Pécs, 7624 Pécs, Hungary
3. Department of Primary Health Care, Faculty of Medicine, University of Pécs, 7623 Pécs, Hungary
4. Doctoral School of Psychology, University of Pécs, 7624 Pécs, Hungary
5. Faculty of Economic Science, School of Management and Organizational Science, The Hungarian University of Agriculture and Life Science, 7400 Kaposvar, Hungary
6. Department of Public Health, Faculty of Health, Universitas Nahdlatul Ulama Surabaya, Surabaya 60237, Indonesia
7. Department of Cultural Theory and Applied Communication Sciences, Faculty of Cultural Studies, Teacher Training and Rural Development, University of Pécs, 7633 Pécs, Hungary
* Correspondence: feher.gergely@pte.hu

Abstract: Background: Occupational accidents are rising, but there is little evidence on the outcomes of patients who received case management during Return to work (RTW) programs. This study examined the case management-based on RTW program features that improve the work ability index (WAI) and quality of life (QoL). Methods: This cross-sectional research involved 230 disabled workers due to an occupational injury in Indonesia, 154 participated in RTW, and 75 did not participate in RTW (non-RTW) during the COVID-19 pandemic. Sociodemographic and occupational factors were used to examine the RTW results. We used the Finnish Institute of Occupational Health's WAI questionnaires to measure the work ability index and World Health Organization Quality of Life Brief Version (WHOQOL-BREF) for quality of life. Results: The study found a statistically significant difference in working duration and preferred treatment for RTW between the groups (*p*-value = 0.039). Furthermore, the quality of life in the domain of environmental health and work ability index score also demonstrated a significant difference between the groups (*p*-value = 0.023 and 0.000, respectively). Conclusions: During the COVID-19 pandemic, this study found that the RTW program improved the quality of life and work abilities of disabled workers.

Keywords: case management; return to work; disabled workers; work ability index; quality of life

1. Introduction

The outbreak of COVID-19 has affected every region of the world since November 2019. To combat the impact of this pandemic, governments have implemented measures such as adjustments to existing occupational accident insurance programs within their social security frameworks. These changes aimed to address the specific challenges posed by COVID-19 [1]. Local government institutions play a crucial role in balancing the need for social distancing to prevent the spread of COVID-19 and the need for economic recovery, as seen in the study of 28 provincial governments in China during the early outbreak of 2020 [2]. Moreover, the World Health Organization issued a series of physical distance-related regulations to ensure that the COVID-19 pandemic would be contained [3]. As a result of the outbreak of COVID-19, plenty of unfavorable things have occurred concerning work all over the globe. More than a hundred individuals have died in Indonesia due to the COVID-19 pandemic, and the bankruptcy of several companies has had a knock-on effect on the country's economy [4] and the quality of life of its workers. It shows that despite their abilities, the pandemic has made it difficult to access a range of activities. As one of the most vulnerable groups affected by the COVID-19 pandemic, people with physical disabilities are at high risk of COVID-19 exposure and have difficulty carrying out daily activities including following COVID-19 prevention protocols [5,6]. During the COVID-19 pandemic, stakeholders focused on ensuring the baseline health of RTW participants and the health and safety considerations for disabled employees, particularly if they had underlying health disorders that increase the risk of COVID-19. Workers with physical disabilities need special equipment or environmental adjustments to carry out the rehabilitation activities as part of the RTW program. Due to constraints on in-person connections and limited resources, implementing these adjustments during a pandemic may be challenging. During the pandemic, some health care providers adopted telemedicine, which may be challenging for disabled workers who need in-person treatment [7]. In addition, the pandemic has made the condition more challenging to return to work after being injured in a workplace accident. This concern has been highlighted because it is imperative for a person whose impairment was caused by a workplace accident to make significant alterations to cope with the new phase of their life.

Indonesia has a unique social security system based on employment, which allows the government to provide a benefit from occupational accident insurance in the form of a specific disability management program called Return To Work (RTW). This program is distinct compared to those offered by other developing nations [8]. The RTW program serves as a complement to in-kind benefit services by providing a comprehensive rehabilitation program. This program included medical, vocational, and psychological rehabilitation with the assistance of case managers [9]. Moreover, in the context of social security and occupational injury insurance, an in-kind benefit is a type of non-cash benefit that is provided to an individual as part of their insurance coverage. These benefits can include things like medical treatment, rehabilitation services, and other forms of assistance that are designed to help an individual recover from an occupational injury or disease. In-kind benefits may be provided directly by the insurance provider, or they may be arranged through third-party providers. For example, an insurance company may cover the cost of medical treatment from a specific hospital or clinic, or they may provide a payment to an individual to cover the cost of rehabilitation services [10].

In this case, BPJS Ketenagakerjaan, the Indonesian social security organization, provides a combination of cash and in-kind benefits to a person who has experienced an occupational injury or occupational disease. A worker could receive a cash payout to compensate lost income due to an occupational accident as well as in-kind benefits to cover the cost of medical care, and rehabilitation services in the form of a case management system and the RTW program [11]. In-kind benefits play an important part in social security and occupational injury insurance systems, supporting those who have been injured or suffered a disease because of their job, and enables individuals to regain their dignity by enhancing their productivity during the course of the RTW program.

The RTW program in Indonesia is designed to support workers who have suffered a disability due to an occupational accident or disease and have been registered as customers of BPJS Ketenagakerjaan. The program provides employees with a range of support services including medical rehabilitation, vocational rehabilitation, and psychosocial rehabilitation to help them regain their physical and mental abilities and to make the transition back to work as smooth as possible. Eligibility for the RTW program is typically determined by BPJS Ketenagakerjaan based on medical indications such as the type of impairment and the employee's ability to perform essential job tasks.

Disability is a complex phenomenon that includes biological functions, activity limits, impediments to participation, and environmental influences, among others [12]. Nonetheless, the social stigma associated with a disability is still widely held in today's culture, which is one of the environmental aspects to consider. Some individuals still have the view that people with disabilities are entirely reliant on the kindness and assistance of others.

Due to this viewpoint, many people with disabilities face discrimination, which prevents them from leading independent lives.

Regulations about equal job opportunities initially sought to enhance the personal well-being of people with disabilities. Unfortunately, the participation of disabled people in the labor market is minimal, and their earnings are meagre. Measuring the quality of life as a kind of individual welfare for employees with disabilities is one way to evaluate the effectiveness of employment restrictions for people with impairments [13]. Disability discrimination in the workplace is a significant issue, and it is important to think about ways to reduce the stigma that disabled people experience at work. Promoting equality and inclusiveness in the workforce requires addressing the stigma faced by disabled individuals [14]. The RTW program for disabled workers can reduce disability discrimination by providing support and accommodation for reintegration into the workforce.

By examining their employment capability, businesses may better accommodate persons with disabilities and provide them with equal chances in the workforce. The work ability index, which accounts for factors such as mental and physical well-being and the capacity to manage obstacles in the physical realm [15,16], may be used for this measurement. On the other hand, quite a few researchers have studied the connection between RTW results and job-related factors such as the quality of life and work ability index among impaired workers. Therefore, this study aims to examine the dynamic relationship between the quality of life and work capability index among disabled workers by analyzing a case management system of disability management through a RTW program experienced by disabled workers during the COVID-19 pandemic.

2. Methods

2.1. Study Setting

This descriptive cross-sectional study measured the QoL and WAI of workers with disabilities after participating in the RTW program. This study was conducted between January and June 2021, identifying the claims for RTW during the outbreak of COVID-19 in Indonesia. Workers who had been registered as customers with the Indonesian National Social Security Agency for Employment (BPJS Ketenagakerjaan) were recruited for participation in this study.

The participants in the study were separated into two groups, RTW and non-RTW, based on their participation in the return to work (RTW) program after receiving workers' compensation benefits from BPJS Ketenagakerjaan. The RTW group consisted of individuals who took part in the program, while the non-RTW group consisted of those who did not. This division aimed to examine the effect of participating in the RTW program on the individuals and compare it to those who did not participate. To be eligible for this study, individuals had to be between 18 and 65 years old, employed during the COVID-19 outbreak, and engaged in the RTW program.

2.2. Data Collection

All data regarding participants in the RTW program were obtained from BPJS Ketenagakerjaan. The authors sent the invitation to potential applicants through a widespread email. A total of 165 individuals in the RTW program who had been asked to participate in the study and met all prerequisites were enrolled at the outset. During the starting procedure, only 154 people agreed to be interviewed and completed our questionnaires. Moreover, we extended invitations to an additional 165 disabled patients who had had an occupational injury but were hesitant to take part in the RTW program. However, only 75 people agreed to participate in this study.

The data were collected by the first and third authors. The lead author conducted a three-hour training session on RTW, WAI, QoL, and instructions for data collection and ethical issues to 11 case managers of BPJS Ketenagakerjaan in 34 provinces throughout Indonesia before commencing the data collection. The case managers involved in this study were employees of BPJS Ketenagakerjaan and were not specifically added for the current study. The case managers acted as enumerators and collected data from patients participating in RTW programs at trauma centers and rehabilitation hospitals, and received training from the lead author on RTW, WAI, QoL, and data collection, and ethical issues. The data collection was carried out by 11 case managers in 34 provinces throughout Indonesia, who were assigned to hospitals based on their location. The data were collected through printed surveys to reduce nonresponse bias. The data collectors analyzed the recovered questionnaires to minimize missing responses and asked for responses in cases of missing items.

The questionnaire included topics on sociodemographic variables as well as disability-related aspects. In addition, a questionnaire assessing the quality of life and work ability index was also included in the research. For the purpose of determining the quality of life (QOL) and the work ability index (WAI), respectively, the WHOQoL-BREF developed by the World Health Organization (WHO) and validated WAI questionnaires developed by the Finnish Institute of Occupational Health were used.

2.3. Data Analysis

The Shapiro–Wilk test was used to check for normality in the data, which was performed by the first author. The purpose of checking for normality in the data is to ensure that the data are normally distributed. A normally distributed dataset is essential for the validity of statistical tests. The categorical patient sociodemographic data were analyzed using frequency statistics. The Mann–Whitney U test was used to compare the RTW and non-RTW groups, while Pearson's correlation was used to analyze the relationship between the free variables and both the dependent and independent variables (r). Free variables are variables that are not controlled by the researcher but can affect the outcome of the study. The Pearson's correlation (r) was used to assess the strength of the relationship between the independent and dependent variables. r ranged from -1 to 1, with negative correlation indicating that one variable decreases as the other increases, and positive correlation indicating both variables increasing or decreasing together. The strength of the relationship was categorized as negligible ($r < 0.2$), low ($r = 0.2$–0.49), moderate ($r = 0.5$–0.69), high ($r = 0.7$–0.85), or very high ($r = 0.86$–1.00), with higher values indicating stronger linear relationships.

For the continuous data, we used independent sample t-tests (t), and for the ordinal data, we utilized Mann–Whitney tests. The Chi-square tests were used in order to investigate the differences in the categorical data. Multivariate logistic regression was used to investigate the association between several predictor factors and the outcome variable. To address the research question of this study in analyzing the relationship between the work ability index and quality of life between the RTW and non-RTW participants, multivariate logistic regression is the most suitable approach since it controls for the effects of other variables.

The study used logistic regression to assess the association between independent and dependent variables while controlling for other factors. The aim of the analysis was to examine the relationships between various factors and the outcome of interest, taking into account the influence of other variables. The independent and dependent variables were determined using a questionnaire that included sociodemographic and disability-related questions as well as assessments of QOL and WAI using validated questionnaires. The logistic regression was performed using SPSS version 26.0, with a p-value of less than 0.05 and a 95% confidence interval.

3. Results

3.1. Return to Work Program as Case Management for Disabled Workers

In accordance with the foregoing concept, this study investigated the aspect of RTW implementation in Indonesia. The research was carried out during the COVID-19 pandemic and we compared the outcomes of the RTW program for employees with impairments and non-RTW participants. The study compared two groups of people: those who participated in the RTW program during COVID-19 and those who did not participate. The research was designed to shed light on the implementation of the RTW program and its outcomes for employees who were impaired due to occupational injuries or occupational diseases during the COVID-19 pandemic. The research began with an assessment of the sociodemographic characteristics of the subjects. The following factors were considered as variables: age, gender, marital status, occupation, level of education, work period, and place of living. In Table 1, we see how the quality of life and work ability index scores of disabled workers are distributed on a general level.

Table 1. Statistic result comparison of RTW and non-RTW participants.

Variables		RTW	Non-RTW	Mann–Whitney, t, and χ^2	Multivariate Logistic Regression	
		N (%) or Mean ± SD	N (%) or Mean ± SD	p-Value	OR (95% CI)	p-Value
Age	69(30.43%) 77(33.48%) 8(3.48%)	39(16.96%) 35(15.22%) 1(0.43%)	39 ± 16.96% 35 ± 15.22% 1 ± 0.43%	0.430	3.726	0.847
Gender	33(14.40%) 121(52.80%)	24(10.50%) 51(22.30%))	24 ± 10.50% 51 ± 22.30%	0.083	0.184	0.125
Marital status	24(10.50%) 130(56.80%)	13(5.70%) 62(27.10%)	13 ± 5.70% 62 ± 27.10%	0.736	4.876	0.585
Job description	146(63.80%) 8(3.50%)	72(31.40%) 3(1.30%)	72 ± 31.40% 3 ± 1.30%	0.692	2.792	0.769
Level of education	132(57.60%) 22(9.60%)	64(27.90%) 11(4.80%)	64 ± 27.90% 11 ± 4.80%	0.939	0.283	0.367
Work Period	8(3.50%) 48(21.00%) 69(30.10%) 29(12.70%)	12(5.20%) 33(14.40%) 22(9.60%) 8(3.50%)	12 ± 5.20% 33 ± 14.40% 22 ± 9.60% 8 ± 3.50%	0.000 *	0.430	0.039 *
Location of residence	83(36.52%) 10(4.35%) 61(26.52%)	36(15.65%) 7(3.04%) 32(13.91%)	36 ± 15.65% 7 ± 3.04% 32 ± 13.91%	0.493	1.143	0.264
Work Ability Index	0(0.00%) 42(18.30%) 84(36.70%) 28(12.20%)	37(16.20%) 20(8.70%) 14(6.10%) 4(1.70%)	37 ± 16.20% 20 ± 8.70% 14 ± 6.10% 4 ± 1.70%	0.000 *	0.692	0.000 *
Quality of Life	72.94 ± 11.94 74.35 ± 10.13 76.14 ± 14.45 69.89 ± 8.78	65.91 ± 10.72 70.84 ± 9.82 74.13 ± 14.17 63.64 ± 8.52	65.91 ± 10.72 70.84 ± 9.82 74.13 ± 14.17 63.64 ± 8.52	0.000 * 0.016 * 0.388 0.000 *	0.988 0.956 1.029 1.062	0.374 0.367 0.055 0.023 *

* $p < 0.05$ indicates a significant difference between the two groups (RTW and Non-RTW) at a level of 95% confidence. * $p < 0.01$ indicates a highly significant difference between the two groups at a level of 99% confidence.

The data in Table 1 are presented in a numerical format (N%) for the nominal and ordinal data and as the mean and standard deviation for the continuous data.

Table 1 shows the results of a study comparing various demographic and health-related variables between two groups: RTW (Return to Work) and Non-RTW (non-Return to Work). The Mann–Whitney test, t-test, and Chi-squared test were used to assess the significance of differences between the two groups for each variable, and multivariate logistic regression was used to determine the odds ratio (OR) and 95% confidence interval (CI) for each variable. The OR (odds ratio) estimate in the multivariate logistic regression captures the relationship between the independent variables and the dependent variables. It measures the odds of an event occurring (i.e., having a certain quality of life or work ability index) given a set of independent variables (i.e., age, gender, marital status, job description, level of education, work period, location of residence). The CI for OR estimates the 95% confidence interval (CI) for the OR estimate represents the range in which the true value of the OR is likely to fall with 95% certainty. It provides information on the precision of the OR estimate.

The results of the Mann–Whitney test, t-test, and Chi-squared test indicated that there were statistically significant differences between the RTW and Non-RTW groups in terms of age (p-value = 0.430), work period (p-value = 0.000 *), quality of life (p-value = 0.000 *) and work ability index (p-value = 0.000 *). The multivariate logistic regression analysis revealed that the odds of RTW were 3.726 times higher in the older age group (95% CI 0.847–15.726) and the odds of RTW were 0.430 times higher for those with a longer work period (95% CI: 0.039–0.737).

The results of the study suggest that age and work period may be important predictors of RTW in injured workers. Additionally, the significant difference in the quality of life between the RTW and non-RTW groups highlights the importance of addressing mental and physical well-being in rehabilitation programs for injured workers.

3.2. A Glimpse of the Quality of Life among Workers with Disabilities

In this study, the quality of life of employees with impairments was evaluated using the WHOQoL-BREF as the standard of measurement. An evaluation of the quality of life involved the domain of physical health, psychological, social bound, and environment respectively, in this research. This research found that when compared to other dimensions of quality of life, the social bound domain had the greatest mean value. However, as shown in Table 1 and Figure 1, the average value of all categories of quality of life for RTW participants was greater than for those who did not engage in the RTW program.

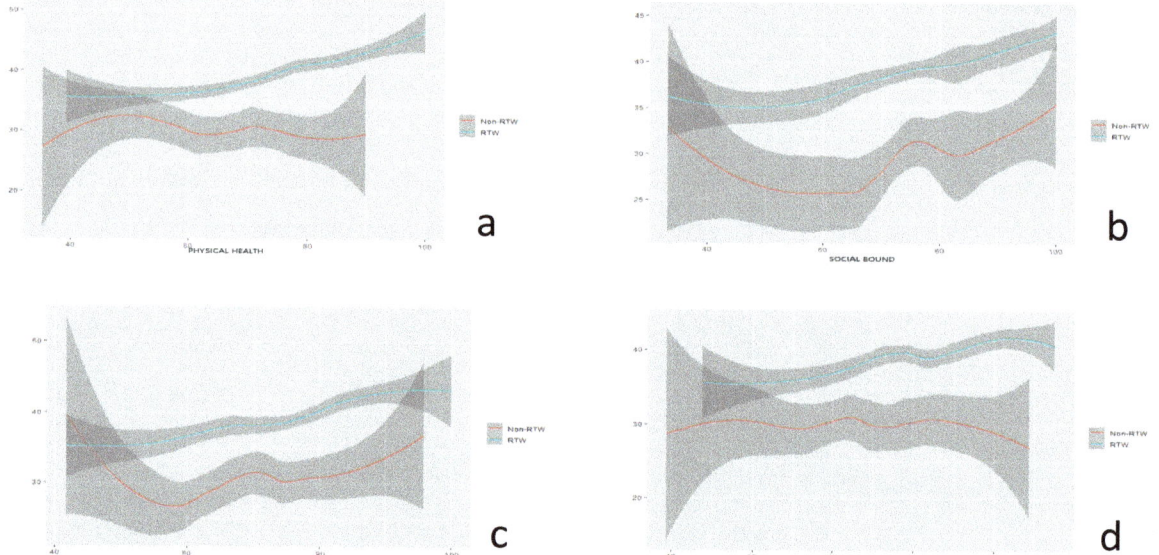

Figure 1. The comparative value of the domains of the disabled employees' QoL in relation to WAI among the RTW and those who did not participate in the RTW. (**a**) Physical health, (**b**) social bound, (**c**) psychological, and (**d**) environmental health.

The data suggest that there may be a noticeable difference in the quality of life for disabled workers, as evidenced by the measurements of QOL and WAI. Moreover, according to Figure 1, which provides a look into the quality of life among workers with disabilities in Indonesia during the COVID-19 outbreak, individuals who participated in RTW program showed a higher level of quality of life in all domains than workers who did not participate in the RTW program. As shown in Figure 1, the horizontal axis represents the domain of QOL of the participants in the study. The vertical axis represents the work ability index (WAI) of the participants in the study. Figure 1a shows that the workers who participated in RTW programs tended to have better physical health) outcomes (OR (0.988), mean S.D. (72.94 ± 11.94)) and WAI score compared to those who did not participate. Additionally, the same pattern of outcomes was seen in other domains including social bound (Figure 1b, OR (1.029), mean S.D. (76.14 + 14.45)), psychological health (Figure 1c, OR (0.956), mean S.D. (74.35 ± 10.13)), and environmental health (Figure 1d, OR (1.062), mean S.D. (69.89 ± 8.78)).

The results of a multivariate logistic regression analysis are shown in Table 1, indicating that the working period, workability index, and the domain of environmental health in the quality of life had a *p*-value of less than 0.05, showing a statistically significant relationship between participation in the RTW program and the variables. In this case, the *p*-value of 0.023 suggests that there is a statistically significant relationship between participation in the RTW program and the environmental health domain of quality of life.

3.3. Work Ability Index of Workers with Disabilities

Both the RTW and non-RTW groups included individuals with a diverse age range from around 26 to 55 years old, as shown in Table 1. Based on the line graph, it was determined that the average work ability index for disabled workers was 39.29. (SD 4.39). Figure 2 provides a detailed illustration of the work ability index based on the age and work period, and the work ability index after research [16] revealed that there was also a correlation between age and the index.

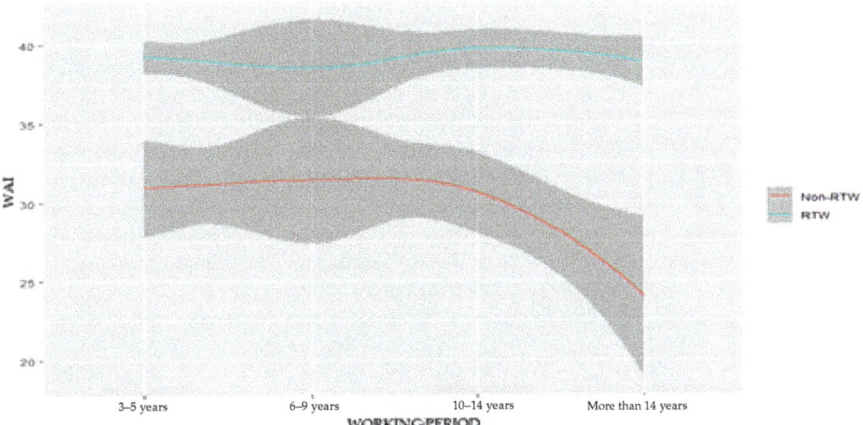

Figure 2. Distribution score of the work ability index based on the age and working period.

According to the description in Figure 2, the distribution score of the work ability index sets the majority of the data in the "good" category for a group of workers participating in the RTW program, which was between 37 and 44 [17]. Conversely, those who were disabled but did not participate in the RTW program showed a lower score of WAI. The use of WAI analysis among employees with disabilities in this research, which were practically in the same context as the study [17,18] of the work ability index in the population of people receiving state insurance, was accomplished.

The results in Figure 3 indicate that the work ability index (WAI) of disabled workers who participated in the return to work (RTW) program appeared to be higher compared to those who did not participate in the RTW program. Specifically, the average WAI score of disabled workers in the non-RTW group was 37%, which is considered poor, while the RTW group had a higher proportion of disabled workers with an excellent WAI score of 28 (12.20%). Furthermore, there were no disabled workers in the poor category after participating in the RTW program, implying that the RTW program is associated with an increased work ability index score of disabled workers, however, it is important to recognize the implication of this research for further study to investigate the causality that the RTW program is effective in enhancing the work ability index of disabled workers.

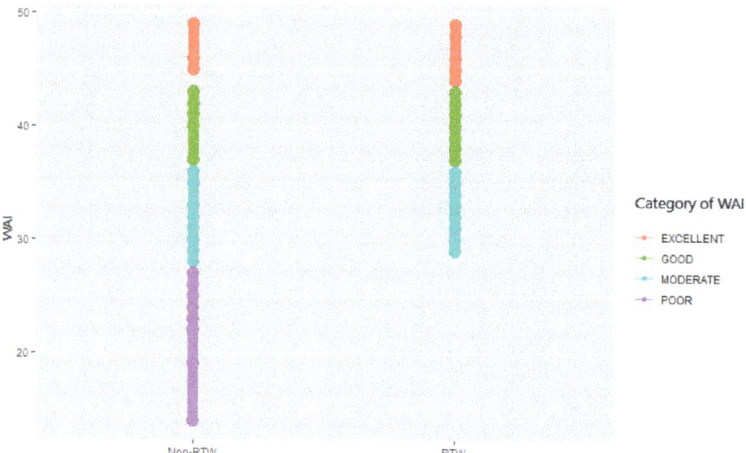

Figure 3. Work ability index dynamic value based on the category.

4. Discussion

4.1. Interpretation of Results in Relation to the Effectiveness of the Return to Work Program

The findings of our study highlight the potential benefits of the return to work program for disabled workers during the pandemic. Our analysis found that workers who participated in the program had significantly higher scores in the measures of quality of life and work ability compared to those who did not participate. There may have been a difference between the participants and non-participants in the RTW program in terms of the severity of their impairments and their motivation to work. It is possible that the participants in the RTW program had less severe injuries or were more motivated to return to work than those who did not participate. This could potentially influence the outcomes of the program and must be taken into account when evaluating the results. This suggests that the RTW program was effective in supporting disabled workers to return to work and maintain their ability to work during the pandemic.

We also observed that the participants who had been out of work for a longer period of time were more likely to prefer the RTW program compared to those who had only been out of work for a shorter period. This may indicate that the longer an individual is out of work, the more likely they are to seek support and resources through the RTW program to return to work. However, it is important to note that there were also a significant number of participants who preferred not to engage in the RTW program, regardless of their working period.

In terms of quality of life, our study found that physical health, psychological health, and environmental health were significantly better among workers who preferred to participate in the RTW program compared to those who preferred not to. This suggests that the RTW program was successful in improving the physical and psychological health outcomes for participants. However, we did not find a significant difference in the domain of social bonds between those who preferred to participate in the RTW program and those who preferred not to participate. This could be due to the fact that the RTW program was focused on supporting individuals to return to work and did not specifically address social connections.

Finally, it is widely believed that participating in return to work programs can have an association with physical health, which is a key component of work ability. RTW programs can support workers in their recovery from injuries or illnesses and promote physical activity and well-being. This study supports these beliefs, as workers who participated in the RTW program tended to have better physical health outcomes compared to those who did not participate.

4.2. The Current State of Information from Findings

This study examined the effectiveness of a return to work (RTW) program for individuals with occupational injuries during the pandemic in Indonesia and provides insights into the support and resources available to disabled workers during this challenging time. To the best of our knowledge, this is the first study of its kind to assess the quality of life (QOL) and work ability index (WAI) among disabled workers who participated in a RTW program during this time.

Our findings suggest that the RTW program was effective in improving the QOL and WAI scores for participants, indicating that it was successful in supporting disabled workers to return to work and maintaining their ability to work during the pandemic. These results have important implications for policy and practice in supporting disabled workers during challenging times such as the COVID-19 pandemic.

4.3. Implications for Supporting Disabled Workers during the Pandemic

Workers who are disabled because of an accident or disease at work are most concerned about their quality of life and their ability to work again after the injury. In order to protect workers from this risk, some countries include occupational injury insurance in their social security programs. Moreover, a study on rural–urban migrants in China highlights the challenges they faced during the COVID-19 pandemic including housing evictions and difficulties with travel [19]. This sheds light on how disabled people, as another disadvantaged population group, may also be impacted by similar issues, and highlights the need for policies to address the needs of various disadvantaged groups. Policy instruments such as occupational health and safety initiatives are necessary to facilitate the work resumption of disadvantaged workers during COVID-19, however, more comprehensive evaluations and implementation details are needed to determine their effectiveness [20]. The implementation of coverage under occupational injury insurance has taken the shape of a case management system which is the Return to Work program [21–25]. Despite the fact that during the pandemic, the state of employment in temporary contracts was related to enhanced well-being and increased performance, the research found that they were also associated with decreased job security [13].

Workers who have been disabled due to an accident or disease might have their dignity restored and their chances of returning to work improved by RTW programs [26]. This is in line with the journey of businesses taking part in the RTW assistance program offered by BPJS Ketenagakerjaan, Indonesia. In addition, there has been an increase in the promotion of career options for those who are either disabled or have a permanent complete handicap. Workers regain their productivity when employers invest in their education and re-entry into the workforce, putting them in a position to compete for better job prospects and, on a larger scale, become one of the elements contributing to good economic development [27]. The success of the RTW program will increase the number of workers engaging in the labor market. The effective management of a disabled workforce can play a critical role in promoting the participation of disabled workers who have suffered from occupational injuries in the labor market. The RTW program supports disabled workers returning to the workforce, promoting their participation in the labor market and effectively managing disabilities. By providing support and accommodation, RTW programs help address the challenges faced by disabled workers. RTW programs are essential for effectively managing disabilities and supporting the workforce [28,29]. This, in turn, will increase the output level, affecting the economy's status in Indonesia.

Our study found that the variable of working period was significantly related to the preference for participating in the return to work (RTW) program, with a *p*-value of

0.000 for the Chi-square test and a p-value of 0.000 in the multivariate logistic regression. This suggests that the length of time an individual has been out of work plays a significant role in their preference for participating in a RTW program. Additionally, we found that the category of working period among workers in the RTW group was dominantly 10–14 years (69 ± 30.10%). In the non RTW group, the dominant category was 5–9 years (69 ± 30.10%). These findings suggest that those who have been out of work for a longer period of time are more likely to prefer the support and resources provided by the RTW program in order to return to work.

It is important to consider the potential implications of these findings for policy and practice. Employers and policy-makers may wish to consider implementing RTW programs that are targeted toward those who have been out of work for longer periods of time, as they may be more likely to benefit from the support and resources provided. Additionally, further research is needed to understand the specific factors that influence an individual's preference for participating in a RTW program such as personal and professional goals, job availability, and health and wellness.

This study shows an identical outcome to a study carried out in Malaysia [22,30] that demonstrated that the outcomes of RTW had a significant correlation with the physical health domain of workers who participated in RTW programs. Under certain situations to turn for equating with a study that followed that sequence, this study shows the results. Research with the same questionnaire was also undertaken for people with disabilities [31], and the results indicated that all means of QOL domains were accordingly lower than this report revealed. Furthermore, this study's setting differed significantly from other studies. Moreover, this research analyzed how the RTW program's comprehensive rehabilitation affects the quality of life for persons with disabilities. It would seem that the RTW program beneficially impacts the practical approach during the COVID-19 pandemic to improve the quality of life among disabled workers.

In addition, regarding the work ability index, this investigation used the work ability index questionnaire developed by the Finnish Institute of Occupational Health [32]. This tool describes the respondents' current work capabilities while also allowing for projections of the health concerns they experience. The results may mean that the category is poor if the score is between 7 and 27 points, and the category is moderate if the result is between 28 and 36 points. In this case, the category is considered good if the score is between 37 and 43 points and excellent if it is between 44 and 49 points. The questionnaire is an instrument for self-evaluation, and its purpose is to determine an individual's job competence by analyzing how that person interacts with the environment in which they are employed. It is flexible enough to be utilized by individual workers and teams [32,33].

The work ability index results classified all participants in a range from moderate to excellent. The broad range of WAI scores in this study ranged from 29 to 49. The results of this study should therefore be seen as a response to specific previous findings [16]. There is some evidence to suggest that there may be a correlation between the WAI and age and working period. Some studies have found that older workers and those with longer working periods tend to have lower WAI scores, while younger workers and those with shorter working periods tend to have higher WAI scores [34]. This may be due to the increased physical and mental demands of work as well as the accumulation of health problems over time.

The purpose of occupational health management that may be achieved by implementing WAI is to consider maintaining and making efforts to improve the quality of work for an inclusive society that includes people with disabilities in accordance with the UN's Sustainable Development Goals (SDGs). It has been revealed that 54.2% (n = 84) of the total number of disabled workers who participated in the RTW program significantly improved their working abilities due to their participation. During the COVID-19 outbreak in Indonesia, it was observed that 27.3% (n = 42) of employees fell into the moderate group, while 18.2% (n = 28) had an exceptionally excellent work ability index.

5. Conclusions

In conclusion, our study found that the return to work program was effective in improving the quality of life and work ability of disabled workers during the COVID-19 pandemic, as seen by the significant difference in scores between the RTW and non-RTW participants. Policy-makers and employers should consider using assessment tools and gathering feedback to regularly assess the program and make necessary improvements.

Limitations and Strengths

There were some flaws in how the study was conducted that need to be pointed out. It is important to consider the limitations of our study including the sample size and specific geographic location. Further research with a larger sample size and diverse location is needed to further understand the effectiveness of RTW programs for disabled workers during the COVID-19 pandemic. The data collection was conducted using a purposive sample, which refers to situations during the pandemic that allowed researchers to approach the subjects through indirect encounters or online, which profoundly affected the willingness of participants to continue with the study, resulting in possible biases. There are, nevertheless, certain advantages to consider. We demonstrated the importance of contextual factors in implementing RTW, especially when examining the program's outcomes in measuring the functional ability and quality of life of workers with disabilities. This was carried out by using various data from very different social and cultural backgrounds and a wide variety of social assistance background frameworks.

Author Contributions: Conceptualization, A.A.K. and G.F.; Methodology, A.A.K., G.F. and K.E.T.; Software, K.E.T.; Formal analysis, A.A.K. and Z.N.; Investigation, A.A.K.; Resources, Z.N.; Data curation, A.A.K. and K.E.T.; Writing—original draft, A.A.K. and E.A.W.; Writing—review & editing, A.A.K.; Visualization, E.A.W.; Supervision, Z.N. and I.Á.; Project administration, G.F. and Z.N.; Funding acquisition, G.F., Z.N. and I.Á. All authors have read and agreed to the published version of the manuscript.

Funding: This research received no external funding.

Institutional Review Board Statement: This research was ethically approved by the Health Research Ethics Committee, Faculty of Public Health Universitas Airlangga, with the number: 58/EA/KEPK/2021. Declared to be ethically appropriate in accordance to 7 (seven) WHO 2011 Standards, (1) Social Values, (2) Scientific Values, (3) Equitable Assessment and Benefits, (4) Risks, (5) Persuasion/Exploitation, (6) Confidentiality and Privacy, and (7) Informed Consent, referring to the 2016 CIOMS Guidelines. This is as indicated by the fulfillment of the indicators of each standard. Informed consent was obtained from all individuals included in the research. Every process was carried out in accordance with the policies, laws, and standards that were in force at the relevant time.

Informed Consent Statement: All individual study participants provided their informed consent.

Data Availability Statement: The authors state that all data validated in the report's findings are included in the document.

Acknowledgments: The authors would like to extend their gratitude to the staff at the YAKKUM Rehabilitation Center and the National Vocational Rehabilitation Center in Indonesia for their cooperation in retrieving data for this study.

Conflicts of Interest: The authors declare no conflict of interest.

References

1. Ståhl, C.; MacEachen, E. Universal Basic Income as a Policy Response to COVID-19 and Precarious Employment: Potential Impacts on Rehabilitation and Return-to-Work. *J. Occup. Rehabil.* **2021**, *31*, 3–6. [CrossRef]
2. Li, X.; Hui, E.; Shen, J. Institutional Development and the Government Response to COVID-19 in China. *Habitat Int.* **2022**, *127*, 102629. [CrossRef] [PubMed]
3. Zhao, T.; Cheng, C.; Liu, H.; Sun, C. Is one- or two-meters social distancing enough for COVID-19? Evidence for reassessing. *Public Health* **2020**, *185*, 87. [CrossRef] [PubMed]

4. Shaw, W.S.; Main, C.J.; Findley, P.A.; Collie, A.; Kristman, V.L.; Gross, D.P. Opening the Workplace After COVID-19: What Lessons Can be Learned from Return-to-Work Research? *J. Occup. Rehabil.* **2020**, *30*, 299–302. [CrossRef]
5. Armitage, R.; Nellums, L.B. The COVID-19 response must be disability inclusive. *Lancet Public Health* **2020**, *5*, e257. [CrossRef]
6. Brown, H.K.; Saha, S.; Chan, T.C.Y.; Cheung, A.M.; Fralick, M.; Ghassemi, M.; Herridge, M.; Kwan, J.; Rawal, S.; Rosella, S.; et al. Outcomes in patients with and without disability admitted to hospital with COVID-19: A retrospective cohort study. *CMAJ Can. Med. Assoc. J.* **2022**, *194*, E112–E121. [CrossRef] [PubMed]
7. Jacka, B.P.; Janssen, T.; Garner, B.R.; Yermash, J.; Yap, K.R.; Ball, E.L.; Hartzler, B.; Becker, S.J. Impact of COVID-19 on OUD management and moudaccess in the us. *J. Addict. Med.* **2021**, *15*, 1–4. [CrossRef]
8. Azhar, M.; Wisnaeni, F.; Solechan Suharso, P.; Setyono, J.; Badriyah, S.M. Strengthening the social security of the indonesian fishermen. *AACL Bioflux* **2020**, *13*, 3721–3726.
9. Casey, P.P.; Guy, L.; Cameron, I.D. Determining return to work in a compensation setting: A review of New South Wales workplace rehabilitation service provider referrals over 5 years. *Work* **2014**, *48*, 11–20. [CrossRef]
10. Kitao, S. A life-cycle model of unemployment and disability insurance. *J. Monet. Econ.* **2014**, *68*, 1–18. [CrossRef]
11. Cheong, E.P.H. Developing the Social Security Organisation (SOCSO) of Malaysia's RTW case management system. *Int. J. Disabil. Manag.* **2014**, *9*, e44. [CrossRef]
12. Cieza, A.; Bickenbach, J.E. Functioning, Disability and Health, International Classification of. *Int. Encycl. Soc. Behav. Sci. Second. Ed.* **2015**, 543–549. [CrossRef]
13. Katsaouni, M.; Constantinidis, T.; Tripsianis, G.; Nena, E. Comparison of job insecurity, quality of life, and work ability between age-matched temporary and permanent workers in the healthcare sector. *Saf. Health Work* **2022**, *13*, S207. [CrossRef]
14. Rapley, C.E. *Accessibility and Development: Environmental Accessibility and Its Implications for Inclusive, Sustainable and Equitable Development for All*; Department of Economic and Social Affairs, United Nations: New York, NY, USA, 2013.
15. Bethge, M.; Gutenbrunner, C.; Neuderth, S. Work ability index predicts application for disability pension after work-related medical rehabilitation for chronic back pain. *Arch. Phys. Med. Rehabil.* **2013**, *94*, 2262–2268. [CrossRef]
16. Godeau, D.; Petit, A.; Richard, I.; Roquelaure, Y.; Descatha, A. Return-to-work, disabilities and occupational health in the age of COVID-19. *Scand. J. Work Environ. Health* **2021**, *47*, 408–409. [CrossRef] [PubMed]
17. Lavasani, S.; Wahat, N.W.A. Work ability index: Validation and model comparison of the Malaysian work ability index (WAI). *Disabil. CBR Incl. Dev.* **2016**, *27*, 37–56. [CrossRef]
18. Jääskeläinen, A. Work ability index and perceived work ability as predictors of disability pension: A prospective study among Finnish municipal employees. *Work Environ. Health* **2016**, *42*, 111–223. [CrossRef]
19. Liu, Q.; Liu, Z.; Kang, T.; Zhu, L.; Zhao, P. Transport inequities through the lens of environmental racism: Rural-urban migrants under COVID-19. *Transp. Policy* **2022**, *122*, 26–38. [CrossRef]
20. Gunn, V.; Kreshpaj, B.; Matilla-Santander, N.; Vignola, E.F.; Wegman, D.H.; Hogstedt, C.; Ahonen, E.Q.; Bodin, T.; Orellana, C.; Baron, S.; et al. Initiatives Addressing Precarious Employment and Its Effects on Workers' Health and Well-Being: A Systematic Review. *Int. J. Environ. Res. Public Health* **2022**, *19*, 2232. [CrossRef]
21. Mont, D. *Social Protection Discussion Paper Series Disability Employment Policy*; The World Bank: Washington, DC, USA, 2004; Volume 413.
22. Murad, M.S.; O'Brien, L.; Farnworth, L.; Chien, C.W. Health status of people with work-related musculoskeletal disorders in return to work programs: A malaysian study. *Occup. Ther. Health Care* **2013**, *27*, 238–255. [CrossRef]
23. Halimatussadiah, A.; Agriva, M.; Nuryakin, C. Persons with Disabilities (PWD) and Labor Force in Indonesia: A Preliminary Study. *Development* **2014**, *17*, 19.
24. Awang, H.; Shahabudin, S.M.; Mansor, N. Return-to-Work Program for Injured Workers: Factors of Successful Return to Employment. *Asia Pac. J. Public Health* **2016**, *28*, 694–702. [CrossRef] [PubMed]
25. Elena, A.; Mehtap, P.; Amir, Z. Return to work following long term sickness absence: A comparative analysis of stakeholders' views and experiences in six European countries. *J. Occup. Rehabil.* **2022**. [CrossRef]
26. Finnes, A.; Hoch, J.S.; Enebrink, P.; Dahl, J.A.; Ghaderi, A.; Nager, A.; Feldman, I. Economic evaluation of return-to-work interventions for mental disorder-related sickness absence: Two years follow-up of a randomized clinical trial. *Scand. J. Work Environ. Health* **2022**, *48*, 264–272. [CrossRef] [PubMed]
27. van Dongen, J.M.; van der Beek, A.J. Economic evaluations in occupational health: What brings the best bang for the buck? *Scand. J. Work Environ. Health* **2022**, *48*, 249–252. [CrossRef] [PubMed]
28. Franche, R.L.; Krause, N. Readiness for return to work following injury or illness: Conceptualizing the interpersonal impact of health care, workplace, and insurance factors. *J. Occup. Rehabil.* **2002**, *12*, 233–256. [CrossRef]
29. Wickizer, T.M.; Franklin, G.M.; Fulton-Kehoe, D. Innovations in Occupational Health Care Delivery Can Prevent Entry into Permanent Disability: 8-Year Follow-up of the Washington State Centers for Occupational Health and Education. *Med. Care* **2018**, *56*, 1018. [CrossRef]
30. Chien, W. The Impact of Return to Work Programs on the Health Status of Injured Workers with Work-Related Musculoskeletal Disorders: A Malaysian Study. *J. Occup. Saf. Health* **2012**, *33*, 1–6.
31. Gnanaselvam, N.A.; Vinoth Kumar, S.P.; Abraham, V.J. Quality of Life of People with Physical Disabilities in a Rural Block of Tamil Nadu, India. *J. Psychosoc. Rehabil. Ment. Health* **2017**, *4*, 171–177. [CrossRef]
32. Tuomi, K.; Ilmarinen, J.; Klockars, M.; Nygård, C.-H.; SJ, P.H. Work ability index. *Saf. Sci.* **1995**, *19*, 71–72. [CrossRef]

53. Morschhäuser, M.; Sochert, R. Healthy work in an ageing Europe: Strategies and instruments for prolonging working life. *Eur. Netw. Workplace Health Promot.* **2006**, 1–76, Imprint Edition.
54. Reeuwijk, K.G.; Robroek, S.J.W.; Niessen, M.A.J.; Kraaijenhagen, R.A.; Vergouwe, Y.; Burdorf, A. The prognostic value of the work ability index for sickness absence among office workers. *PLoS ONE* **2015**, *10*, e0126969. [CrossRef] [PubMed]

Disclaimer/Publisher's Note: The statements, opinions and data contained in all publications are solely those of the individual author(s) and contributor(s) and not of MDPI and/or the editor(s). MDPI and/or the editor(s) disclaim responsibility for any injury to people or property resulting from any ideas, methods, instructions or products referred to in the content.

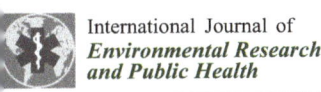

Article

Green Jobs: Bibliometric Review

Łukasz Jarosław Kozar [1],* and Adam Sulich [2,3],*

1. Department of Labour and Social Policy, Faculty of Economics and Sociology, University of Lodz, ul. Rewolucji 1905 r. No 37, 90-214 Lodz, Poland
2. Department of Advanced Research in Management, Faculty of Business Management, Wroclaw University of Economics and Business, ul. Komandorska 118/120, 53-345 Wroclaw, Poland
3. Schulich School of Business, York University, 4700 Keele Street, Toronto, ON M3J 1P3, Canada
* Correspondence: lukasz.kozar@uni.lodz.pl (Ł.J.K.); adam.sulich@ue.wroc.pl (A.S.)

Abstract: Among the visible effects as Sustainable Development (SD) transitions from theory into practice, there are Green Jobs (GJs). There are multiple variants in naming this phenomenon in the labor market. Among them are green collars, green employment, and sustainable employment, all indicating a profound inconsistency in the GJ definition. This article aims to identify keyword-specified areas around which the topic of GJs revolves in the scientific literature indexed in the Scopus database. The usage of two methods has achieved this goal. First is the Structured Literature Review (SLR) variation with queries, and it is used to explore the scientific database to determine GJ's definition consistency by the queries syntax. The second method is the search results analysis performed in the Scopus database online to identify the most cited publications and most contributing authors. Then the bibliometric analysis was performed to create bibliometric maps of the most critical keywords in VOSviewer software. The combination of those two approaches allowed this research to indicate the most influential research directions on GJs. The results are presented in graphical forms, and tables with main co-occurring keyword clusters were identified. GJs are a key part of green economy development, where green self-employment and green entrepreneurship play a pivotal role. The presented results can inspire other researchers who are looking for a research gap or describing the state of the art. Politicians and decision-makers can be influenced by the presented contextualization of green job's meaning in the labor market.

Keywords: green jobs; green labor market; green economy; sustainable development

Citation: Kozar, Ł.J.; Sulich, A. Green Jobs: Bibliometric Review. *Int. J. Environ. Res. Public Health* **2023**, *20*, 2886. https://doi.org/10.3390/ijerph20042886

Academic Editor: Delfina G. Ramos

Received: 15 January 2023
Revised: 3 February 2023
Accepted: 6 February 2023
Published: 7 February 2023

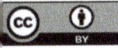

Copyright: © 2023 by the authors. Licensee MDPI, Basel, Switzerland. This article is an open access article distributed under the terms and conditions of the Creative Commons Attribution (CC BY) license (https://creativecommons.org/licenses/by/4.0/).

1. Introduction

The technological transition from a brown economy (based mainly on the exploitation of fossil fuels) to a green economy (based on renewable energy sources) is a multidimensional, worldwide process [1,2] that involves all sectors of the modern economy [3,4]. This process is the result of the need to implement the idea of Sustainable Development (SD) in socio-economic practice [5,6]. The assumption is that the green economy is about conducting all economic activities with respect for nature's assets and in such a way as to prevent irreversible changes to the environment [7]. Therefore, there are changes taking place in all business processes and decision-making aiming at a low-carbon, and a resource-efficient economy based on green technologies [8,9]. The examples of the changes towards SD are visible in all economic sectors and there is a gradual green transformation of the whole economy taking place [10,11]. This shift towards a green economy is particularly visible in the labor market [12,13]. In this economic area, there is the creation of new jobs or the change of existing jobs for the needs of a gradually greening or circular economy [14,15]. Such jobs created as a result of pro-environmental transformations of activities undertaken by various types of entities are called green jobs (GJs) [9,16,17]. GJs are the result of the ongoing transformation focused on SD [18] and are an important part of the scientific analyses raised around the topic of a green economy [19,20]. In particular, the scientific literature emphasizes that employees employed in GJs should be characterized by appropriate levels of knowledge [21,22], skills [23,24], attitudes [25], and pro-environmental behavior [26,27]. Hence, there are a growing number of scientific studies addressing the issue of the green competence of employees [28,29]. Based on previous research on the issue of GJs, it is possible not only to point out how they differ from non-green jobs [30,31], but also to draw the conclusion that it is on the degree of development of human capital in the context of sustainability issues that progress aimed at greening modern economies depends [32]. GJs can be characterized by both quality and degree of greening [9,33]. Thus, GJs can be called a kind of litmus test of the greening of modern economies of both the countries concerned and international communities [34].

There is an ongoing scientific discussion on the question of defining what GJs are [9,15]. This discussion is triggered by diverse scientific and research approaches to such specific positions [35,36]. The result of the considerations undertaken by researchers is the identification of GJs with given economic sectors [37,38], which are called green sectors [39,40], or with specific jobs [41,42]. According to the most popular definition of GJs, they represent "work in agricultural, manufacturing, research and development, administrative, and service activities that contribute substantially to preserving or restoring environmental quality" [43]. Recently, special attention has been paid to the energy sector [44,45], where it is indicated that the transformation of this sector towards renewable energy sources contributes to the creation of GJs [4,33]. In addition, researchers on the subject recognize another important aspect resulting from the indicated transformation, namely that the renewable energy sector creates more jobs per unit of energy than the fossil fuel-based sector [46,47]. Thus, what is occurring in this area is not only a qualitative change in jobs but also the creation of new GJs [48,49]. In light of the research conducted to date on the topic of GJs, a view directed toward qualitative research of all jobs in the economy in terms of their greening is also evident [9,50].

The aim of this article is to identify key areas around which the topic of GJs revolves in the literature. Such an area-based systematization is important since a significant systematic research gap is still apparent in this field. Previous literature studies aimed at this goal primarily ignore the issue of the different nomenclature of GJs [51], or analyze the indicated issues in rather narrow periods [52], and thus make the undertaken deductions incomplete. The research problems observed are the main reason for this study. The purpose of the article presented above is accompanied by verification of the statement that GJs and their nomenclature are constantly evolving, which in itself is an important field for researchers and management theory development.

To achieve a such goal to identify key areas and keywords, around which GJs are developed in the scientific literature, the bibliometric analysis was performed. The adopted method was Structured Literature Review (SLR) variation method with queries. The scientific database explored in this bibliometric study is the Scopus collection of peer-reviewed articles, conference proceedings, book chapters, etc. In this study, the whole collection was analyzed according to the presented in the Materials and Methods section methodology. Using the VOSviewer software (version 1.6.18) the co-occurrences networks were generated to identify associations between frequently occurring keywords in scientific articles indexed in Scopus.

Following the logic adopted in this paper as a bibliometric review, the presentation of the GJs subject is divided into four interrelated sections. After presenting in the first section the reasons for bibliometric research and explaining the purpose of the work, a description of the research methodology is presented in the second section. The results of the research are presented in the third section with the support of bibliometric maps and their descriptions. The article concludes with a discussion of the results, along with recommendations and directions for future research on the GJs subject.

2. Materials and Methods

There are two complementary methods used in this research. First is the SLR variation with queries (Figure 1, path no. 1), and it is used to explore the scientific database to determine GJ's definition consistency by the queries syntax. The second method is the search results analysis performed in the Scopus database online to identify the most cited publications and most contributing authors (Figure 1, path no. 2). The first method results are analyzed in VOSviewer in form of bibliometric maps. The second method is the analysis of the results in Scopus and is a development of the first used in this paper method, the SLR results method. Therefore, this section is divided into two subchapters.

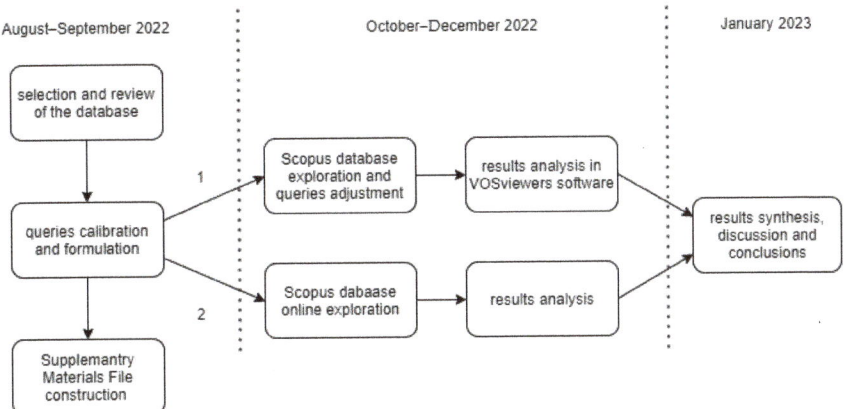

Figure 1. Methods and stages of the research. Source: Authors' elaboration.

The stages of the research covered 5 months of the bibliometric study. In the first period, based on the initial query formulation and calibration, observations have been made. In this stage, Supplementary Materials File S1 has been constructed. The conclusions and remarks have been gathered after all stages were completed and have been introduced into proper sections of this paper.

2.1. Structured Literature Review Method Variation

The SLR method variation is supported by the research queries exploring the Scopus database. The SLR has its own procedure, which is not presented in detail in this paper [53,54]. In this study, the SLR method is used as a tool for the identification of knowledge gaps and the future direction of the research collected in bibliographic databases [55]. The SLR method variation is based on the research queries, which are used to explore the Scopus database. In this paper, the whole Scopus database was researched without any limitation to specific years or periods. The subject of this study is metadata of scientific literature collected in the Scopus database. This database was selected due to its broad scientific recognition and wider collection of content than other databases [55,56]. The information related to the bibliometric records of the Scopus database were explored by the bibliometric visualization tool software. The results of this method are presented in form of bibliometric maps with the use of the VOSviewer program (version 1.6.18). This software is commonly used by researchers in bibliometric studies in different research areas [57,58]. The method used in this research is to perform bibliometric analysis to produce a network visualization of keywords for the queries. In the variation of the SLR method, the three original queries were formulated and developed as presented in Table 1. There are differences in the formulated queries, although the queries have a syntax that corresponds with the database on which they are used. There are different numbers of results depending on the number of used green job equivalents and variants such as green employment, green collar, environmental job, or sustainable job.

Table 1. Queries focused on typologies used in the Scopus scientific database exploration on 20 August 2022.

Symbol	Query Syntax	No. of Results (20 August 2022)
Q1	TITLE-ABS-KEY ("green job" OR "green employment" OR "green collar" OR "sustainable job" OR "sustainable employment" OR "sustainability job" OR "eco-friendly employment" OR "eco employment" OR "environmental job" OR "environmental employment")	1094
Q2	TITLE-ABS-KEY ("green job" OR "green employment" OR "green collar" OR "sustainability job" OR "eco-friendly employment" OR "eco employment" OR "environmental job" OR "environmental employment")	702
Q3	TITLE-ABS-KEY ("green job" OR "green employment" OR "green collar" OR "sustainability job" OR "environmental job")	684

Source: Authors' elaboration.

The data presented in Tables 1 and 2 queries' construction and calibration are presented in Supplementary Materials File S1 in detail. These queries are focused on the GJs typologies visible in Scopus database-indexed publications. The subject areas in this research were not chosen automatically by the selection in the Scopus database but each paper was carefully reviewed to exclude misleading results to be further analyzed. This time-consuming operation explains the different dates presented in Tables 1 and 2 results. There are differences in the formulated queries in Table 2, although the queries have a syntax that corresponds with the database on which they are used [59].

Table 2. Syntaxes used in Queries after calibration for the Scopus scientific database exploration GJs concept.

No.	Query Syntax	No. of Results (31 December 2022)
Q4	TITLE-ABS-KEY ({green job} OR {green jobs} OR {green-jobs} OR {'green' job} OR {'green' jobs} OR {'green job'} OR {'green jobs'} OR {green collar} OR {green-collar} OR {'green-collar'} OR {'green collar'} OR {green employment} OR {green employments} OR {environmental job} OR {environmental jobs} OR {'environmental job'} OR {sustainability job})	671
Q5	TITLE-ABS-KEY ({green job} OR {green jobs} OR {*green job*} OR {green-jobs} OR {'green' job} OR {'green' jobs} OR {'green job} OR {'green jobs'}) OR ({green collar} OR {green collars} OR {*green collar*} OR {green-collar} OR {'green-collar'} OR {'green collar'} OR {green employment} OR {*green employment*} OR {green employments}) OR ({environmental job} OR {environmental jobs} OR {*environmental job*} OR {'environmental job'} OR {environm* employment}) OR ({sustainab* job} OR {sustainab* employment} OR {environm* employment})	611

Source: Authors' elaboration.

Presented queries do not differ in the publication type, years, or category, because such filters were not used to explore the Scopus database. The results obtained from Queries 4 and 5 (Q4 and Q5, respectively) were downloaded each time as a set of files in .csv format and during the export procedure, all fields on the publication were marked. Further analyses were carried out on the collected data in the VOSviewer program and the results are shown in bibliometric maps [60].

This research has its own limitations because the choice of the number of co-occurrences determines the result obtained in its graphical presentation and bibliometric map clarity. Therefore, a minimum number of 10 keyword co-occurrences was set for each bibliometric map initially, then it was changed and indicated specifically before each figure with the bibliometric map. The VOSviewer program allows researchers to define the research gaps covered by the published paper and indicate the directions of scientific development [55]. The exploration of the scientific database, presented in Table 2 Q4 and Q5, leads to the comparison of the GJ variants in two sets of query results.

2.2. Search Results Analysis in Scopus

Search results analysis in Scopus is a continuation of the SLR method. This analysis was based on Query 1 (symbol Q1 in Table 1), 1094 results, and was performed on the Scopus database online website after the option "analyze search results" was selected. The years 1966–2022 were the time frame for this online analysis. There were no other fields selected or deselected on the Scopus website.

3. Results

This section is divided into two subsections and reflects the two methods used in this research. The first subsection presents the bibliometric analysis which is gaining in popularity and is based on the SLR modification with queries and VOSviewer software. The second subsection contains the simple search results analysis offered by the Scopus database among the results of the indexed documents.

3.1. Bibliometric Analysis of SLR Method Results

Queries 4 and 5 (Table 2) were used for studying the Scopus database with different results for the same time point. The obtained results of those two queries were 671 and 611 publications, respectively (Table 2). Those results were analyzed in the VOSviewer software in form of bibliometric maps representing the keywords frequently occurring together.

Figure 2 is a bibliometric map of keyword co-occurrences of indexed keywords from publications index in Scopus distinguished as the Q4 results (Table 2). The method used to generate Figure 2 was full counting, and in this method 2418 indexed keywords were identified, among them 67 indexed keywords met the threshold of 10 co-occurrences. Among those results, keywords were referring to the countries and organizations' names that were deselected from the proposed keywords list. Additionally deselected keywords from the proposed in VOSviewer list were: "human", "humans", "article", "female", "male", and "adult". Then from 67 keywords, 11 were deselected. Finally, there are 56 keywords collected in four clusters automatically colored and identified by the VOSviewer software. Figure 2 presents the keywords most often used in the scientific publications dedicated to green jobs, green collars, green employment, and sustainable employment and their combinations explored by the Q4 syntax. As a result, only two keywords representing "green jobs" and "green job" were placed in the bibliometric map (Figure 2).

There are four clusters presented in Figure 2 and Table 3, and those clusters were automatically organized by the VOSviewer software. There are different numbers of keywords in each of the four clusters. In the first red-colored cluster there are 23 items and this is the most numerous group of keywords. The second is marked in green in Figure 3; this cluster consists of 15 keywords. The third cluster consists of 13 keywords presented in blue in Figure 2. There is also a yellow cluster with 5 automatically distinguished keywords. At this aggregate level, it is possible to identify themes of clusters of keywords based on the co-occurrence's frequency. The size of nodes presented in Figure 2 is proportional to the number of occurrences of indexed keywords. Another important feature of the presented bibliometric map is the fact that closer proximity between nodes indicates a closer relationship between keywords. These characteristics allow aggregate keywords into clusters presented in Table 3. The number of occurrences for each keyword is indicated in parentheses, after each keyword.

Based on the generated results of Q4 there was also an overlay map generated (Figure 3). The purpose of this figure is to present the evolution of the scientific interests represented by the keywords related to the GJs. Figure 3 has automatically generated a time scale by VOSviewer. Figure 3 is similar to Figure 2 in shape and represents the same nodes, and edges as in Figure 2 and occurrences in Table 3.

In Figure 3 there are visible darker and lighter elements. The dark blue color represents the oldest keywords and this group reflexes the fourth cluster in Table 3. Keywords represented by the yellow nodes in Figure 3 represent the newest and still actual fields of interest in the subject of green jobs, and even the keyword "green job" is still in yellow in Figure 3. The importance of these yellow-marked keywords is the basis of the discussion and conclusions for future research directions in respective sections of this paper.

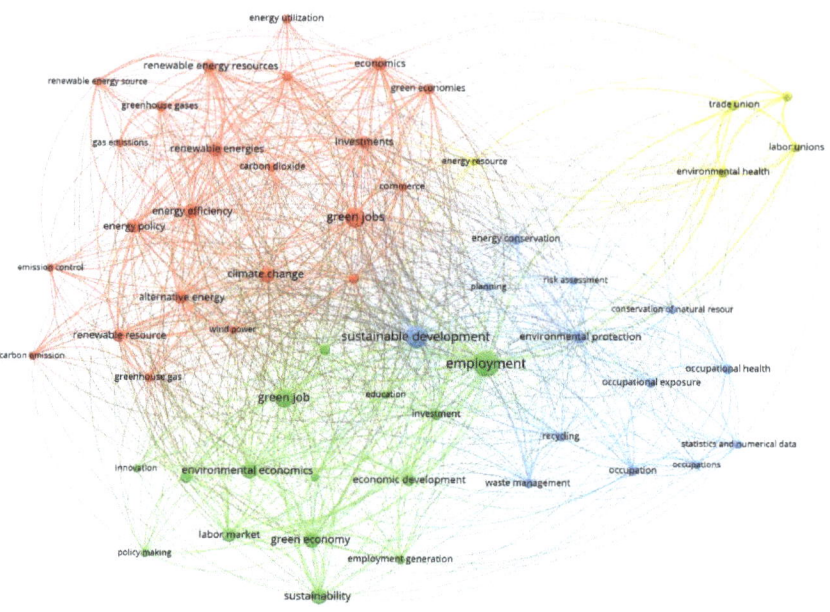

Figure 2. Bibliometric map of keywords co-occurrences Q4 results analysis in Scopus. Source: Authors' elaboration.

Table 3. Clusters of keyword co-occurrences presented in Figure 2 for Scopus Q4.

Cluster	Color	Keywords
1	Red	alternative energy (23), carbon dioxide (12), carbon emission (10), climate change (34), commerce (13), economic and social effects (14), economics (28), emission control (10), energy efficiency (28), energy policy (24), energy utilization (12), fossil fuels (14), gas emissions (11), green economies (18), green jobs (59), greenhouse gas (13), greenhouse gases (17), investments (21), renewable energies (28), renewable energy resources (21), renewable energy source (10), renewable resource (22), wind power (11)
2	Green	economic development (23), economic growth (11), education (10), employment (96), employment generation (13), environmental economics (36), environmental impact (17), environmental policy (20), green economy (33), green job (48), innovation (11) investment (18), labor market (27), policy making (10), sustainability (36)
3	Blue	conservation of natural resources (10), energy conservation (16), environmental protection (21), occupation (15), occupational exposure (14), occupational health (15), occupations (11), planning (11), recycling (15), risk assessment (11), statistics and numerical data (10), sustainable development (72), waste management (14)
4	Yellow	energy resource (10), environmental health (17), labor unions (15), organization and management (14), trade union (16)

Source: Authors' elaboration.

Figure 4 is a bibliometric map of keywords co-occurrences of indexed keywords from publications index in Scopus distinguished as the Q5 results (Table 2). The method used to generate Figure 4 was full counting of indexed keywords co-occurrences, and in this method, 2213 indexed keywords were identified, among them 58 indexed keywords met the threshold of 10 co-occurrences. Among those results, keywords were referring to the countries and organizations' names that were deselected from the proposed keywords list. Additionally deselected keywords from the proposed in VOSviewer list were: "human", "humans", and "article". Then from 58 keywords, 7 were deselected. Finally, there are 51 keywords collected in four clusters, automatically colored and identified by the VOSviewer software. Figure 4 presents the keywords most often used in the scientific publications dedicated to green jobs, green collars, green employment, and sustainable employment and their combinations explored by the Q5 syntax. As result, only two keywords representing "green jobs" and "green job" were placed in the bibliometric map (Figure 4).

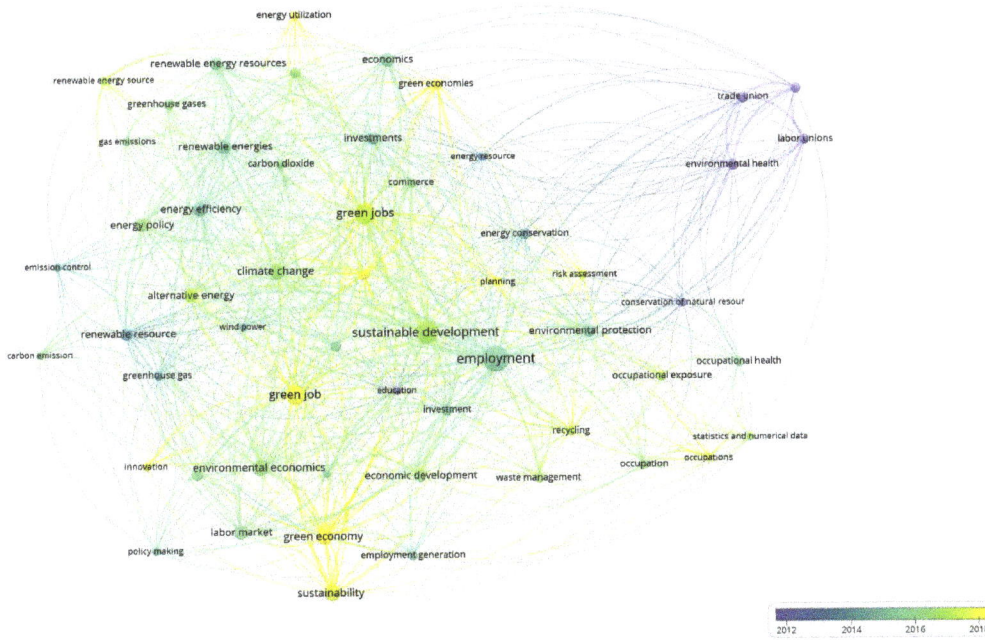

Figure 3. Overlay Visualization of keywords co-occurrences Q4 results analysis in Scopus. Source: Authors' elaboration.

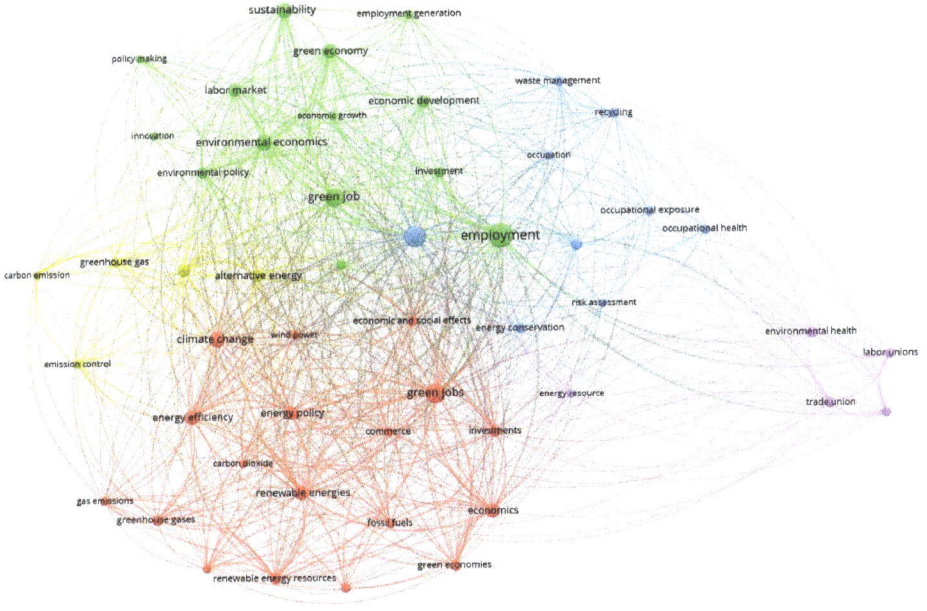

Figure 4. Bibliometric map of keywords co-occurrences Q5 results analysis in Scopus. Source: Authors' elaboration.

There are five clusters presented in Figure 4 and described in Table 4 which are automatically colored by VOSviewer software. There is the most numerous of all clusters colored in red the first cluster with 18 items. Second is the green cluster with 14 distinguished keywords. The third is a blue cluster consists of 9 items and collects the keywords: "recycling", "waste management", "risk assessment", "occupational exposure", "occupational health", occupation", "environmental health", "energy conservation", and "sustainable development". There is also a fourth yellow cluster with 5 items. The fifth cluster in Table 4, consists also of 5 keywords but it is colored purple. The number of occurrences for each keyword is indicated in parentheses, after each keyword, in Table 4.

Table 4. Clusters of keywords co-occurrences visible in Figure 4 for Scopus Q5 results.

Cluster	Color	Keywords
1	Red	carbon dioxide (11), climate change (33), commerce (13), economic and social effects (14), economics (27), energy efficiency (27), energy policy (22), energy utilization (12), fossil fuels (13), gas emissions (18), green economies (18), green jobs (59), greenhouse gases (17), investments (19), renewable energies (28), renewable energy resource (20), renewable energy sources (21), wind power (11)
2	Green	economic development (22), economic growth (11), employment (88), employment generation (13), environmental economics (35), environmental impact (14), environmental policy (19), green economy (31), green job (48), innovation (11), investment (18), labor market (26), policy making (10), sustainability (33)
3	Blue	energy conservation (15), environmental protection (19), occupation (11), occupational exposure (13), occupational health (12), recycling (14), risk assessment (11), sustainable development (67), waste management (14)
4	Yellow	alternative energy (23), carbon emission (10), emission control (10), greenhouse gas (13), renewable resource (22)
5	Purple	energy resource (10), environmental health (17), labor unions (15), organization and management (14), trade union (16)

Source: Authors' elaboration.

There are similarities between the presented two tables with VOSviewer results automatically divided into clusters, although Table 3 consists of more keywords than Table 4. The number of clusters in Table 4 is also smaller than in Table 3. The first cluster in Table 4 revolves around negative aspects of the GJs definition expressed in human activities' pressure on the natural environment measures. The second cluster presented in Table 4 consists of positive aspects of the GJs definition expressed in progress, economic development, and sustainability. There is also a third cluster in Table 4 and this cluster revolves around employee health protection and conservation of the resources. The fourth cluster presented in Table 4 represents the rules or regulations associated with the GJs which influence "energy resources", "environmental health", "labor unions", "organization and management", and "trade union".

There are the same similarities between Figures 4 and 5 as the described similarities between Figures 2 and 3, in terms of the shape and connections. In Figure 5 there is also an automatically distinguished time scale of co-occurring keywords evolution. The oldest keywords marked in darker colors correspond with the fifth subnetwork of the created map and parts of the other clusters. The distribution of those older keywords is then complex. However, the lighter keywords representing the relatively newest scientific interests are scattered. In Figure 5, attention is deserved for two centrally located keywords "green job" and "green jobs" marked in lighter colors, which indicates the ongoing debate which revolves around those terms. Based on Figure 5, the view on the perspective and emerging future directions of studies are developed in the discussion and conclusion sections.

The order of keywords in each cluster is automatically proposed by the VOSviewer software. Their complex relations prove that the concept of GJs emerged from the concept of sustainable development and the assumption that greening the economy or creating a green economy, would generate GJs [61]. Therefore, the most important and biggest node in Figures 2 and 3 is the "employment" keyword. Its central place in the bibliometric map reflects the research results, which claim that with GJs it is possible to fight unemployment as well as to counteract environmental degradation [62].

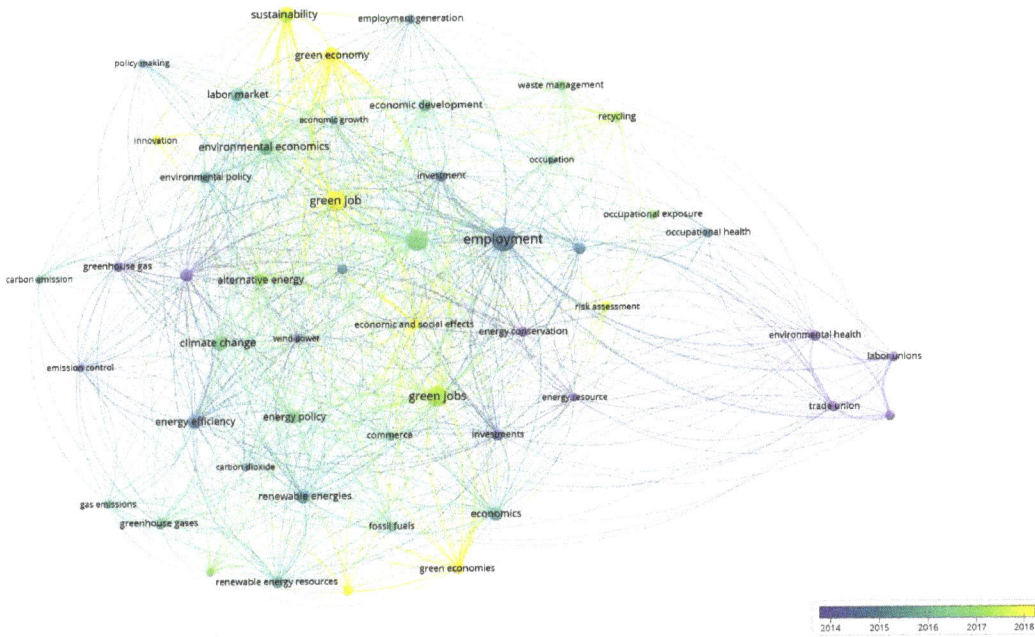

Figure 5. Overlay Visualization of keywords co-occurrences Q5 results analysis in Scopus. Source: Authors' elaboration.

There are not only quantitative differences in Q4 and Q5 results but also qualitative, related to the GJs definition. The broad definition of GJs has raised concerns among the expert teams and created the need to clarify the direction of further work on the definition of GJs. As part of their work on the GJs definition, the teams identified their specific sectors for their regions that meet the condition of respecting nature's assets and residents [63,64]. The colors presented in Figures 2 and 4 are also different, although the keywords in Tables 3 and 4 are similar. The shapes of Figures 2 and 4 are also matching. The most interesting feature of both figures is separated on the right side of the area of the figures which consists of five keywords. These nodes are as follows: "energy resource", "environmental health", "labor unions", "organization and management", and "trade union". These keywords are mainly related to the green labor market or labor conditions and are the same in both bibliometric maps.

3.2. Search Results Analysis in Scopus

The analysis performed online on the Scopus website was based on 1094 documents indexed in Scopus scientific database, which are Q1 results (Table 1). The first publication among these results and related to the GJs was an article by Ronald J. Burke, titled *Are Herzberg's motivators and hygienes unidimensional?* published in the 1966 Journal of Applied Psychology [65]. This publication used the term "environmental job" and research revolved around job satisfaction or dissatisfaction in a such-named green job [65]. Therefore, the time frame of the Scopus exploration starts in 1966.

Figure 6 presents the rapid growth in the amount of indexed publications dedicated to GJs or their variant names (as indicated in Q1 syntax) that occurred in 2008 (with 26 publications). Since then, the linear trend is growing, and 2022 was the year in which the highest number of publications (119 documents in Scopus) dedicated to GJs were published.

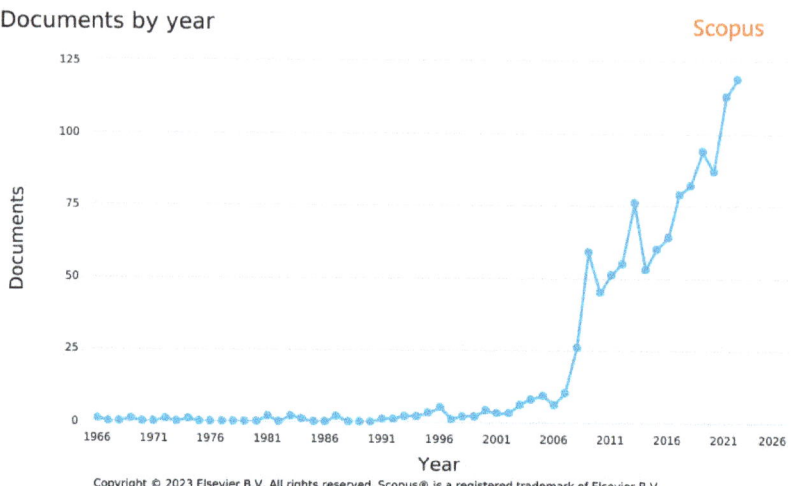

Figure 6. Documents results of Q1 in Scopus. Source: Authors' elaboration.

The analysis of the Q1 result allowed for identification of the main quantitatively contributing authors in the field of GJs by a number of authored documents collected in Scopus. In Figure 7 are presented selected authors with six and more publications indexed in Scopus. There is a similar analysis result for the other queries [66].

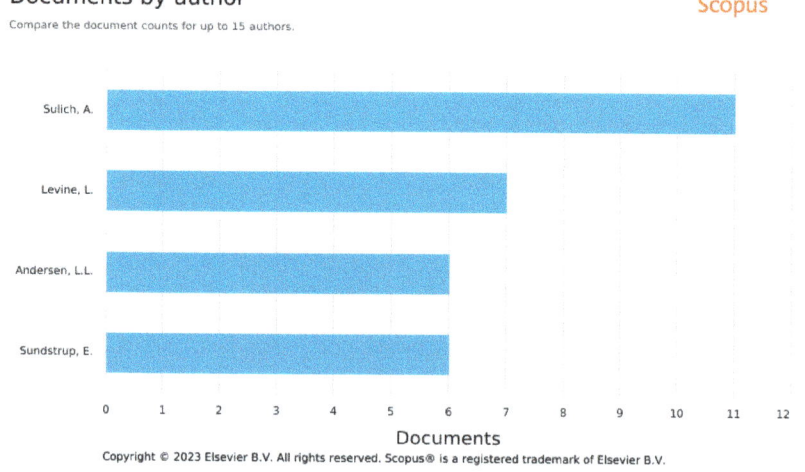

Figure 7. Documents by authors. Analysis of the results of Q1 in Scopus. Source: Authors elaboration.

The authors who contributed most to the subject of GJs (Figure 7) are not the most-cited authors. Those are presented in Table 5, where the most cited publications (over 400 citations in Scopus) among results of Q1 are also listed.

The Publications presented in Table 5 revolve around different name variants for GJs. The first publication titled *Comparing structural and index decomposition analysis* uses the term environmental employment [67]. The second publication is related to sustainable jobs and explores smart manufacturing subjects [68]. The only book among the most cited publications is dedicated to the GJs concept and labor market issues. In his book, Ross surveys "the new topography of the global workplace and finds an emerging pattern of labor instability and uneven development on a massive scale" [69]. The fourth of the most cited publications indexed in Scopus does not refer to any of explored GJs variants proposed in queries employed in this article. The article published in the Energy Policy journal presents an analytical job creation model for the USA power sector from 2009 to 2030 [46]. Therefore, all works gathered in Table 5 combine non-fossil fuels technologies, resource-efficient economy, and technologies of carbon capture and storage with positive changes in the labor market expressed by GJs creation [37,70]. The different qualitative approaches lead to new implications in the number of created jobs related to green and sustainable economic transformation.

Table 5. Top Four most cited publications dedicated to the subject of GJs.

Document Type	Document Title	Authors	Source	Cited by
Journal article	Comparing structural and index decomposition analysis [67]	Hoekstra, R., van der Bergh, J.J.C.J.M.	Energy Economics, 2003, 25(1), pp. 39–64	620
Journal article	Smart manufacturing, manufacturing intelligence and demand-dynamic performance [68]	Davis, J., Edgar, T., Porter, J., Bernaden, J., Sarli, M.	Computers and Chemical Engineering, 2012, 47, pp. 145–156	481
Book	Nice work if you can get it: Life and labor in precarious times [69]	Ross, A.	Nice work if you can get it: Life and labor in precarious times, New York University Press, New York, 2009, pp. 1–263	432
Journal article	Putting renewables and energy efficiency to work: How many jobs can the clean energy industry generate in the US? [46]	Wei, M., Patadia, S., Kammen, D.M.	Energy Policy, 2010, 38(2), pp. 919–931	418

Source: Authors' elaboration.

4. Discussion

Based on the analyses carried out, it is important to note the lack of uniform naming of GJs, which is overlooked by some of the researchers of this problem. As a result, the resulting analyses are not fully comprehensive; however, they present the most popular keywords associated with the GJs. The existing used terms of GJs, which are presented in the third part, indicate the evolution of this concept and the slowly establishing pattern in the literature of the name GJs, which is the most frequently cited name of the explored phenomenon. Nevertheless, there are still many researchers who use quotation marks to refer to this type of job or a completely different name in the form of various equivalents of the names: green employment [71,72], green collar [73,74], environmental job [75], or sustainability job [76]. The results show that the use of terms equivalent to green jobs depends on the context of their use. Green collars appear in engineering articles on renewable energy technologies. Sustainability jobs, on the other hand, appear in articles related to strategy formulation. Authors of publications seeking scientific novelty create new names for already defined terms, which is why constructs such as "ecojobs" appear [77].

Emerging new concepts make it difficult to carry out a comprehensive analysis of the concept of green jobs and expand the context for searching databases. Therefore, the analysis undertaken focuses on commonly occurring synonyms for green jobs. The analysis undertaken is devoid of the mantle of linguistic research or somatic analysis of words as undertaken by the authors of the publications under investigation. At the same time, it may be an interesting new direction for future research, which may show the different perceptions of researchers regarding green jobs. Such different nomenclature forces researchers on the subject of GJs to analyze the content of individual articles quite meticulously at the stage of selection for analysis, which is carried out using programs such as VOSviewer. Researchers should especially pay attention to "green collar", a name that also appears concerning issues related to military areas (with the absence here of any reference to sustainability issues). This forces researchers to perform an in-depth qualitative analysis of the surveyed publications when qualifying them for analysis using VOSviewer. Only after such a qualitative analysis that leads to the exclusion of articles not related to the topic of sustainability the procedure presented in Figure 1 can be applied.

The year 2008 was linked to the global economic crisis [78]. The study observed a multidimensionality of social economic and environmental problems, which were closely interlinked. In this context, solutions were sought to find a way out of the crisis. It was noted that the current paradigm of economic development, which is mainly based on non-renewable resources, is unreliable and does not provide opportunities for future generations [77,79]. The researchers, therefore, drew attention to the need to implement sustainable development and related green jobs into economic practice [80,81]. This explains the growing interest in green jobs, not only from a scientific but also from a practical point of view [82].

A limitation of this study is the lack of a detailed dynamic analysis performed in VOSviewer which addresses the strength of the connections between individual keywords. Such a dynamic analysis is only possible when using the VOSviewer program and its graphical representation is impossible, due to a large number of identified connections (graph edges). However, the lack of such an analysis does not affect the quality of the presented research results and conclusions.

It should be recognized that GJs are a key element of the green economy. They bind numerous areas of the economy together with their issues. Based on the analysis carried out, it can be concluded that when discussing the issue of GJs, an important emphasis is placed on the "education" keyword, which is located close to "employment" in a green cluster in Figure 2. To the "education" keyword there are other related terms such as knowledge, skills, attitudes [83,84], and pro-environmental behavior of employees researched deeply in Green Humans Resources [29,85]. These are the elements of complex business activities that indicate whether or not an employee employed at a given green job will contribute to minimizing the negative impact of a given economic entity on the environment [84]. This area was indicated also automatically by the bibliometric software as the first and most numerous cluster in both analyses of Queries 4 and 5.

5. Conclusions

In this paper 671 (Q4 in Table 2) and 611 (Q5 in Table 2) peer-reviewed academic publications associated with green jobs (GJs) using Scopus were identified. This study used the VOSviewer software to present a bibliometric analysis and to identify key areas around which the topic of GJs revolves in the literature. Then, identified clusters of keywords were associated with different aspects of green jobs. The very separation of GJs from the total number of jobs contributes to the segmentation of the labor market. The authors would like to emphasize that GJs form a key element of the green labor market [86]. At the same time, based on the analyzed scientific studies, it can be seen that due to the fact of gradual greening of the economy, not all employees who would like to work in GJs will find such employment, despite having the appropriate green competencies and qualifications, as well as being characterized by pro-environmental behavior and attitudes. Hence, to ensure that their green capital is not depreciated based on non-GJs, an alternative is to take up green self-employment. This area should be recognized by policymakers influencing the creation of national policies on labor market issues [87]. The active labor market policy instruments should be developed in the context of supporting green self-employment [63].

The creation of GJs contributes to the need to implement an appropriate management process in business entities so that green human capital is properly used to achieve competitive advantages [88]. In addition, proper management of green human capital in business entities is aimed at preventing its depreciation. Hence, one should notice the emerging theme of green human resource management, or sustainable human resource management, in the scientific studies analyzed. Thus, the emergence of GJs not only causes effects of an economic nature (the need to commit adequate capital to green existing jobs or create new GJs), but also strictly organizational in terms of the need to develop a new model of human capital management in the organization.

Supplementary Materials: The following supporting information can be downloaded at https://www.mdpi.com/article/10.3390/ijerph20042886/s1. Table S1. Syntaxes used in Queries calibration for the Scopus scientific database exploration variants of naming green job; Table S2. Syntaxes used in Queries calibration for the Scopus scientific database exploration variants of naming green collar; Table S3. Syntaxes used in Queries calibration for the Scopus scientific database exploration variants of naming green employment; Table S4. Syntaxes used in Queries calibration for the Scopus scientific database exploration variants of naming environmental job; Table S5. Syntaxes used in Queries calibration for the Scopus scientific database exploration variants of naming sustainability job.

Author Contributions: Conceptualization, Ł.J.K. and A.S.; methodology, Ł.J.K. and A.S.; software, Ł.J.K. and A.S.; validation Ł.J.K. and A.S.; formal analysis, Ł.J.K. and A.S.; investigation, Ł.J.K. and A.S.; resources, Ł.J.K. and A.S.; data curation, Ł.J.K. and A.S.; writing—original draft preparation, Ł.J.K. and A.S.; writing—review and editing, Ł.J.K. and A.S.; visualization, Ł.J.K. and A.S.; supervision, Ł.J.K. and A.S.; project administration, Ł.J.K. and A.S.; funding acquisition, Ł.J.K. and A.S. All authors have read and agreed to the published version of the manuscript.

Funding: (A.S.) This article has been written within the framework of the PROM Programme for International Exchange of Doctoral Students and Academic Staff Contract No. PPI/PRO/2019/1/00049/U/00001. (Ł.J.K.) This project is financed by the Faculty of Economics and Sociology, University of Lodz; Internal Research Grant title: "Green self-employment as a method of professional activation for the unemployed and economically inactive", project no. B2211201000090.07, decision number 10/2021; total funding amount PLN 21,930.00.

Institutional Review Board Statement: Not applicable.

Informed Consent Statement: Not applicable.

Data Availability Statement: Not applicable.

Acknowledgments: The authors thank the anonymous reviewers who attended the double double-round blind review and editors for their valuable contributions that improved this manuscript. The authors would like to thank Marcin Hernes, Letycja Sołoducho-Pelc, and Tomasz Zema (Wrocław University of Economics and Business, Poland) for their consultation on the selection of calibration keywords and the construction of queries.

Conflicts of Interest: The authors declare no conflict of interest. The funders had no role in the design of the study; in the collection, analyses, or interpretation of data; in the writing of the manuscript, or in the decision to publish the results.

References

1. Wang, C. The assessment of the green transformation capacity in low carbon economy of China. *Open Cybern. Syst. J.* **2015**, *9*, 2030–2034. [CrossRef]
2. Cheba, K.; Bąk, I.; Szopik-Depczyńska, K.; Ioppolo, G. Directions of green transformation of the European Union countries. *Ecol. Indic.* **2022**, *136*, 108601. [CrossRef]
3. Sulich, A.; Sołoducho-Pelc, L. The circular economy and the Green Jobs creation. *Environ. Sci. Pollut. Res.* **2022**, *29*, 14231–14247. [CrossRef] [PubMed]
4. Lehr, U.; Lutz, C.; Edler, D. Green jobs? Economic impacts of renewable energy in Germany. *Energy Policy* **2012**, *47*, 358–364. [CrossRef]
5. Mohan Das Gandhi, N.; Selladurai, V.; Santhi, P. Unsustainable development to sustainable development: A conceptual model. *Manag. Environ. Qual. An Int. J.* **2006**, *17*, 654–672. [CrossRef]
6. Agbedahin, A.V. Sustainable development, Education for Sustainable Development, and the 2030 Agenda for Sustainable Development: Emergence, efficacy, eminence, and future. *Sustain. Dev.* **2019**, *27*, 669–680. [CrossRef]
7. Rutkowska-Podołowska, M.; Sulich, A. Zielone miejsca pracy w gospodarce [Green Jobs in Economy]. In *Improving the Efficiency in Eterprise—Selected Aspects*; Howaniec, H., Malara, Z., Wyród-Wróbel, J., Eds.; The University of Bielsko-Biała [Akademia Techniczno-Humanistyczna w Bielsku-Białej]: Bielsko-Biała, Poland, 2016; pp. 165–176.
8. Mróz-Gorgoń, B.; Wodo, W.; Andrych, A.; Caban-Piaskowska, K.; Kozyra, C. Biometrics Innovation and Payment Sector Perception. *Sustainability* **2022**, *14*, 9374. [CrossRef]
9. Kozar, Ł.J. *Zielone Miejsca Pracy. Uwarunkowania–Identyfikacja–Oddziaływanie na Lokalny Rynek Pracy; [Green Jobs. Determinants-Identification-Impact on the Local Labour Market]*; Wydawnictwo Uniwersytetu Łódzkiego: Łódź, Poland, 2019; ISBN 978-83-8142-836-1.
10. Hou, J.; Teo, T.S.H.; Zhou, F.; Lim, M.K.; Chen, H. Does industrial green transformation successfully facilitate a decrease in carbon intensity in China? An environmental regulation perspective. *J. Clean. Prod.* **2018**, *184*, 1060–1071. [CrossRef]
11. Sulich, A.; Sołoducho-Pelc, L. Changes in Energy Sector Strategies: A Literature Review. *Energies* **2022**, *15*, 7068. [CrossRef]

12. Sulich, A.; Zema, T. Green jobs, a new measure of public management and sustainable development. *Eur. J. Environ. Sci.* **2018**, *8*, 69–75. [CrossRef]
13. DeVries, H.; Tripoli, L. Corporate progress: What are green jobs paying? *Sustainability* **2010**, *3*, 276–282. [CrossRef]
14. Pavlović, M.; Vulić, M.; Pavlović, A. *Circular Economy in Republic of Serbia and Region*; Springer: Singapore, 2019; ISBN 9789811510526/9789811510519.
15. Dordmond, G.; de Oliveira, H.C.; Silva, I.R.; Swart, J. The complexity of green job creation: An analysis of green job development in Brazil. *Environ. Dev. Sustain.* **2021**, *23*, 723–746. [CrossRef]
16. Sulich, A.; Rutkowska, M.; Popławski, Ł. Green jobs, definitional issues, and the employment of young people: An analysis of three European Union countries. *J. Environ. Manag.* **2020**, *262*, 110314. [CrossRef]
17. Luca, F.-A.; Epuran, G.; Ciobanu, C.-I.; Horodnic, A.V. Green jobs creation—Main element in the implementation of bioeconomic mechanisms | Crearea de locuri de muncă ecologice—Componentă de bază pentru implementarea mecanismelor bioeconomice. *Amfiteatru Econ.* **2019**, *21*, 60–74. [CrossRef]
18. Pop, O.; Dina, G.C.; Martin, C. Promoting the corporate social responsibility for a Green Economy and innovative jobs. *Procedia Soc. Behav. Sci.* **2011**, *15*, 1020–1023. [CrossRef]
19. Aceleanu, M.I. Green jobs in a green economy: Support for a sustainable development. *Prog. Ind. Ecol.* **2015**, *9*, 341–355. [CrossRef]
20. van der Ree, K. Promoting Green Jobs: Decent Work in the Transition to Low-Carbon, Green Economies. *Rev. Int. Polit. Développement* **2019**, *11*, 248–271. [CrossRef]
21. Falxa-Raymond, N.; Svendsen, E.; Campbell, L.K. From job training to green jobs: A case study of a young adult employment program centered on environmental restoration in New York City, USA. *Urban For. Urban Green.* **2013**, *12*, 287–295. [CrossRef]
22. Wagner, C. Adult Learning Meets the Green Economy: Lessons From a Green Jobs Education Project. *Adult Learn.* **2013**, *24*, 14–21. [CrossRef]
23. Heong, Y.M.; Sern, L.C.; Kiong, T.T.; Binti Mohamad, M.M. The Role of Higher Order Thinking Skills in Green Skill Development. *MATEC Web Conf.* **2016**, *70*, 05001. [CrossRef]
24. Cabral, C.; Dhar, R.L. Green competencies: Insights and recommendations from a systematic literature review. *Benchmarking* **2021**, *28*, 66–105. [CrossRef]
25. Ibrahim, Z.; Lai, C.S.; Zaime, A.F.; Lee, M.F.; Othman, N.M. Green skills in knowledge and attitude dimensions from the industrial perspective. *IOP Conf. Ser. Mater. Sci. Eng.* **2020**, *917*, 012025. [CrossRef]
26. Renwick, D.W.S.; Jabbour, C.J.C.; Muller-Camen, M.; Redman, T.; Wilkinson, A. Contemporary developments in Green (environmental) HRM scholarship. *Int. J. Hum. Resour. Manag.* **2016**, *27*, 114–128. [CrossRef]
27. Piwowar-Sulej, K.; Mroziewski, R. Management by Values and Socially Responsible HRM as Success Factors in the Time of the COVID-19 Crisis. In *Corporate Social Responsibility and Sustainability*; Bachnik, K., Kaźmierczak, M., Rojek-Nowosielska, M., Stefańska, M., Szumniak-Samolej, J., Eds.; Routledge: New York, NY, USA, 2022; ISBN 9781000595192/9781003270768.
28. Murga-Menoyo, M.Á. Learning for a sustainable economy: Teaching of green competencies in the university. *Sustainability.* **2014**, *6*, 2974–2992. [CrossRef]
29. Kozar, Ł. Shaping the Green Competence of Employees in an Economy Aimed at Sustainable Development. *Green Hum. Resour. Manag.* **2017**, *6*, 55–67.
30. Consoli, D.; Marin, G.; Marzucchi, A.; Vona, F. Do green jobs differ from non-green jobs in terms of skills and human capital? *Res. Policy* **2016**, *45*, 1046–1060. [CrossRef]
31. Bowen, A.; Kuralbayeva, K.; Tipoe, E.L. Characterising green employment: The impacts of 'greening' on workforce composition. *Energy Econ.* **2018**, *72*, 263–275. [CrossRef]
32. Stukalo, N.; Simakhova, A. Social Dimensions of Green Economy. *Filos. Sociol.* **2019**, *30*, 91–99. [CrossRef]
33. Kozar, Ł.J.; Matusiak, R.; Paduszyńska, M.; Sulich, A. Green Jobs in the EU Renewable Energy Sector: Quantile Regression Approach. *Energies* **2022**, *15*, 6578. [CrossRef]
34. Sulich, A. The Green Economy Development Factors. In *Vision 2020: Sustainable Economic Development and Application of Innovation Management from Regional Expansion to Global Growth. Proceedings of the 32nd International Business Information Management Association Conference, Sevilla, Hiszpania, 15–16 November 2018*; Soliman, K.S., Ed.; International Business Information Management Association (IBIMA): King of Prussia, PA, USA, 2018; pp. 6861–6869.
35. Burger, M.; Stavropoulos, S.; Ramkumar, S.; Dufourmont, J.; van Oort, F. The heterogeneous skill-base of circular economy employment. *Res. Policy* **2019**, *48*, 248–261. [CrossRef]
36. Dell'Anna, F. Green jobs and energy efficiency as strategies for economic growth and the reduction of environmental impacts. *Energy Policy* **2021**, *149*, 112031. [CrossRef]
37. Kozar, Ł. "Green" jobs by sector of the economy; ["Zielone" miejsca pracy w ujęciu sektorowym gospodarki]. In *Ekonomia Zrównoważonego Rozwoju. Społeczeństwo, Środowisko, Innowacje w Gospodarce*; Wydawnictwo Uniwersytetu Łódzkiego: Łódź, Poland, 2016.
38. Unay-Gailhard, İ.; Bojnec, Š. The impact of green economy measures on rural employment: Green jobs in farms. *J. Clean. Prod.* **2019**, *208*, 541–551. [CrossRef]
39. Annandale, D.; Morrison-saunders, A.; Duxbury, L. Regional sustainability initiatives: The growth of green jobs in Australia. *Local Environ.* **2004**, *9*, 81–87. [CrossRef]
40. Stoyanova, Z.; Harizanova, H. Analysis of the External Environment of Green Jobs in Bulgaria. *Econ. Altern.* **2017**, 122–136.

1. Ones, D.S.; Dilchert, S. Measuring, Understanding, and Influencing Employee Green Behaviors. In *Green Organizations: Driving Change with I-O Psychology*; Huffman, A.H., Klein, S.R., Eds.; Routledge: New York, NY, USA, 2013; pp. 115–148. ISBN 9781136499234. Available online: https://labordoc.ilo.org/discovery/fulldisplay?docid=alma995074693502676&context=L&vid=41ILO_INST:41ILO_V1&lang=en&search_scope=MyInst_and_CI&adaptor=Local%20Search%20Engine&tab=Everything&query=sub,exact,%20Csr%20 (accessed on 30 December 2022).
2. Kozar, Ł. Która ze stosowanych metod identyfikacji zielonych miejsc pracy w gospodarce jest najefektywniejsza? [Which of the methods used to identify green jobs in the economy is the most effective?]. In *W Poszukiwaniu Zielonego Ładu*; Wydawnictwo Uniwersytetu Łódzkiego: Łódź, Poland, 2022.
3. Bowen, A.; Kuralbayeva, K. Looking for Green Jobs: The Impact of Green Growth on Employment. Grantham Research Institute on Climate Change and the Environment and Global Green Growth Institute Working Papers. 2015. Available online: http://www.lse.ac.uk/grantham/ (accessed on 2 December 2022).
4. Böhringer, C.; Rivers, N.J.; Rutherford, T.F.; Wigle, R. Green jobs and renewable electricity policies: Employment impacts of Ontario's feed-in tariff. *B.E. J. Econ. Anal. Policy* **2012**, *12*, 25. [CrossRef]
5. Tănasie, A.V.; Năstase, L.L.; Vochița, L.L.; Manda, A.M.; Boțoteanu, G.I.; Sitnikov, C.S. Green Economy—Green Jobs in the Context of Sustainable Development. *Sustainability* **2022**, *14*, 4796. [CrossRef]
6. Wei, M.; Patadia, S.; Kammen, D.M. Putting renewables and energy efficiency to work: How many jobs can the clean energy industry generate in the US? *Energy Policy* **2010**, *38*, 919–931. [CrossRef]
7. Kammen, D.M.; Engel, D. Green Jobs and the Clean Energy Economy. In Proceedings of the 2009 UN Climate Change Conference (COP15), Copenhagen, Denmark, 7–18 December 2009; pp. 160–171.
8. Ge, Y.; Zhi, Q. Literature Review: The Green Economy, Clean Energy Policy and Employment. *Energy Procedia* **2016**, *88*, 257–264. [CrossRef]
9. Stevis, D. Green jobs? Good Jobs? Just Jobs? US Labour Unions Confront Climate Change1. In *Trade Unions in the Green Economy. Working for the Environment*; Räthzel, N., Jackson, T., Uzzell, D., Eds.; Routledge: London, UK, 2012; ISBN 9780203109670. Available online: https://www.taylorfrancis.com/books/edit/10.4324/9780203109670/trade-unions-green-economy-nora-r%C3%A4thzel-david-uzzell-tim-jackson?refId=ec8168d0-2286-4b3d-bd4b-98880b44d751&context=ubx (accessed on 30 December 2022).
10. Bogusz, K.; Sulich, A. The Sustainable Development Strategies in Mining Industry. In *Education Excellence and Innovation Management through Vision 2020*; Soliman, K.S., Ed.; International Business Information Management Association (IBIMA): King of Prussia, PA, USA, 2019; pp. 6893–6911.
11. García Vaquero, M.; Sánchez-Bayón, A.; Lominchar, J. European Green Deal and Recovery Plan: Green Jobs, Skills and Wellbeing Economics in Spain. *Energies* **2021**, *14*, 4145. [CrossRef]
12. Stanef-Puică, M.-R.; Badea, L.; Șerban-Oprescu, G.-L.; Șerban-Oprescu, A.-T.; Frâncu, L.-G.; Crețu, A. Green Jobs—A Literature Review. *Int. J. Environ. Res. Public Health* **2022**, *19*, 7998. [CrossRef]
13. Zema, T.; Sulich, A.; Grzesiak, S. Charging Stations and Electromobility Development: A Cross-Country Comparative Analysis. *Energies* **2022**, *16*, 32. [CrossRef]
14. Boyack, K.; Glänzel, W.; Gläser, J.; Havemann, F.; Scharnhorst, A.; Thijs, B.; van Eck, N.J.; Velden, T.; Waltmann, L. Topic identification challenge. *Scientometrics* **2017**, *111*, 1223–1224. [CrossRef]
15. Zema, T.; Sulich, A. Models of Electricity Price Forecasting: Bibliometric Research. *Energies* **2022**, *15*, 5642. [CrossRef]
16. Weron, R. Electricity price forecasting: A review of the state-of-the-art with a look into the future. *Int. J. Forecast.* **2014**, *30*, 1030–1081. [CrossRef]
17. Bertocci, F.; Mannino, G. Can Agri-Food Waste Be a Sustainable Alternative in Aquaculture? A Bibliometric and Meta-Analytic Study on Growth Performance, Innate Immune System, and Antioxidant Defenses. *Foods* **2022**, *11*, 1861. [CrossRef]
18. Gizzi, F.T. Worldwide trends in research on the San Andreas Fault System. *Arab. J. Geosci.* **2015**, *8*, 10893–10909. [CrossRef]
19. Elsevier. How Can I Best Use the Advanced Search?—Scopus: Access and Use Support Center. Available online: https://service.elsevier.com/app/answers/detail/a_id/11365/supporthub/scopus/#tips (accessed on 30 December 2022).
20. van Eck, N.J.; Waltman, L. Software survey: VOSviewer, a computer program for bibliometric mapping. *Scientometrics* **2010**, *84*, 523–538. [CrossRef]
21. Baer, P.; Brown, M.A.; Kim, G. The job generation impacts of expanding industrial cogeneration. *Ecol. Econ.* **2015**, *110*, 141–153. [CrossRef]
22. Manijean, L.; Saffache, P. Geothermal energy: The pool of jobs!! *Trans. Geotherm. Resour. Counc.* **2017**, *41*, 636–646.
23. Ramos, D.; Afonso, P.; Rodrigues, M.A. Integrated management systems as a key facilitator of occupational health and safety risk management: A case study in a medium sized waste management firm. *J. Clean. Prod.* **2020**, *262*, 121346. [CrossRef]
24. Rutkowska, M.; Sulich, A.; Szczygieł, N. Green jobs. In Proceedings of the 3rd International Conference on European Integration 2016, ICEI 2016, Ostrava, Czechia, 19–20 May 2016; Kovářová, E., Melecký, L., Staníčková, M., Eds.; VŠB—Technical University of Ostrava: Ostrava, Czechy, 2016; pp. 822–829.
25. Burke, R.J. Are Herzberg's motivators and hygienes unidimensional? *J. Appl. Psychol.* **1966**, *50*, 317–321. [CrossRef] [PubMed]
26. Sulich, A. Green Jobs Impact by Adam Sulich. Available online: https://www.researchgate.net/publication/366445592_Green_jobs_impact_by_Adam_Sulich?channel=doi&linkId=63a217ed9835ef259035a189&showFulltext=true (accessed on 9 January 2023).
27. Hoekstra, R.; van der Bergh, J.J.C.J.M. Comparing structural and index decomposition analysis. *Energy Econ.* **2003**, *25*, 39–64. [CrossRef]
28. Davis, J.; Edgar, T.; Porter, J.; Bernaden, J.; Sarli, M. Smart manufacturing, manufacturing intelligence and demand-dynamic performance. *Comput. Chem. Eng.* **2012**, *47*, 145–156. [CrossRef]

69. Ross, A. *Nice Work If You Can Get It: Life and Labor in Precarious Times*; New York University Press: New York, NY, USA, 2009; ISBN 0814776299/9780814776292.
70. Kulhanek, L.; Sulich, A.; Zema, T. European integration and real convergence in V4 Group: Transformation towards green economy. In Proceedings of the 6th International Conference on European Integration, Ostrava, Czechia, 18–20 May 2022; Stanickova, M., Melecky, L., Eds.; VSB—Technical University of Ostrava: Ostrava, Czechia, 2022; pp. 363–371.
71. Elliott, R.J.R.; Lindley, J.K. Environmental Jobs and Growth in the United States. *Ecol. Econ.* **2017**, *132*, 232–244. [CrossRef]
72. Hersh, M. *Ethical Engineering for International Development and Environmental Sustainability*; Springer Ltd.: London, UK, 2015; ISBN 9781447166184/9781447166177.
73. Sullivan, J.; Lee, C.-Y. (Eds.) *A New Era in Democratic Taiwan: Trajectories and Turning Points in Politics and Cross-Strait Relations*; Routledge: New York, NY, USA, 2018; ISBN 9781315161648/9781138062429.
74. Lee, J.-H.; Lee, W.; Yoon, J.-H.; Seok, H.; Roh, J.; Won, J.-U. Relationship between symptoms of dry eye syndrome and occupational characteristics: The Korean National Health and Nutrition Examination Survey 2010–2012. *BMC Ophthalmol.* **2015**, *15*, 147. [CrossRef] [PubMed]
75. Ben Cheikh, N.; Ben Zaied, Y. Nonlinear analysis of employment in waste management. *Appl. Econ. Lett.* **2020**, *27*, 477–483. [CrossRef]
76. Rempel, G.; Moshiri, M.; Milligan, C.; Bittner, J.; Montufar, J. Options for Hauling Fully Loaded ISO Containers in the United States. *J. Transp. Eng.* **2012**, *138*, 760–767. [CrossRef]
77. Song, K.; Kim, H.; Cha, J.; Lee, T. Matching and Mismatching of Green Jobs: A Big Data Analysis of Job Recruiting and Searching. *Sustainability* **2021**, *13*, 4074. [CrossRef]
78. Baciu, E.-L. Employment Outcomes of Higher Education Graduates from during and after the 2007–2008 Financial Crisis: Evidence from a Romanian University. *Sustainability* **2022**, *14*, 11160. [CrossRef]
79. Bracarense, N.; Bracarense Costa, P.A. Green Jobs: Sustainable Path for Environmental Conservation and Socio-Economic Stability and Inclusion. *Rev. Polit. Econ.* **2022**, 1–22. [CrossRef]
80. Sylvan, A.M. *Social Innovation, Entrepreneurship and New Green Jobs: Successful Experiences in Mexico*; World Scientific Publishing Co.: Singapore, 2014; ISBN 9789814596619/9789814596602.
81. Saba, A. Five year review: Evolving environmental law and advice to green lawyers. *Environ. Claims J.* **2017**, *29*, 194–207. [CrossRef]
82. Knuth, S. Whatever Happened to Green Collar Jobs? Populism and Clean Energy Transition. *Ann. Am. Assoc. Geogr.* **2019**, *109*, 634–643. [CrossRef]
83. Junhong, W. Education model of guiding college students to find employment in environmental company. *J. Environ. Prot. Ecol.* **2021**, *22*, 2634–2642.
84. Kozar, Ł.; Oleksiak, P. *Organizacje Wobec Wyzwań Zrównoważonego Rozwoju—Wybrane Aspekty [Organisations Facing the Challenges of Sustainable Development—Selected Aspects]*; Wydawnictwo Uniwersytetu Łódzkiego: Łódź, Poland, 2022; ISBN 9788382208191.
85. Sulich, A.; Rutkowska-Podołowska, M. Green jobs and changes in modern economy on the labour market. In *The Propensity To Changes in the Competitive and Innovative Economic Environment: Processes–Structures–Concepts*; Borowiecki, R., Kaczmarek, J., Eds.; Foundation of the Cracow University of Economics: Kraków, Poland, 2017; pp. 87–94.
86. Rutkowska, M.; Sulich, A. Green Jobs on the background of Industry 4.0. *Procedia Comput. Sci.* **2020**, *176*, 1231–1240. [CrossRef]
87. Budur, T.; Demir, A. The Relationship Between Transformational Leadership and Employee Performance: Mediating Effects of Organizational Citizenship Behaviors. *Iran. J. Manag. Stud.* **2022**, *15*, 899–921. [CrossRef]
88. Sołoducho-Pelc, L.; Sulich, A. Between Sustainable and Temporary Competitive Advantages in the Unstable Business Environment. *Sustainability* **2020**, *12*, 8832. [CrossRef]

Disclaimer/Publisher's Note: The statements, opinions and data contained in all publications are solely those of the individual author(s) and contributor(s) and not of MDPI and/or the editor(s). MDPI and/or the editor(s) disclaim responsibility for any injury to people or property resulting from any ideas, methods, instructions or products referred to in the content.

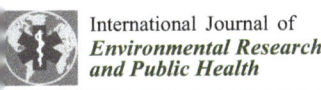

International Journal of
Environmental Research and Public Health

Article

Occupational Exposure to Incidental Nanomaterials in Metal Additive Manufacturing: An Innovative Approach for Risk Management

Marta Sousa [1,2,*], Pedro Arezes [1] and Francisco Silva [1,3]

1. ALGORITMI Research Center/LASI, University of Minho, 4800-058 Guimarães, Portugal
2. CATIM—Technological Center for the Metal Working Industry, 4100-414 Porto, Portugal
3. CTCV—Technological Center for Ceramic and Glass, 3040-540 Coimbra, Portugal
* Correspondence: marta.sousa@dps.uminho.pt

Citation: Sousa, M.; Arezes, P.; Silva, F. Occupational Exposure to Incidental Nanomaterials in Metal Additive Manufacturing: An Innovative Approach for Risk Management. *Int. J. Environ. Res. Public Health* **2023**, *20*, 2519. https://doi.org/10.3390/ijerph20032519

Academic Editors: Delfina G. Ramos and Paul B. Tchounwou

Received: 20 October 2022
Revised: 27 January 2023
Accepted: 29 January 2023
Published: 31 January 2023

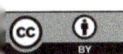

Copyright: © 2023 by the authors. Licensee MDPI, Basel, Switzerland. This article is an open access article distributed under the terms and conditions of the Creative Commons Attribution (CC BY) license (https://creativecommons.org/licenses/by/4.0/).

Abstract: The benefits of metal 3D printing seem unquestionable. However, this additive manufacturing technology brings concerns to occupational safety and health professionals, since recent studies show the existence of airborne nanomaterials in these workplaces. This article explores different approaches to manage the risk of exposure to these incidental nanomaterials, on a case study conducted in a Portuguese organization using Selective Laser Melting (SLM) technology. A monitoring campaign was performed using a condensation particle counter, a canning mobility particle sizer and air sampling for later scanning electron microscopy and energy dispersive X-ray analysis, proving the emission of nano-scale particles and providing insights on number particle concentration, size, shape and chemical composition of airborne matter. Additionally, Control Banding Nanotool v2.0 and Stoffenmanager Nano v1.0 were applied in this case study as qualitative tools, although designed for engineered nanomaterials. This article highlights the limitations of using these quantitative and qualitative approaches when studying metal 3D Printing workstations. As a result, this article proposes the IN Nanotool, a risk management method for incidental nanomaterials designed to overcome the limitations of other existing approaches and to allow non-experts to manage this risk and act preventively to guarantee the safety and health conditions of exposed workers.

Keywords: incidental nanoparticles; control banding; risk management; occupational exposure; metal additive manufacturing

1. Introduction

Freedom of design, time efficiency, reduction of labor and machine costs are a few examples of the several advantages mentioned when the subject is metal 3D Printing, also known as metal Additive Manufacturing (AM) [1]. Regardless of its considerable potential, metal AM has been raising some concerns regarding occupational health and safety [2]. Among other occupational risks, it is known that during these processes incidental metal nano-objects are emitted and it is essential to manage the risk of exposure to this airborne matter to reduce possible negative ill-health effects on workers [3].

Different approaches have been used to assess and/or manage the occupational risk of exposure to incidental nanomaterials in AM processes, but the definition of standardized methods still remains an urgent need [4]. Looking at this occupational risk from the point of view of the common industrial hygiene approach, it is possible to monitor and to quantify the airborne matter released during metal 3D printing. Recent publications in this field endorse the use of direct-reading instruments (for example condensation particle counter—CPC, optical particle counter—OPC and scanning mobility particle sizer—SMPS) and/or the collection of samples and subsequent structural and chemical analysis, by using scanning electron microscopy (SEM), transmission electron microscopy (TEM) and/or energy dispersive X-ray analyzers (EDS) [2,3,5–8]. However, this attempt at a more industrial hygiene conservative approach has limitations that cross all these studies: The lack of clearly defined and standardized occupational exposure limits for metal incidental nanomaterials and the lack of standardized sampling strategies. Some of these studies use as comparison reference values for nanomaterials proposed by different competent local entities and institutes, but so far, no specific limits have been proposed for metal incidental nanomaterials. The most common approach is to compare the results to the recommended benchmarks defined by the Nanosafety Research Centre of the Finnish Institute of Occupational Health (FIOH), i.e., 20,000 nanoparticles/cm^3 (with a density higher than 6000 kg/m^3) for an 8-h exposure time. This limit was later adopted by the Institute for Occupational Safety and Health of the German Social Accident Insurance (IFA DGUV) and the IVAM Environmental Research UVA BV in the Netherlands [5,9]. Even if this value is assumed to be an appropriate reference for metal AM case studies, the quantitative risk assessment still has limitations, namely the possible lack of access to equipment and laboratory analysis for these monitoring campaigns and also the lack of experts to perform them and interpret the results.

Another possibility to assess this risk during metal AM has been to apply qualitative methods originally designed for engineered nanomaterials (ENM), namely control banding based ones. Sousa et al. [8] and Dugheri et al. [5] applied Control Banding Nanotool v2.0 to assess the risk of exposure to ultrafine particles during metal 3D printing operations. Sousa et al. [8] highlight some difficulties on using this approach for incidental nanoparticles, especially the lack of background information on the particles (such as size, shape, and solubility, among others). These authors suggest the design of new methods for incidental nanomaterials, with different inputs than the ones for ENM, to reduce the uncertainty associated with the assessment. Dugheri et al. [5] also emphasize the importance of searching different strategies to assess this occupational risk.

This article aims to explore different approaches to study the potential exposure to incidental nanomaterials during metal AM, through a case study conducted in an organization using Selective Laser Melting (SLM) technology. The main purpose of this article is to propose a risk management tool, entitled IN Nanotool, designed for incidental metal nanomaterials originated from metal AM processes to overcome the limitations of other existing approaches.

2. Materials and Methods

2.1. Facility, Operation Conditions and Materials

This study was conducted in an organization that uses Selective Laser Melting (SLM) technology for metal additive manufacturing. The SLM printer is located in a room dedicated to prototyping, with approximately 85 m^2 and 3 m in height. On the data collection day, no other equipment besides the printer was operating.

The printing process consists in the deposition of layers of a metal powder, usually 20 to 70 microns depending on materials, followed by the application of an infrared laser light scan (1064 nm) of 250 W that melts the powder to reproduce a three-dimensional part, previously defined in a CAD program. The material used was a nitrogen gas atomized spherical powder for additive manufacturing: Stainless steel 316L, with particle size between 20 and 53 µm. Stainless steel 316L is an alloy of iron (>75%) and chromium ($\approx$17%) which also contains nickel ($\approx$12.5%), molybdenum ($\approx$2.5%) and other elements in less significant amount. In this case study, 59.15 cm^3 of this powder were used during the printing process but the final part only had 0.35 cm^3 (approximately 0.59%).

In addition to the initial preparation for printing (which includes CAD design and filling the powder in the printer), the worker's tasks can be divided into 3 distinct phases, as described in Table 1.

Table 1. Description of the tasks under study.

Task 1	Supervision of printing process
Task 2	Removing the part from the printer and cleaning it with a brush
Task 3	Removing the remains of powder, sieving it for reuse and cleaning the powder container

Data gathering included a sample of powder before and after the printing process, technical and material safety data sheets of the powder, information on operation conditions and on-site measurements.

2.2. Quantitative Approach

In the attempt to study the risk of exposure to airborne nanomaterials using a quantitative assessment, the following equipment was used:

- A thermo-hygrometer, TSI® Model 9545 (TSI Incorporated, MN, USA), to measure air velocity, room temperature and relative humidity.
- Portable condensation particle counter (CPC), TSI® model 3007, to measure the total particle number concentration from 10 nm to >1000 nm in 1-s time resolution.
- A scanning mobility particle sizer (SMPS), TSI® Model 3910, to measure nanoparticle size distributions and concentrations, with a size distribution from 10 to 420 nm. The number of particles per size was measured by an internal CPC which counts single particles to provide accurate counts, even at low concentrations.
- A personal air sampling pump, SKC AirChek® TOUCH (SKC, PA, USA), to collect samples for subsequent Scanning Electron Microscopy (SEM) and Energy-dispersive X-ray spectroscopy (EDS) analysis. The samples were collect using a polycarbonate membrane filter (with 25 mm diameter and 0.4 µm porosity) and a heat-treated quartz filter (DPM Cassette with 0.8 µm Impactor), since these types of filters were used in previous studies and proved to be effective for nanomaterials [10–12].

The monitoring campaign started with background measurements before any printing activity. Then, measurements were performed during three different tasks, previously described in Table 1.

Even though the printer works closed and has an exhausting system working during the printing activity to avoid emissions, the operator stands frequently near the control panel. For that reason, measurements were carried out during this task, to better know the risk of exposure to potential emissions while parts are being printed.

2.3. Qualitative Approach

Control Banding has been often used for studying the risk of exposure to ENM and has been suggested as a potential approach to assess the risk of exposure to incidental nanomaterials [8]. In 2021, Sousa, Silva and Arezes [13] published a review on control band, focusing the occupational exposure to incidental nanoparticles. This study provided an overview on different Control Banding approaches designed for ENM and their potential to be used for incidental nanomaterials, highlighting CB Nanotool and Stoffenmanager Nano as potential methods in this field, considering some adaptations. Therefore, Control Banding Nanotool (version 2.0) and Stoffenmanager Nano (version 1.0) were used in this case study. While both methods are control banding based, their approach is significantly different, especially regarding the inputs for the determination of bands and the risk control considerations.

CB Nanotool 2.0 was proposed in 2009 [14] and revalidated by its authors 10 years later [15]. Applying this method, it is possible to determine the risk level of a particular operation using a four-by-four matrix, based on severity and probability scores. The severity score depends on factors associated with the nanomaterial (70% of the severity score) and with the parent material (30% of the severity score). Nanomaterial (NM) factors include: Surface chemistry; particle shape; particle diameter; solubility; carcinogenicity;

reproductive toxicity; mutagenicity; dermal toxicity; and asthmagen. The parent material (PM) factors are scored considering: Occupational Exposure Limit (OEL); carcinogenicity; Reproductive Toxicity; Mutagenicity; Dermal Toxicity; and Asthmagen. The second step is to reach the probability score, for which the following factors are considered: estimated amount of material used; dustiness/mistiness; number of employees with similar exposure; frequency of operation; and duration of operation. Finally, after reaching a severity and probability score, this tool leads to one of four risk levels (RL), which correspond to a certain control measure: RL 1—general ventilation; RL 2—fume hoods or local exhaust ventilation; RL 3—containment; and RL 4—seeking specialist advice.

However, Stoffenmanager Nano 1.0 is a risk-banding tool created to prioritize the risk of exposure to manufactured nano-objects and to help defining control measures [16]. This tool defines five hazard bands (A being the least hazardous until E which is the most hazardous), considering hazardous characteristics of the nano-object under study, such as particle size, water solubility, persistent fibers or other structure and classification based on data available on the nano-object or on the hazardous potential of its parental material. Four exposure bands are also determined (1 to 4, with 1 being the lowest exposure), considering nine modifying factors related to source emission, transmission, and immission (receptor) Substance emission potential, handling (activity emission potential), localized controls segregation, dilution/dispersion, personal behavior, separation (personal enclosure), surface contamination, and respiratory protective equipment. The online tool guides the user through six steps:

- Step 1—General: Allows the user to select the source domain of potential release of nanomaterials, among four options: release of primary particles during actual synthesis; handling of bulk aggregated/agglomerated nanopowders; spraying or dispersion of a ready-to-use nanoproducts; or fracturing and abrasion of manufactured nano-objects-embedded end products.
- Step 2—Product characteristics: Includes information provided by product information sheets and/or material safety data sheets (if available), such as dustiness, moisture content, concentration, presence of fibers, and inhalation hazard.
- Step 3—Handling/process: Considers information to characterize tasks such as the way the product is handled, duration and frequency of the task, distance to the breathing zone of employees and number of employees performing the task.
- Step 4—Working area: Takes into account information on frequency of room cleaning, inspections and maintenance, as well as volume and ventilation conditions of the working room.
- Step 5—Local control measures and personal protective equipment (PPE): Includes information regarding control measures, location of the employees and type of PPE used during the task.
- Step 6—Risk assessment: Inputs of the 5 previous steps are considered to calculate the exposure-hazard-class and show the risk priority band using the risk matrix. Overall, 1 represents the highest priority and 3 the lowest priority.

2.4. Semi-Quantitative Approach—Proposal for a New Risk Management Method

After applying the previously mentioned qualitative and quantitative approaches in this case study, a different approach was designed. As highlighted by Sousa et al. [13], the existing qualitative and quantitative approaches have significant limitations when aiming to manage the risk of exposure to incidental nanomaterials, mainly during metal 3D printing. Therefore, in this study, a new semi-quantitative risk management tool was designed and verified.

The IN Nanotool is based on control banding and aims to enable the risk management of exposure to incidental metal nanomaterials released in AM processes. The existing control banding methods for studying the risk associated with exposure to nanomaterials in workplaces were designed for engineered nanomaterials [13]. However, there is a need to create methods to study the risk of exposure to incidental ones, since the number of workers exposed to them is significantly higher than the ones exposed to ENM [17].

Therefore, IN Nanotool was designed taking into consideration the limitations and opportunities already identified in previous studies regarding exposure to incidental nanomaterials in addition to the results of this particular case study.

3. Results
3.1. Quantitative Assessment
3.1.1. On-Site Measurements

Temperature, relative humidity, and air velocity were determined to characterize the background environmental conditions of the prototyping room and the conditions near the 3D printer while it was printing, as shown in Table 2.

Table 2. Environmental characterization provided by the thermo-hygrometer: Air velocity, room temperature and relative humidity.

Measured Parameters	Background (before Printing)	Near the Printer (Close to the Door)
Temperature [°C]	27.4	28.1
Relative Humidity [%]	54.2	53.7
Air Velocity [m/s]	<0.01	0.17

The CPC provided the particle number concentration, from 10 nm to >1000 nm, during the three tasks under study, in addition to the background measurement. Table 3 indicates the mean particle number concentration for these four distinct periods. Additionally, Figure 1 illustrates how the concentration of this airborne particle changed over time during the trial.

Table 3. Results provided by the CPC.

	Background	Task 1	Task 2	Task 3
Time [min]	15	105	8	15
Mean particle number concentration [particles/cm^3]	6003.07	12,636.92	12,734.70	11,121.98

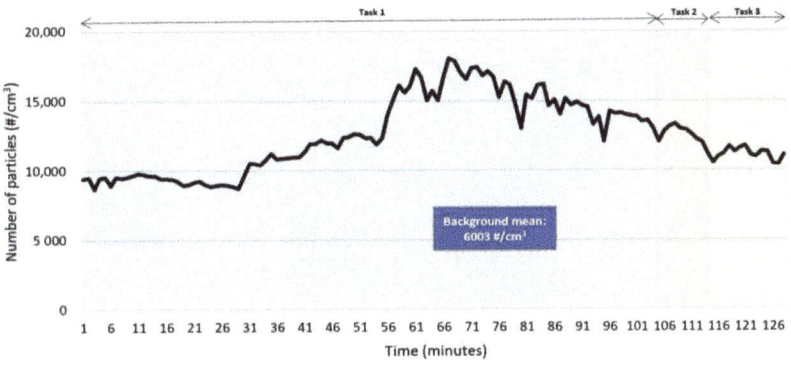

Figure 1. Number particle concentration (#/cm^3) over time measured by the CPC.

The SMPS allowed us to better understand the potential exposure to smaller particles, by providing the size distributions from 10 to 420 nm. The corresponding results are presented in Table 4 and Figure 2.

Table 4. Results provided by the SMPS: Mean particle number concentration (particles/cm^3) by particle size.

	11.5	15.4	20.5	27.4	36.5	48.7	64.9	86.6	115.5	154.0	205.4	273.8	365.2	Total	GSD [1]
Background	219.69	461.75	458.70	630.35	709.28	684.59	602.07	502.39	347.25	153.61	3.89	0.00	0.00	4773.58	40.63
Task 1	1080.31	1379.35	788.44	1129.41	1250.13	1010.95	654.65	430.89	278.75	129.33	13.35	0.00	0.12	8145.38	30.66
Task 2	883.65	1611.25	1146.33	1365.82	1430.65	1206.07	836.94	527.58	274.65	72.86	0.00	0.00	0.00	9355.81	30.27
Task 3	714.64	1436.72	1118.46	1292.11	1353.58	1177.73	856.14	543.37	266.28	54.00	0.00	0.00	0.00	8813.04	31.19

[1] Geometric Standard Deviation.

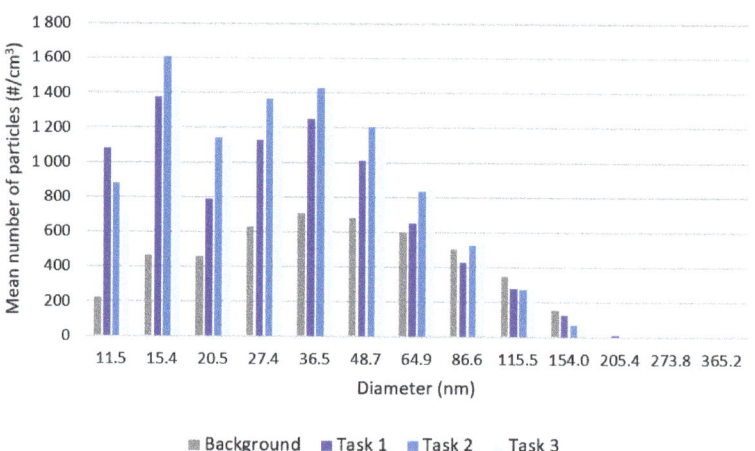

Figure 2. Results provided by the SMPS: Mean particle number concentration (particles/cm^3) by particle size range.

3.1.2. SEM and EDS

The data collection included two samples of stainless steel 316L: One of the raw powder before printing and other of the powder after the laser action, which is collected after printing to be reused in future prints. Scanning electron microscopy and energy-dispersive X-ray spectroscopy analysis were performed to these two samples, to study possible changes in size, shape and/or chemical composition. The results are shown in Figures 3–6.

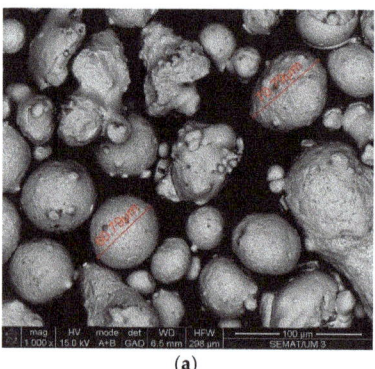
(**a**)

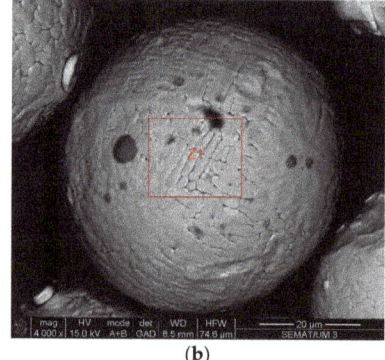
(**b**)

Figure 3. SEM analysis results: Stainless steel 316L raw powder, before any AM process. (**a**) Size and shape of particles in the sample; (**b**) image of the particle analyzed by EDS (results in Figure 4).

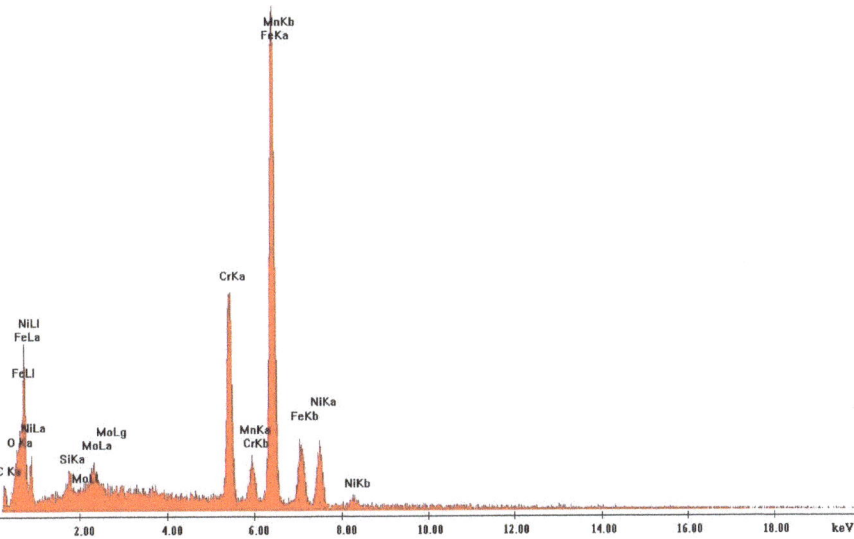

Figure 4. EDS analysis results: Stainless steel 316L raw powder, before any AM process.

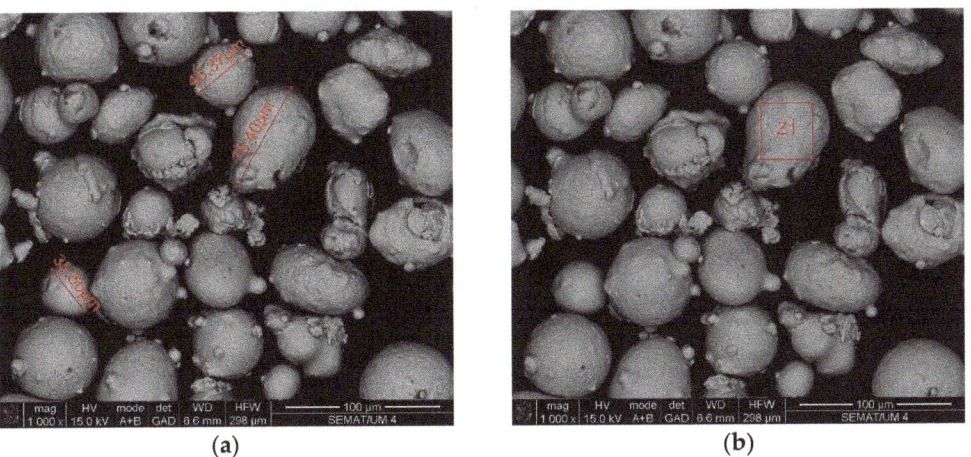

Figure 5. SEM analysis results: Stainless steel 316L powder after AM process. (**a**) Size and shape of particles in the sample; (**b**) image of the particle analyzed by EDS (results in Figure 6).

To better characterize the size and shape of the particles released to the work atmosphere during this AM process, the air samples collected on the polycarbonate membrane filter and on the heat-treated quartz filter were subjected to SEM. EDS analysis was also carried out to verify the elementary composition of these samples. Figures 7–10 illustrate these results.

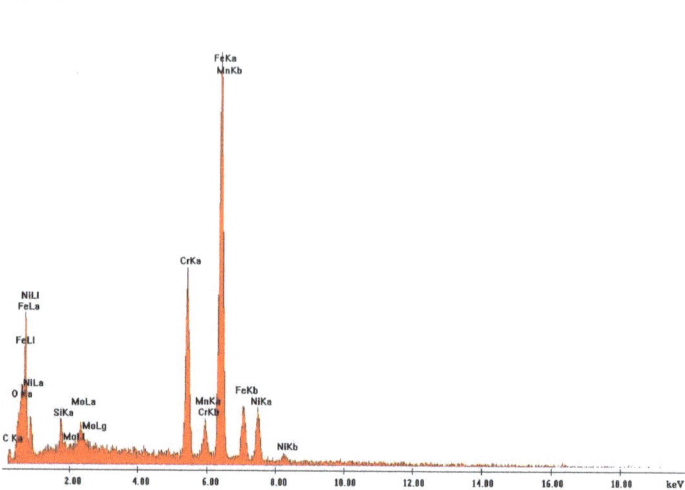

Figure 6. EDS analysis results: Stainless steel 316L powder after printing.

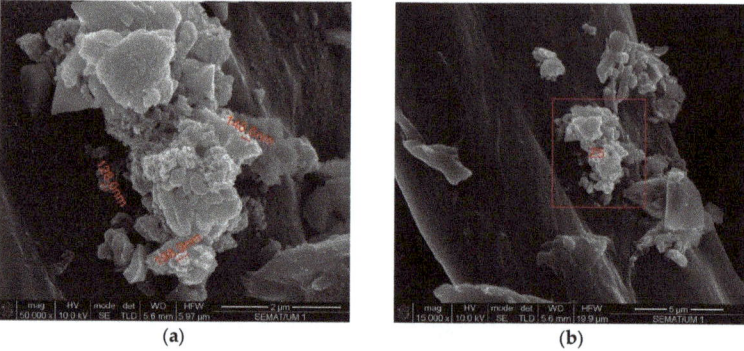

Figure 7. SEM analysis results: airborne sample collected on quartz filter. (**a**) Size and shape of particles in the sample; (**b**) image of the particle analyzed by EDS (results in Figure 8).

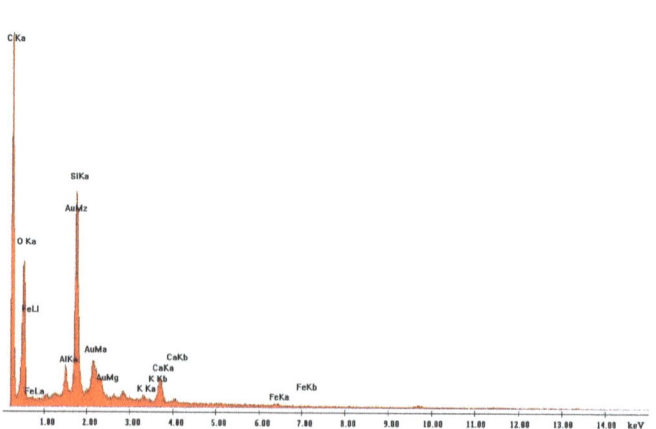

Figure 8. EDS analysis results: Airborne sample collected on quartz filter.

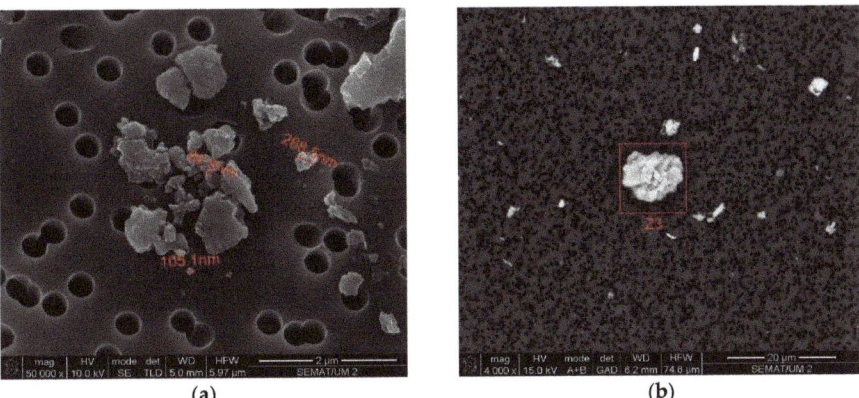

Figure 9. SEM analysis results: airborne sample collected on polycarbonate filter. (**a**) Size and shape of particles in the sample; (**b**) image of the particle analyzed by EDS (results in Figure 10).

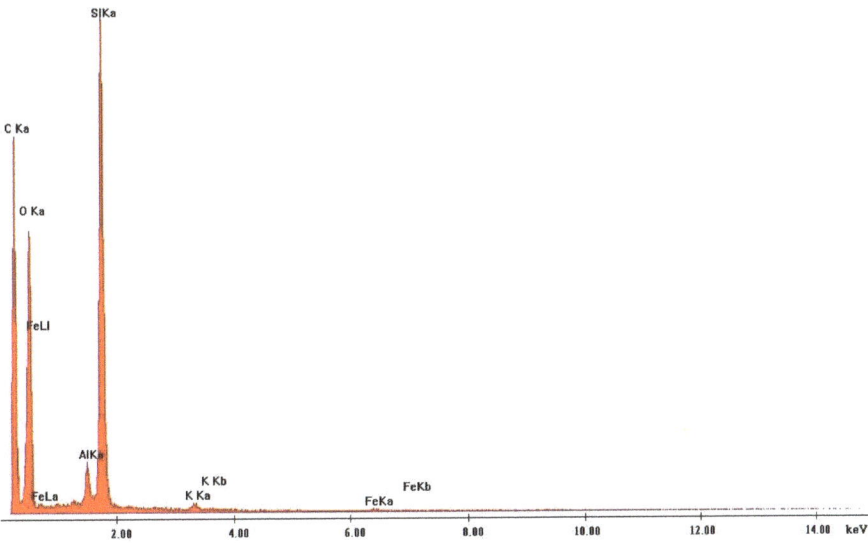

Figure 10. EDS analysis results: Airborne sample collected on polycarbonate filter.

3.2. Qualitative Assessment

3.2.1. Control Banding Nanotool 2.0

As mentioned before, CB Nanotool 2.0 was one of the methods used to qualitatively assess the risk of exposure to incidental nanoparticles during the tasks understudy. Table 5 summarizes the considerations and results of the application of this qualitative method.

Table 5. Results of the application of CB Nanotool version 2.0.

CB Factors	Task 1	Task 2	Task 3
PM OEL	200 µg/m³ [1]	200 µg/m³ [1]	200 µg/m³ [1]
PM Carcinogenicity	yes [2]	yes [2]	yes [2]
PM Reproductive Toxicity	no	no	no
PM Mutagenicity	no	no	no
PM Dermal Toxicity	yes [3]	yes [3]	yes [3]
PM Asthmagen	no	no	no
NM Surface Chemistry	unknown	unknown	unknown
NM Particle Shape	unknown	unknown	unknown
NM Particle Diameter	unknown	unknown	unknown
NM Solubility	unknown	unknown	unknown
NM Carcinogenicity	unknown	unknown	unknown
NM Reproductive Toxicity	unknown	unknown	unknown
NM Mutagenicity	unknown	unknown	unknown
NM Dermal Toxicity	unknown	unknown	unknown
NM Asthmagen	unknown	unknown	unknown
**Severity Score	Band**	63	High	63	High	63	High
Estimated amount of material used	>100 mg	>100 mg	>100 mg
Dustiness/mistiness	high	high	high
Number of employees with similar exposure	1–5	1–5	1–5
Frequency of operation	daily	daily	daily
Duration of operation	>4 h	<30 min	<30 min
**Probability Score	Band**	85	Probable	70	Likely	70	Likely
Risk Level and recommended controls	RL 4—Seek specialist advice	RL 3—Containment	RL 3—Containment

[1] Considering the lowest OEL recommended in Portugal: Nickel inorganic compounds (Portuguese Institute of Quality, 2014). [2] Carc. 2, H351 according to the material safety data sheet. [3] Skin Sens. 1, H317 according to the material safety data sheet.

3.2.2. Stoffenmanager Nano 1.0

The results of the application of Stoffenmanager Nano 1.0 to assess qualitatively the risk of exposure to incidental nanoparticles during the tasks understudy are in Table 6.

3.3. IN Nanotool—Design

3.3.1. Framework

As previously mentioned, one of the main goals of this study was to design a more accurate control banding based method to manage the risk of exposure to incidental nano-scale matter in metal AM workplaces. This was only possible after studying and understanding the limitations and potential of the currently used methods.

The IN Nanotool redefined inputs by adapting them to incidental nanomaterials originating from metal powders. Additionally, this tool added quantitative data as a potential input, given the possibility to include information on shape and size of nanomaterials, taking into consideration that many authors consider this information fundamental to classify hazards [16].

The IN Nanotool defines four hazard bands, considering metal powder properties and airborne nanomaterials properties, and four exposure bands, considering materials and operation conditions and existing control measures. Then, it allows for the determination of the risk level associated with the exposure to nanomaterials during metal AM, according to previously determined hazard and exposure bands, using a four-by-four matrix. Finally, this method recommends additional control measures depending on the risk level, as an increment to the existing ones.

Table 6. Results of the application of Stoffenmanager Nano 1.0.

CB Factors	Task 1	Task 2	Task 3
Product appearance	powder	powder	powder
Dustiness	very high	very high	very high
Moisture content	dry product	dry product	dry product
Exact concentration of the nano component	unknown	unknown	unknown
Concentration	small (1–10%)	small (1–10%)	small (1–10%)
Fibers or fiber like particles in the product	no	no	no
Inhalation hazard	unknown	unknown	unknown
OECD components	other MNOs	other MNOs	other MNOs
PM with one or more of the R phrases: R40, R42, R43, R45, R46, R49, R68 [1]	yes	yes	yes
Hazard Band	**E**	**E**	**E**
Task characterization	Handling of products in closed containers	Handling of products with low speed or little force	Handling of products with low speed or little force
Duration task	30–120 min/day	1–30 min/day	1–30 min/day
Frequency task	≈4 to 5 days/week	≈4 to 5 days/week	≈4 to 5 days/week
Distance head-product (breathing zone)	>1 m	<1 m	<1 m
More than one employee performing the task simultaneously	no	no	no
Room cleaned daily	yes	yes	yes
Inspections and maintenance of machines/ancillary equipment performed at least monthly	no	no	no
Volume of the working room	100–1000 m^3	100–1000 m^3	100–1000 m^3
Ventilation of the working room	Mechanical and/or natural ventilation	Mechanical and/or natural ventilation	Mechanical and/or natural ventilation
Local control measures	Containment of the source with local exhaust ventilation	none	none
The employee is situated in a cabin	no	no	no
Personal Protective Equipment used	none	Filter mask P3 (FFP3)	Filter mask P3 (FFP3)
Exposure Band	**1**	**2**	**2**
Risk Level	**RL 1—Highest priority**	**RL 1—Highest priority**	**RL 1—Highest priority**
Recommended controls	• Product elimination • Task elimination • Product substitution • Automation of tasks • Enclosure of the source • Local exhaust ventilation • Enclosure of the source in combination with local exhaust ventilation • Wetting of powders/substance • Applying glove boxes/bags • Use of a spraying booth • Use of work cabins with clean air supply • Use of work cabins without clean air supply • Respiratory protection		• Product elimination • Task elimination • Process adaptations • Product substitution • Automation of tasks • Enclosure of the source • Local exhaust ventilation • Enclosure of the source in combination with local exhaust ventilation • Wetting of powders/substance • Applying glove boxes/bags • Use of a spraying booth • Use of work cabins with clean air supply • Use of work cabins without clean air supply • Respiratory protection

[1] Defined in Annex III of European Union Directive 67/548/EEC, no longer in force; replaced by CLP Regulation No 1272/2008.

IN Nanotool was thought to be used by occupational safety and health (OSH) professionals, including non-experts. Therefore, it aims to be an intuitive and user-friendly tool maintaining the necessary accuracy for an assertive risk management, guaranteeing the safety and health conditions of exposed workers. The assessment steps are described in detail on the following subsubsections.

3.3.2. Hazard Band Determination

The hazard band is determined by the sum of all points from 11 different factors related to the metal powder characteristics (50 possible points out of 100) and the airborne nanomaterials characteristics (50 possible point out of 100), as summarized in Table 7.

Table 7. Hazard factors and points per factor.

Metal Powder Characteristics
1. Powder Carcinogenicity: score is assigned based on whether the material is carcinogenic or not. It is possible to confirm this information on the material safety data sheet, for example, by checking if any of these hazard statements are included in its hazard identification: H350, H351 (according to CLP Regulation). yes: 6   no: 0   unknown: 4.5
2. Powder Reproductive Toxicity: score is assigned based on whether the material is a reproductive hazard or not. It is possible to confirm this information on the material safety data sheet, for example, by checking if any of these hazard statements are included in its hazard identification: H360, H361, H362 (according to CLP Regulation). yes: 6   no: 0   unknown: 4.5
3. Powder Mutagenicity Toxicity: score is assigned based on whether the material is a mutagenic or not. It is possible to confirm this information on the material safety data sheet, for example, by checking if any of these hazard statements are included in its hazard identification: H340, H341 (according to CLP Regulation). yes: 6   no: 0   unknown: 4.5
4. Powder Dermal Toxicity: score is assigned based on whether the material is a dermal hazard or not. It is possible to confirm this information on the material safety data sheet, for example, by checking if any of these hazard statements are included in its hazard identification: H310, H311, H312 (according to CLP Regulation). yes: 6   no: 0   unknown: 4.5
5. Powder Inhalation Toxicity: score is assigned based on whether the material is toxic if inhaled or not. It is possible to confirm this information on the material safety data sheet, for example, by checking if any of these hazard statements are included in its hazard identification: H330, H331, H332, H333 (according to CLP Regulation). yes: 6   no: 0   unknown: 4.5
6. Other health hazards of the powder: score is assigned based on other hazards of the material besides the ones already scored in factors 1 to 5. It is possible to confirm this information on the material safety data sheet, for example, by checking if any hazard statement starting with H3 is included in its hazard identification (besides the ones already mentioned in factors 1 to 5). yes: 4   no: 0   unknown: 3
7. Lowest OEL applicable to powder [$\mu g/m^3$]: a different score is given depending on the lowest OEL defined for the metal powder's components. <$100\ \mu g/m^3$: 8 100–$1000\ \mu g/m^3$: 4 1001–$10{,}000\ \mu g/m^3$: 2   >$10{,}000\ \mu g/m^3$: 0   unknown: 6
8. Powder Solubility: score is given depending on the water-solubility of the material, considering it is soluble if the solubility higher than 1 g/L. If this property is unknown, 3 points are given. insoluble (<1 g/L): 4   soluble (>1 g/L): 0   unknown: 3
9. Powder Average particle size [μm]: the score is assigned according to the available information or analyzes performed. If unknown, 3 points are given. <50 μm: 4   50–1000 μm: 3   >100 μm: 1   unknown: 3
Airborne nanomaterials characteristics
10. Shape: the score is assigned according to available information, for example, to SEM or TEM analyzes results, considering the most common shape verified. If unknown, 18.75 points are given. tubular, fibrous: 25   anisotropic: 12.5   compact/spherical: 6.25   unknown: 18.75
11. Size: the score is assigned according to available information, for example, to SEM or TEM analyzes results, considering the main size of airborne materials. If unknown, 18.75 points are given. <100 nm: 25   100–500 nm: 12.5   >500: 6.25   unknown: 18.75

Regarding the properties of the metal powder, the first six factors are related with the hazard classification of the powder: Carcinogenicity, reproductive toxicity, mutagenicity, dermal toxicity, inhalation toxicity and/or other significant health hazards. These properties can be verified, for example, on the second section of the material safety data sheet (MSDS) of the product (hazard identification), confirming if any of the related hazard statements are included. Other CB methods for ENM also include some of this information [14,16,18]. Regardless, IN Nanotool attempts to better catalog these hazards in different factors and also to simplify the process of classification by using as guideline the related hazard statements, according to European Classification, Labelling and Packaging (CLP) Regulation. Many authors considerer that standardized communication, such as MSDS, should be the source of hazard information, including Stoffenmanager authors [19].

There are three more factors for the characteristics of the metal powder: Lowest Occupational Exposure Limit (OEL) applicable, solubility, and average particle size. The first one is based on the CB Nanotool factor Parent Material OEL, considering that it is important to take into account the known and already established occupational exposure limits. These limits may originate from bibliography, legislation, standardization or other reliable source. Next factor, solubility, is a physicochemical property considered in most CB approaches to study exposure to ENM [20]. A material is not considered water-soluble unless the solubility limit exceeds 1 g/L or is listed as soluble or highly water-soluble. Points are given considering that even if the material is soluble does not mean there is no hazard; thus nano-specific properties are expected to be lost when particles are in solution [16]. Finally, the average particle size factor is taken into account, since the size of the primary particles is an important input for a precautionary approach [21]. The particle size can sometimes be found in the material safety data sheet of the product or in its technical sheet. Alternatively, it is possible to obtain this information by performing a SEM or TEM analysis. The points are given depending on a range of sizes, that goes from smaller than 50 µm to higher that 100 µm. Even though, in SLM technology it is very common to use metal powders with a typical particle size of 40 µm [7], there are other technologies that use different size ranges. For instance, several AM technologies use metal powder between 15 to 100 µm [22].

To complete the hazard band determination, there are two significant factors related to the properties of airborne nanomaterials: Shape and size. Shape is also an input in CB Nanotool 2.0 for the severity band of ENM [14] and it was also considered in IN Nanotool given its relevance. It can be scored considering, for example, results of a SEM or TEM analysis. Regarding size, despite the definition of nanomaterial, cells and organisms are also affected by particles whose external dimensions are bigger than 100 nm, since cells are capable of absorbing particles of up to approximately 500 nm [21]. Therefore, it is possible to assign different scores in this last factor, depending on the main size range: Lower than 100 nm, between 100 and 500 nm or higher than 500 nm. This factor can be scored considering, for example, results of a SEM or TEM analysis. If it is not possible to obtain accurate information on the shape and size of airborne matter, the IN Nanotool allows the user to assign 18.75 points to each factor, assuming it is unknown. In fact, for all 11 factors it is possible to classify the factor as unknown, giving the uncertainty in these studies.

After assigning scores to all 11 factors, the hazard band is determined depending on the sum of these points. There are four different hazard bands: low (0–25), medium (26–50), high (51–75) or very high (76–100).

3.3.3. Exposure Band Determination

The exposure band is determined by the sum of all points from five distinct factors related to material operation conditions (60 possible points out of 100) and four factors associated with existing control measures (40 possible points out of 100), as presented in Table 8.

Table 8. Exposure factors and points per factor.

Operation Conditions			
1. Powder Dustiness: points are provided based on a judgment of whether the material's dustiness is high, medium, or low. If unknown, 11.5 points are given.			
high: 15	medium: 10	low: 5	unknown: 11.25
2. Frequency of operation: points are provided depending on the regularity of the procedure.			
daily: 10	weekly: 5	monthly: 2.5	>monthly: 0 — unknown: 7.5
3. Duration of operation (per day): score is assigned based on the daily time dedicated to the operation.			
>4 h: 10	1–4 h: 5	30–60 min: 2.5	<30 min: 0 — unknown: 7.5
4. Task characterization: points are provided based on a judgment of whether the quantity of dust generated and dispersed during the task is large, low or negligible during manual handling. If there is no manual handling or it is performed in a closed container (for example printing operation in a closed printer), 0 points are assigned to this factor.			
manual handling the powder where large quantities of dust are generated and dispersed: 15	manual handling the powder where low quantities of dust are generated and dispersed: 10	manual handling the powder where negligible quantities of dust are generated and dispersed: 5	no manual handling or handling in closed containers: 0
Existing control measures			
5. Working room control measures: points are provided by confirming on-site ventilation conditions.			
no general ventilation: 10	natural ventilation: 5	mechanical ventilation (alone or combined with natural ventilation): 0	unknown: 7.5
6. Source control measures: score is given by confirming the control measures on the source of emissions.			
no control measures at the source: 15	use of a product that limits the emission: 10	local exhaust ventilation or fume hood: 5	containment of the source or glove box or glove bag: 0
7. Preventive procedures: score is assigned according to the existing cleaning and maintenance routines.			
room cleaned daily and printer maintenance performed at least monthly: 0	cleaning and maintenance procedures less frequent than previous option: 10		unknown: 7.5
8. Worker related control measures: points are chosen considering the personal protective equipment (PPE) used by the worker.			
The worker does not work in a separate room/cabin and does not use any PPE: 5			
The worker uses eye protection and/or protective clothing (including gloves): 4			
The worker uses filter mask P2/FFP2: 4			
The worker uses filter mask P2/FFP2 and protective clothing (including gloves) or eye protection: 3			
The worker uses filter mask P2/FFP2, protective clothing (including gloves) and eye protection: 2.5			
The worker uses filter mask P3/FFP3: 3			
The worker uses filter mask P3/FFP3 and protective clothing (including gloves) or eye protection: 2.5			
The worker uses filter mask P3/FFP3, protective clothing (including gloves) and eye protection: 1			
The worker uses powered/supplied air respirator: 1			
The worker uses powered/supplied air respirator and protective clothing (including gloves) or eye protection: 0.5			
The worker uses powered/supplied air respirator, protective clothing (including gloves) and eye protection: 0			
The worker works in a separate room/cabin with independent ventilation system: 0			

The first five factors are related with the material and operation conditions: Dustiness, frequency of operation, duration of operation per day, task characterization and estimated amount of powder used in that task. When handling a powdered material, the main factor for intrinsic emission potential is dustiness [23], therefore this is factor number one in the exposure band factors of the IN Nanotool. Points are given based on a judgment of whether the material's dustiness is high, medium, or low. Most of these five factors are also considered in the other nano CB approaches, since they are essential to study exposure to nanomaterials [24]. In IN Nanotool, the number of employees exposure was not considered, since 3D printers usually are operated by only one or two workers, which means this is not a very relevant input to determine exposure in these workplaces.

The last four factors are related to existing control actions. Considering the already implemented control measures, it is possible to assess the actual exposure of the worker. Therefore, IN Nanotool follows a similar approach to Stoffenmanger Nano [16], which does not compromise the subsequent proposal for additional control measures that can be implemented and effectively reduce the risk.

After summing the scores of the nine factors, the exposure band is defined according to the following criteria: low if the score is under 25, medium if the score is between 26 and 50, high if between 51 and 75 or very high if the sum is 76 or higher.

3.3.4. Risk Level Determination

After defining the hazard and exposure bands, IN Nanotool allows the user to determine the risk level using a four-by-four matrix, as commonly used in other CB strategies [25]. This risk matrix is presented in Figure 11, and it is based on the matrix of the CB Nanotool 2.0.

		EXPOSURE BAND			
		Low	Medium	High	Very High
		0–25	26–50	51–75	76–100
HAZARD BAND	Very High 76–100	RL 3	RL 3	RL 4	RL 4
	High 51–75	RL 2	RL 2	RL 3	RL 4
	Medium 26–50	RL 1	RL 1	RL 2	RL 3
	Low 0–25	RL 1	RL 1	RL 1	RL 2

Figure 11. IN Nanotool risk matrix. The darker the color the higher the risk level.

3.3.5. Risk Control

The IN Nanotool aims not only to assess the risk of exposure to incidental metal nanomaterials, but also to help users to properly manage this risk by providing recommendations for risk control. These recommendations depend on the risk level and on the control measures already implemented. They aim to be an increment to the already existing measures. For each risk level, there is more than one recommendation. The user must analyze the options and select one (or more) that is not yet implemented and that can ideally have an impact on the higher scored factors. A new risk assessment may be performed after the implementation of the recommended controls, to validate the risk level decrease. However, when selecting the control, the user can take advantage of the tool to assess the impact of that measure in the risk level, helping to choose the more effective control measure. Table 9 shows the list of recommended additional control measures based on risk level.

3.4. IN Nanotool—Case Study Application

To experiment and verify the potential of IN Nanotool concept, this tool was applied to the SLM printer case study. The inputs had in consideration the MSDS and the technical sheet of the powder, the Portuguese Standard NP 1796:2014 (regarding the lowest OEL) [26], SEM results presented in Section 3.1, printer manufacturer information and in situ observation and consultation of workers. Table 10 shows the results of the application of the IN Nanotool to this case study.

Table 9. Recommended additional control measures based on risk level.

Risk Level	Total Score	Recommended Additional Control Measures Based on Risk Level
RL 4	151–200	Seek specialist advice Product replacement Task elimination or automatization Containment/Glove box/Glove bag Worker isolation (separate room/cabin)
RL 3	101–150	Task elimination or automatization Containment/Glove box/Glove bag Worker isolation (separate room/cabin) Local exhaust ventilation or fume hood Change operation conditions
RL 2	51–100	Worker isolation (separate room/cabin) Local exhaust ventilation or fume hood Change operation conditions Mechanical ventilation Change Personal Protective Equipment
RL 1	≤50	Change operation conditions Mechanical ventilation Change Personal Protective Equipment Improve internal preventive procedures

Table 10. Results of the application of the IN Nanotool.

CB Factors	Task 1	Task 2	Task 3
Powder Carcinogenicity	yes [1]	yes [1]	yes [1]
Powder Reproductive Toxicity	no	no	no
Powder Mutagenicity	no	no	no
Powder Dermal Toxicity	no	no	no
Powder Inhalation Toxicity	no	no	no
Other Hazards of the powder	yes [2]	yes [2]	yes [2]
Lowest OEL applicable to powder	200 µg/m^3 [3]	200 µg/m^3 [3]	200 µg/m^3 [3]
Powder Solubility	insoluble	insoluble	insoluble
Powder Average particle size	<50 µm	<50 µm	<50 µm
Airborne NM Shape	anisotropic	anisotropic	anisotropic
Airborne NM Size	100–500 nm	100–500 nm	100–500 nm
**Hazard Score	Band**	**47	Medium**	**47	Medium**	**47	Medium**
Powder Dustiness	high	high	high
Frequency of operation	daily	daily	daily
Duration of operation (per day)	1–4 h	<30 min	<30 min
Task characterization	No manual handing	Manual handling the powder where large quantities of dust are generated and dispersed	Manual handling the powder where large quantities of dust are generated and dispersed
Estimated amount powder used	100–1000 g	100–1000 g	100–1000 g
Local control measure—Working room	Natural ventilation	Natural ventilation	Natural ventilation
Local control measures—Source	Containment of the source	No control measures at the source	No control measures at the source
Local control measures—Preventive procedures	Room cleaned daily and printer maintenance performed at least	Room cleaned daily and printer maintenance performed at least	Room cleaned daily and printer maintenance performed at least
Local control measures—Worker	The worker uses protective clothing	The worker uses filter mask P3/FFP3 and protective clothing	The worker uses filter mask P3/FFP3 and protective clothing

Table 10. *Cont.*

Exposure Score | Band	46.5 | Medium	70 | High	70 | High
Risk Level	RL 1	RL 3	RL 3
Recommended controls	• Change operation conditions • Mechanical ventilation • Change Personal Protective Equipment • Improve internal preventive procedures	• Task elimination or automatization • Containment/Glove box/Glove bag • Worker isolation (separate room/cabin) • Local exhaust ventilation or fume hood • Change operation conditions	

[1] Carc. 2, H351 according to the material safety data sheet. [2] Skin Sens. 1, H317 and Stop RE 1, H372 according to the material safety data sheet. [3] Considering the lowest OEL recommended in Portugal: Nickel inorganic compounds (Portuguese Institute of Quality, 2014).

4. Discussion

4.1. Quantitative Assessment

On-site measurements showed the lowest mean number particle concentration on the background trial, as expected, since the printer was not yet operating. After the AM operation started, the highest mean number particle concentration was obtained while the worker removed the part from the printer and cleaned it with a brush (task 2), as shown in Table 3. This number is very close to the one measured during the first task (printing). In reality, when analyzing Figure 1, it is possible to verify that the highest values of the number of particles occurred during the printing process, and not during the subsequent tasks. This result may be an indicator that, although the metal parts are printed in a closed chamber, there is still emission of matter during the process that may be released into the work atmosphere. In fact, the real-time measurement of air velocity near the door of the printer indicated 0.17 m/s, as shown in Table 2, endorses this possibility, since it is significantly higher than the background measurement (<0.01 m/s). Regardless this finding, several studies showing results of workplace airborne matter measurements during metal 3D printing do not consider the printing process [5,6,8]. In view of these results, further investigation is needed in this field, to verify if currently containment conditions are enough to prevent workers' exposure to nanomaterials during printing processes, or if containment improvement is required and/or if safety-by-design measures are needed at the printer manufacturing stage.

The results of the SMPS shown in Table 4 are consistent with the ones from the CPC (Table 3). When comparing these results to the previously mentioned recommended value of 20,000 nanoparticles/cm^3 for an 8-h exposure time (mean number of particles between 10 and 100 nm lower than 9300 particles/cm^3 for all tasks), it is possible to conclude that the results are consistently lower, which does not mean an absence of risk. In Figure 2, it is possible to confirm that SMPS measurements indicate that the smaller particles are released during the printing activity.

Another finding of this quantitative approach, by using the EDS technology, was that there was no significant change in the chemical composition of the powder after laser action (Figures 4 and 6). The same results were achieved in similar studies [7]. The results of SEM analysis to the airborne samples (Figures 7 and 9) indicate the presence of agglomerates/aggregates of nanometer-scale particles, with an anisotropic shape.

This quantitative approach gives good insights on number particle concentration, size and shape of airborne matter, chemical composition, and environmental conditions.

4.2. Qualitative Assessment

Qualitative assessments present risk levels as a result and allow the user to access information on recommended controls. Additionally, opposite to quantitative analysis, this approach does not require access to measuring equipment.

Table 5 summarizes the application of CB Nanotool 2.0 to this case study. Since stainless steel 316L is an alloy of iron and chromium and contains a significant quantity of nickel ($\approx$12.5%), nickel inorganic compounds' OEL was considered as PM OEL, since it is the lowest one amount the significant components of this alloy. According to the material safety data sheet, the metal powder used is carcinogenic (H351) and skin sensitizing (H317), so PM carcinogenicity and PM dermal toxicity factors were scored as yes (this last one considering a precautionary approach). All nanomaterial related factors were classified as "unknown" since there is no information available for these airborne incidental nanomaterials. These considerations lead to a severity score of 63 (high band) for all tasks performed.

Regarding probability band, the amount of powder used in each task is similar (always more than 100 mg). So is the number of employees exposure and the frequency of the operation, thus scores were the same. Only the duration of the operation is different, so the probability score for task 1 (the longest one) is 85 (Probable band) and for task 2 and 3 the score is 70 (Likely band). According to these results, for task 1 it is recommended to seek specialist advice since risk level is the highest possible. For task 2 and 3 the recommendation is containment since the Risk Level is 3.

These results may be considered unexpected, since the highest risk level is usually associated with handling tasks, like sieving and cleaning [27]. Another observation of the CB Nanotool results is related to the recommended controls. Containment may not be adequate for task 2 and 3 since it may not be viable when carrying the part to remove it from the chamber of the machine and when removing the remains of powder.

However, Stoffenmanager Nano 1.0 lead to different results, as presented in Table 6 since it is a source-receptor model [28]. The criteria for the hazard band were the same for all tasks: dry powder with very high dustiness, small concentration of nanocomponents and unknown characteristics of the nanomaterials (concentration and inhalation hazard). In the factor related to OECD components, the option "other MNOs" was selected in the absence of another specific for incidental NM and, in the last factor, it was necessary to establish a relation between the current hazard identification and the one considered in this method, defined in Annex III of European Union Directive 67/548/EEC, which is no longer in force (replaced by CLP Regulation No 1272/2008). Hazard band E, the hazardous one, was therefore the result for the 3 tasks. In this method, hazard band E is assigned when the parental material is classified for carcinogenicity, mutagenicity, reproduction toxicity, or sensitization [16].

Concerning the exposure band, the duration of each task was considered, as well as distance to the breathing zone of the worker and specific existing local control measures for each operation. Thus, exposure band 1 was the result for task 1 (lowest band) and exposure band 2 for the other tasks. Despite the different exposure bands, the overall risk level for all tasks was RL 1 (highest priority).

Subsequent controls recommended for each task are listed in Table 6 and they are different for tasks 1 as it shows lower exposure. The recommendations for printing operation include automation of tasks and enclosure of the source, which are already implemented. It also mentions controls that are not viable for this operation, such as wetting the powder or eliminating this task, since it would compromise all the manufacturing process. For task 2 and 3, recommendations also mention already implemented controls, such as respiratory protection, and not suitable solutions, like using a spraying booth or wetting the powder.

When applying Stoffenmanager Nano 1.0 to this case study, the hazard band E was obtained for all tasks, therefore risk level 1 was the corresponding final result by default. In view of these results, it is possible to conclude that, although this method considers relevant inputs for incidental NM and considers some control measures already implemented, it is not a suitable method for metal AM workstations, since it does not differentiate the level of risk of different tasks performed and it does not provide tailored control actions aiming at the reduction of the exposure risk in these workplaces.

4.3. IN Nanotool

Considering all results and limitations from the previous described qualitative and quantitative approaches, IN Nanotool was designed for managing the exposure to incidental NM in metal 3D printing workstations and it was applied in this case study. The results of this application are presented in Table 10, in which it is possible to verify that the results obtained by using the IN Nanotool are significantly different from the ones achieved by the other approaches.

When analyzing the hazard band, the first six factors were provided by the properties of the metal powder present in the MSDS of the product, being clear that it is a powder with carcinogenicity and other associated health hazards. The lowest OEL criteria was the same as the one used for CB Nanotool 2.0 application. According to its MSDS the powder is water insoluble, and the average particle size range is between 20 and 53 μm. The two remaining factors to define the hazard band (shape and size) were possible to score due to the results of SEM analysis (Figures 7 and 9). If these SEM results would not be available, the score of these two factors would be 18.75 (unknown), which would increase the hazard band, since a precautionary approach is intended. The hazard band obtained for all three tasks is Medium (47 points), since the material used is the same throughout all 3D printing process.

Regarding the exposure band in this case study, material and operation conditions were determined by observing the conditions in situ and consulting the organization and the workers involved. The outcome was an exposure score of 46.5 (medium band) for task 1, mainly because it was considered that there is containment of the source and high dustiness, even though the time of exposure is higher, and no PPE were used during this period. For tasks 2 and 3 the exposure score was 70, meaning the exposure band is high. In this case, although the worker uses filter mask FFP3 and protective clothing, no eye protection is used and there is no containment of the source or isolation of the worker, when dustiness is high.

Using the risk matrix from Figure 11, it is possible to conclude that the printing process represents a Risk Level 1 and the other two tasks a Risk Level 3. These results are different from the ones obtained by applying CB Nanotool 2.0 and Stoffenmanager Nano 1.0. Using IN Nanotool, distinct risk levels are obtained for considerably different operations and the results seem to support the belief that not contained manual handling processes are the ones with higher risk [26].

It should be highlighted that in this case study using IN Nanotool the highest risk level (RL4) was not assigned to any of the tasks under study. This is aligned with the quantitative results, that show that the measured number particle concentration was not high when comparing to other metal 3D printing case studies [6,8] and to previously mentioned nano reference values.

Finally, according to the IN Nanotool, additional risk control measures should be considered. Critically analyzing the recommended controls for task 1 (see Table 10), in addition to the already containment of source, mechanical ventilation can be installed in the room, the operation conditions can change (for example, by reducing the frequency and/or duration), additional PPE can be used by precaution and/or internal procedures can be improved. For tasks 2 and 3, it is possible to clean the part with a brush and to sieve the powder in a glove box or bag, to install local exhaust ventilation or fume hood and/or to change operation conditions.

5. Conclusions

The difficulties to manage the risk of exposure to incidental nanomaterials and the lack of information on this matter have been recently discussed and are a cause of concern. Quantitative assessments require access to specific measurement equipment and don't provide control recommendations, requiring expert knowledge to assess and control the risk. On the other hand, limiting the risk management approach to the existing qualitative tools focused on ENM may be biased. Using those methods for incidental NM represents a significant difficulty in background data gathering, as shown in this case study.

The main objective of this study was to explore and highlight these difficulties and to design and test a tool to manage the risk of exposure to metal incidental NM in 3D printing processes. IN Nanotool redefined the inputs of CB approaches for incidental NM and added quantitative ones. Unlike quantitative approaches, this method does not necessary require special measurement equipment and it is not dependent from reference or limit values. Moreover, this method culminates in risk control recommendations, allowing to manage the risk of exposure to airborne incidental NM originated in metal AM processes, without the need to resort to a specialist. This tool was designed to enable this risk management, by providing a comprehensive and accessible approach to OSH professionals, including non-experts. However, there are limitations to this method. For instance, if the user does not have access to majority of background information, the method allows to score factors as unknown, resulting in a high risk level. This precautionary result may lead to the suggestion of exaggerated control measures in relation to the real risk. Additionally, this tool requires additional testing and further validation. Regardless of its limitations, the IN Nanotool application to the present case study led to reliable results that are more in line with the state-of-the-art, showing its potential to fill the lack of methods for incidental NM.

Author Contributions: Conceptualization, M.S., P.A. and F.S.; methodology, M.S., P.A. and F.S.; validation, P.A. and F.S.; investigation, M.S.; writing—review and editing, M.S., P.A. and F.S.; supervision, P.A. and F.S. All authors have read and agreed to the published version of the manuscript.

Funding: This research received no external funding.

Institutional Review Board Statement: Not applicable.

Informed Consent Statement: Not applicable.

Data Availability Statement: No new data were created or analyzed in this study. Data sharing is not applicable to this article.

Acknowledgments: The results of this study would not be possible to obtain without the support of the organization where measurements were performed. We wish to acknowledge the help provided by the board of the organization and the workers involved in the study. Additionally, we express our acknowledgments to CTCV (Technological Center of Ceramics and Glass) for the measuring equipment providing during the monitoring campaign.

Conflicts of Interest: The authors declare no conflict of interest.

References

1. Duda, T.; Raghavan, L.V. 3D Metal Printing Technology. *IFAC-PapersOnLine* **2016**, *49*, 103–110. [CrossRef]
2. Graff, P.; Ståhlbom, B.; Nordenberg, E.; Graichen, A.; Johansson, P.; Karlsson, H. Evaluating Measuring Techniques for Occupational Exposure during Additive Manufacturing of Metals: A Pilot Study. *J. Ind. Ecol.* **2017**, *21*, S120–S129. [CrossRef]
3. Ljunggren, S.A.; Karlsson, H.; Ståhlbom, B.; Krapi, B.; Fornander, L.; Karlsson, L.E.; Bergström, B.; Nordenberg, E.; Ervik, T.K.; Graff, P. Biomonitoring of Metal Exposure during Additive Manufacturing (3D Printing). *Saf. Health Work* **2019**, *10*, 518–526. [CrossRef] [PubMed]
4. Leso, V.; Ercolano, M.L.; Mazzotta, I.; Romano, M.; Cannavacciuolo, F.; Iavicoli, I. Three-Dimensional (3D) Printing: Implications for Risk Assessment and Management in Occupational Settings. *Ann. Work Expo. Health* **2021**, *65*, 617–634. [CrossRef] [PubMed]
5. Dugheri, S.; Cappelli, G.; Trevisani, L.; Kemble, S.; Paone, F.; Rigacci, M.; Bucaletti, E.; Squillaci, D.; Mucci, N.; Arcangeli, G. A Qualitative and Quantitative Occupational Exposure Risk Assessment to Hazardous Substances during Powder-Bed Fusion Processes in Metal-Additive Manufacturing. *Safety* **2022**, *8*, 32. [CrossRef]
6. Jensen, A.C.; Harboe, H.; Brostrøm, A.; Jensen, K.A.; Fonseca, A.S. Nanoparticle Exposure and Workplace Measurements during Processes Related to 3D Printing of a Metal Object. *Front. Public Health* **2020**, *8*, 608718. [CrossRef]
7. Mellin, P.; Jönsson, C.; Åkermo, M.; Fernberg, P.; Nordenberg, E.; Brodin, H.; Strondl, A. Nano-sized by-products from metal 3D printing, composite manufacturing and fabric production. *J. Clean. Prod.* **2016**, *139*, 1224–1233. [CrossRef]
8. Sousa, M.; Arezes, P.; Silva, F. Occupational exposure to ultrafine particles in metal additive manufacturing: A qualitative and quantitative risk assessment. *Int. J. Environ. Res. Public Health* **2021**, *18*, 9788. [CrossRef]
9. Hendrikx, B.; Van Broekhuizen, P. Nano reference values in the Netherlands. *Gefahrst.–Reinhalt Luft* **2013**, *10*, 407–414.

10. Dewalle, P.; Sirven, J.B.; Roynette, A.; Gensdarmes, F.; Golanski, L.; Motellier, S. Airborne nanoparticle detection by sampling on filters and laser-induced breakdown spectroscopy analysis. *J. Phys. Conf. Ser.* **2011**, *304*, 012008. [CrossRef]
11. Tsai, C.S.J.; Hofmann, M.; Hallock, M.; Ellenbecker, M.; Kong, J. Assessment of exhaust emissions from carbon nanotube production and particle collection by sampling filters. *J. Air Waste Manag. Assoc.* **2015**, *65*, 1376–1385. [CrossRef] [PubMed]
12. Tsai, S.J.; Ada, E.; Isaacs, J.A.; Ellenbecker, M.J. Airborne nanoparticle exposures associated with the manual handling of nanoalumina and nanosilver in fume hoods. *J. Nanopart. Res.* **2009**, *11*, 147–161. [CrossRef]
13. Sousa, M.; Arezes, P.; Silva, F. Occupational exposure to incidental nanoparticles: A review on control banding. *J. Phys. Conf. Ser.* **2021**, *1953*, 012008. [CrossRef]
14. Zalk, D.M.; Paik, S.Y.; Swuste, P. Evaluating the Control Banding Nanotool: A qualitative risk assessment method for controlling nanoparticle exposures. *J. Nanopart. Res.* **2009**, *11*, 1685–1704. [CrossRef]
15. Zalk, D.M.; Paik, S.Y.; Chase, W.D. A Quantitative Validation of the Control Banding Nanotool. *Ann. Work Expo. Health* **2019**, *63*, 898–917. [CrossRef]
16. Van Duuren-Stuurman, B.; Vink, S.R.; Verbist, K.J.M.; Heussen, H.G.A.; Brouwer, D.H.; Kroese, D.E.D.; Van Niftrik, M.F.J.; Tielemans, E.; Fransman, W. Stoffenmanager nano version 1.0: A web-based tool for risk prioritization of airborne manufactured nano objects. *Ann. Occup. Hyg.* **2012**, *56*, 525–541.
17. Viitanen, A.K.; Uuksulainen, S.; Koivisto, A.J.; Hämeri, K.; Kauppinen, T. Workplace measurements of ultrafine particles-A literature review. *Ann. Work Expo. Health* **2017**, *61*, 749–758. [CrossRef]
18. Paik, S.Y.; Zalk, D.M.; Swuste, P. Application of a pilot control banding tool for risk level assessment and control of nanoparticle exposures. *Ann. Occup. Hyg.* **2008**, *52*, 419–428.
19. Juric, A.; Meldrum, R.; Liberda, E.N. Achieving Control of Occupational Exposures to Engineered Nanomaterials. *J. Occup. Environ. Hyg.* **2015**, *12*, 501–508. [CrossRef]
20. Lamon, L.; Aschberger, K.; Asturiol, D.; Richarz, A.; Worth, A. Grouping of nanomaterials to read-across hazard endpoints: A review. *Nanotoxicology* **2019**, *13*, 100–118. [CrossRef]
21. Höck, J.; Behra, R.; Bergamin, L.; Bourqui-Pittet, M.; Bosshard, C.; Epprecht, T.; Furrer, V.; Frey, S.; Gautschi, M.; Hofmann, H.; et al. *Guidelines on the Precautionary Matrix for Synthetic Nanomaterials*; Federal Office of Public Health and Federal Office for the Environment: Berne, Switzerland, 2018; pp. 1–46.
22. Tang, J.C.; Luo, J.P.; Huang, Y.J.; Sun, J.F.; Zhu, Z.Y.; Xu, J.Y.; Dargusch, M.S.; Yan, M. Immunological response triggered by metallic 3D printing powders. *Addit. Manuf.* **2020**, *35*, 101392. [CrossRef]
23. Schneider, T.; Brouwer, D.H.; Koponen, I.K.; Jensen, K.A.; Fransman, W.; Van Duuren-Stuurman, B.; Van Tongeren, M.; Tielemans, E. Conceptual model for assessment of inhalation exposure to manufactured nanoparticles. *J. Expo. Sci. Environ. Epidemiol.* **2011**, *21*, 450–463. [CrossRef] [PubMed]
24. Groso, A.; Petri-Fink, A.; Magrez, A.; Riediker, M.; Meyer, T. Management of nanomaterials safety in research environment. *Part. Fibre Toxicol.* **2010**, *7*, 40. [CrossRef]
25. Dimou, K.; Emond, C. Nanomaterials, and Occupational Health and Safety—A Literature Review about Control Banding and a Semi-Quantitative Method Proposed for Hazard Assessment. *J. Phys. Conf. Ser.* **2017**, *838*, 012020. [CrossRef]
26. CT042. *Standard NP 1796:2014*; Occupational Health and Safety: Occupational Exposure Limits and Biological Exposure Indices to Chemical Agents. Portuguese Institute of Quality: Lisbon, Portugal, 2014.
27. Chen, R.; Yin, H.; Cole, I.S.; Shen, S.; Zhou, X.; Wang, Y.; Tang, S. Exposure, assessment and health hazards of particulate matter in metal additive manufacturing: A review. *Chemosphere* **2020**, *259*, 127452. [CrossRef]
28. Brouwer, D.H. Control banding approaches for nanomaterials. *Ann. Occup. Hyg.* **2012**, *56*, 506–514.

Disclaimer/Publisher's Note: The statements, opinions and data contained in all publications are solely those of the individual author(s) and contributor(s) and not of MDPI and/or the editor(s). MDPI and/or the editor(s) disclaim responsibility for any injury to people or property resulting from any ideas, methods, instructions or products referred to in the content.

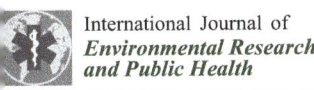

Article

Safety Management and Safety Performance Nexus: Role of Safety Consciousness, Safety Climate, and Responsible Leadership

Farida Saleem [1,*] and Muhammad Imran Malik [2]

[1] Department of Management, College of Business Administration, Prince Sultan University, Riyadh 11586, Saudi Arabia
[2] Department of Management Sciences, COMSATS University Islamabad, Attock Campus, Attock 43600, Pakistan
* Correspondence: fsaleem@psu.edu.sa

Abstract: Drawing from social system theory, social identity theory, and social exchange theory, this study examines how safety management practices are linked with employee safety performance through safety consciousness and safety climate. Furthermore, responsible leadership is introduced as a boundary condition in the safety consciousness—safety performance and safety climate—safety performance relationships. Data were collected from employees belonging to pharmaceutical firms located in different industrial zones of Lahore, Pakistan. The support is found for full mediation of safety consciousness and safety climate for the safety management and safety performance relationships. Responsible leadership moderates the safety consciousness—safety performance and safety climate—safety performance relationships so that when the safety climate is weak or the safety consciousness is low, a high level of responsible leadership enhances safety performance.

Keywords: safety performance; safety climate; safety consciousness; responsible leadership; industrial safety

1. Introduction

Occupational safety and safety performance can provide competitive advantage to the firms [1] and have has become a prominent area of research in the last three decades [2,3]. The focus of this research is to identify safety-related outcomes and to provide guidance for improving health and safety in organizations. An inadequate safety management system is the root cause of the majority of industrial disasters [4]. Hence, organizations' adoption of safety management systems is linked with their attempt to achieve performance excellence. Safety performance is one of the key factors for gaining a competitive advantage in today's rapidly globalizing world. Effective preventive measures like safety management systems or behavior-based system approaches can help in the reduction in occupational accidents.

According to the most recent data on workplace health and safety, there are currently 2 million people who believe their illnesses were made worse by their employment, and each employee loses an average of 30 million days (1.3 days) every year because of illness or injury [5,6]. This is a result of potential carelessness on the part of the companies in maintaining safety procedures. Some businesses fail to give health and safety the priority it needs, despite the clear necessity for proactive management. This could be the result of insufficient staff resources or a lack of expertise, skills, and motivation. However, employee safety management and alertness are the keys to reducing the ratio of work-related illnesses and accidents at work. Safety management relates to the real procedures, duties, and responsibilities involved in staying safe [7,8]. Safety consciousness, on the other hand, is the awareness of risks and the vigilance for danger. It has a strong

influence on the actions of an individual because of his desire to remain alive and uninjured. There is always a need to develop safety consciousness because most injuries can be traced to someone's lack of safety consciousness [3,9]. It is a key predictor of safety outcomes that has attracted limited attention.

According to Kirwan [8], safety management is related to all practices that are associated with remaining safe, which includes actual practices, roles, and functions. Safety management is a sub-system of organizational management systems that are integrated into the organization and has a focus on controlling the hazards that can negatively affect the health and safety of employees [4]. Safety management systems not only implement policies and procedures, activities that are required to control the hazards, but also comply with the existing legislation applicable to the organization. The safety management system is an important antecedent of a safety climate [3,4] and the development of safety consciousness in employees. A safety climate is the shared perception of employees regarding the state of safety of their organization [10]. Similarly, safety consciousness is the awareness of an individual regarding the safety issues and concerns of an organization [11]; this awareness can be at both cognitive and behavioral levels [4]. Neal et al. [12], and Vinod kumar and Bhasi [4], have considered safety climate as a factor that influences the safety performance (including safety compliance and safety participation) of an organization. de Koster et al. [13] identified safety consciousness as an antecedent of the safety performance of employees in an organization. Based on social system theory (SST), social identity theory (SIT), and social exchange theory (SET), safety consciousness and safety climate are both proposed as mediators for the safety management and safety performance relationship.

A responsible leadership role in safety management and performance relationship is implicit as the majority of organizations' central goal is to ensure the value of safety is in the minds of employees [14]. The personality, values, and choices that employees make the people they trust, the appeals they respond to, and the way they invest their time and energy in an organization are the outcomes of the values of leadership [14,15]. Based on social identity theory (SIT) and social exchange theory (SET), responsible leadership is proposed as moderator for the safety consciousness and safety performance and safety climate and safety performance relationships.

The importance of small and medium-sized enterprises (SMEs), especially in developing countries, cannot be denied. SMEs are considered a major contributing sector to the economic development of emerging and developing economies. Similar to other developing and emerging economies, most businesses in Pakistan are SMEs [16,17]. According to one report, about 99% of economic establishments are SMEs and their GDP contribution is 40% with 26% exports from the manufacturing sector [18]. The majority of firms in the pharmaceutical industry of Pakistan are SMEs [19]. Even though safety management and its outcomes have been researched and reported from various parts of the world, there is not much evidence available from small and medium-sized pharmaceutical firms in Pakistan, where safety performance is yet to get the priority it deserves.

The aim of the current investigation is to identify the impact of safety management practices on safety performance while taking safety consciousness and safety climate as mediators and responsible leadership as the moderator in pharmaceutical firms in Pakistan. This investigation is attempting to contribute to the literature in three ways first, by empirically investigating a comprehensive mediated moderation model of safety management and safety performance; second, by generalizing the safety management and safety performance investigations that are majorly focused on developed countries to a developing country; and last, by focusing on the pharmaceutical industry of Pakistan.

Theoretical Framework

The theoretical foundations for this study come from three theories, namely social systems theory, social identity theory, and social exchange theory. The social system theory [20] holds social behavior as the result of the interaction of the institution's role and expectations and individual personality and needs [21,22]. In an organization, organizational behaviors are products of interaction between the organizational factors and individual factors. The safety management practices adopted by the organizations in terms of safety-policy making, safety training, safety communication, and preventive planning lead to developing a safety climate that further boosts safety performance. Skyttner [23] stated that the emergence of anything results from the interaction of independent parts when they stop being independent and start to influence each other; therefore, it is posited that when individuals come together (the leader and employees) and develop a common sense of implementing safety in the organization it creates a safety climate in the organization, thus satisfying the social systems approach. It is noted that when individuals adopt safety practices, they try to achieve safety synergy [24], reflecting the social systems approach. Individual after individual following the safety standards combine together and make it a success.

Similarly, according to social identity theory, positive CSR perceptions (safety management, safety consciousness, safety climate, and safety performance) enhance organizational identification. This leads to the desire to maintain this positive identity and group membership, which later on translates into commitment. In safety-oriented organizations, the people feel safe and tend to retain their jobs for longer times.

The theory of social exchange [25] postulates that in any social interaction where one party acts in a manner that benefits a second party, a mutual expectation will emerge that obligates the second party to reciprocate, at some later stage, by acting in a way that benefits the first party [26]. The social exchange theory (SET) is a theory that describes relationships as result-oriented social behavior. It is based on the reciprocity of the behaviors. The social behavior in the interaction of organization and employees is used for a cost–benefit analysis to create a win–win situation [27]. In this situation of give and take, this study argues that responsible leaders, by virtue of taking care of the stakeholders [28], will ensure the formulation of effective health and safety policies and procedures, provide the necessary knowledge, skills, and abilities, provide support on such policies and procedures, communicate performance standards, and promote a safety climate. As suggested by the social exchange theory [25], responsible leaders will be fostering a trusting relationship among employees (as stakeholders) through their proactive participation in ensuring the implementation of health and safety procedures, thereby acting as role models of health and safety rules and regulations [29]. Moreover, it is noted that socially responsible behaviors such as safety behaviors cannot be implemented without the influence of the leaders [30]. Under such arguments, it is posited that when employees get something of value from their leaders, they try to give it back through their hard work and by following the practices they require from them to ensure performance targets. The employees who take training from their responsible leaders tend to stand with them and try their best to practice safety at the workplace, thus enforcing the social exchange. The proposed research framework is presented in Figure 1.

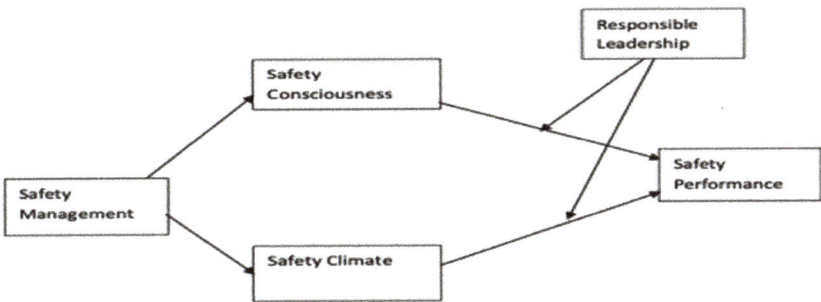

Figure 1. Proposed Research Framework.

2. Literature Review
2.1. Safety Management and Safety Consciousness

According to Barling et al. [11], safety consciousness consists of two components: the cognitive component and the behavioral component. This indicates that the idea goes beyond only being aware of safety risks and that taking necessary action is important too [31,32]. Furthermore, in the organizations, the modeling of behaviors depends upon demands put forth by the top managers. The managers emphasize the importance of health and safety policies and procedures and will inspire subordinates to ponder safety, hence increasing their safety consciousness [33]. Similarly, safety management requires clear communication of the health and safety policies. This requires the provision of training to the employees to enhance their subordinates' consciousness. Studies suggest that consciousness is an important predictor of safety behaviors.

The main goal of safety management is to prevent workplace injuries, illnesses, and deaths, as well as the suffering and financial hardships of the organizations [34]. The recommended practices use a proactive approach to managing workplace safety and health, instead of using the reactive ones, i.e., problems are addressed only after a worker is injured or becomes sick. These recommended practices recognize that finding and fixing hazards before they cause injury or illness is a far more effective approach [35].

The rate of accidents can be minimized through safety management and consciousness. This relationship forms a pattern that affects the well-being of all workers. The factor of luck may distort the pattern, but over a long period of time the pattern remains unchanged [36]. The employees are required to perform in a safer way that would not harm themselves and their co-workers [37]. Common causes of error may include time pressure, mental pressure, fatigue, being new to the task, distractions, and overconfidence.

The safety management practices enforced through safety policies, plans, procedures, training, and frequent safety communication enable people to avoid accidents [13,38]. The push to follow the safety practices from the managers adds to the consciousness. This consciousness as mindfulness brings positive results for individuals and organizations. Safety-conscious workers are more likely to notice potential risks, make unbiased judgments, and control their unsafe or risky behaviors [39,40]. Bahari [41] conducted a safety-related study and found that the employees' safety can be improved by employees' understanding of safety, knowledge about safety, and the skills necessary to ensure safety. Moreover, the management's attitude and actions toward safety were found to be crucial in improving organizational safety.

Accidents at work generally occur because of deficient knowledge or training, deficient supervision, and deficient procedures to carry out task safety [42]. The organizations can prevent the dangers via a safety policy implementation across the organization by setting safety objectives. This enables employees to achieve the set safety objectives, which directly means facing low risks and damage [43]. At the same time, preventive planning is a key to ensuring safety in organizations [44].

An effective way to promote safety management is safety communication. Pandit et al. [45] found safety communication to be an effective way of promoting safety management in the organization and poor safety communication can lead to disasters. It is also noted that when not only the managers but also the employees do not communicate frequently about the hazards involved in their work and possible preventive measures to be taken, this leads them to unexpected injuries. Safety training is equally important and enables employees to learn the relevant knowledge, skills, and abilities to tackle possible dangers [9]. The social systems theory posits that when components of a system combine and work in the same direction, they achieve a synergetic safety working (see Figure 1). Therefore, the hypothesis developed is:

Hypothesis 1. *There is a positive impact of safety management on safety consciousness.*

2.2. Safety Management and Safety Climate

Management concern for safety develops the safety climate. The safety climate is the perceptions and attitudes of the organization's workforce about surface features of the culture of safety in the organization at a given point in time [46]. Safety management is the adoption of practices to reduce errors, which fosters a safe climate in the organization. A better safety climate in an organization is associated with committing fewer errors and better outcomes.

Anticipated benefits would stem from the ability of organizations (use of safety practices) with strong safety climates to cultivate behaviors that enhance collective learning by addressing unproductive beliefs and attitudes about errors, their cause and cure [47].

According to Mearns et al. [48], the organizations that want safe operations have to ensure a safe climate. Research has focused on supervisors as role models for instilling safety awareness and supporting safe behavior [48]. Involvement of the workforce in safety-decision-making has also received attention [49]. These things require a consideration of the safety philosophy of upper management and the safety management system of the organization. Organizations with lower accident rates were characterized by the presence of upper managers who were personally involved in safety activities, the prioritization of safety in meetings and in decisions concerning work practices, and the thorough investigation of incidents [48,50]. The accumulation of the safety practices and compelling employees to follow the safety measures while at work makes a safety climate in the organization.

Guo et al. [51] noted that the climate can be developed through management emphasizing safety practices. A safety climate consists of social support, management safety commitment, knowledge of safety, and pressure of production. Management's commitment to safety has a direct relationship with social support [52]. Hence, management should establish clear policies on safety and safety issues that encourage people to follow safety standards. The present study posits that the managers with safety concerns will ensure the formulation of effective health and safety policies and procedures, provide necessary training on such policies and procedures, communicate performance standards, and promote a safety culture [53].

The safety climate is the shared perceptions of employees about the importance of safety within the organization. This is developed when the individual parts work together and develop a common sense of safety in the organization to make a system, as per social systems theory (see Figure 1). In the light of such arguments the hypothesis developed is:

Hypothesis 2. *There is a positive impact of safety management on safety climate.*

2.3. Safety Climate and Safety Performance

Griffin and Neal [54] argued that employees' perceptions of the policies, procedures, and practices relating to safety comprise the safety climate. The safety climate acts as a frame of reference for the behavior and attitudes of individuals and groups of employees, and it is argued that it will also affect their accident involvement. The employees with more favorable safety perceptions (indicating a positive safety climate) are less likely to engage in unsafe acts [55]. Safety performance is defined by Neal et al. [12] as the level of safety compliance and safety participation. Safety compliance means "adhering to safety procedures and carrying out work in a safe manner", and safety participation means "helping co-workers, promoting the safety program within the workplace, demonstrating initiative and putting effort into improving safety in the workplace" (p. 101).

Humans play an important role in the occurrence of workplace accidents, but the safety climate can achieve excellence in prevention [56]. At the individual level, the safety climate is concerned with employees' understanding of safety stimuli such as practices, procedures, and policies in the workplace. The safety climate, in fact, serves as a benchmark for directing and guiding suitable and adaptive safety behavior [57].

Guo et al. [51] believe that if individuals have favorable perceptions of safety, they are less likely to act unsafely on site. As a result, accident rates are likely to decline. As such, a safety climate can cause a profound change in employees' behavior and mentality, leading to true safety implementation, thus enhancing safety performance. Borgheipour et al. [52] found a positive result for a safety climate influencing safety performance. The safety climate inculcates danger-avoiding practices and improves safety performance. The safety climate encourages employees to learn safety practices, thus fostering safety performance.

Jafari et al. [58] worked on the development of the safety climate scale and found 10 dimensions, namely management commitment, workers' empowerment, communication, blame culture, safety training, job satisfaction, an interpersonal relationship, supervision, continuous improvement, and a reward system, to be effective in making the safety climate. Management commitment to safety and safety training make people capable of better safety performance. Eskandari et al. [59] developed a scale for measuring safety performance. They considered three factors for their examination, such as the organizational factors, the environmental factors, and the individual factors. They found organizational factors had the highest contribution toward safety performance. A safe climate is rightly considered an organizational factor that encompasses a common understanding of safety among employees.

A safety climate, that is, the common perceptions and attitudes of the employees about ensuring safety practices in the organization at a given point in time [46], leads to minimizing errors at work. This further leads to efficient working and low waste-age of resources, thus ensuring safety performance in the organization. Clarke [60] stated that the assumption underlying the link between an organizational safety climate and the accident rate is that climate provides guidance on suitable organizational behavior, so that a more positive climate encourages safe behaviors through organizational rewards (e.g., recognition and feedback for making safety suggestions), while a more negative safety climate reinforces unsafe behaviors by removing incentives to improve safety (e.g., prioritizing production over safety), which, in turn, are related to the occurrence of workplace accidents.

The social identity theory posits that positive corporate responsibility perceptions like providing safety training to the stakeholders, i.e., employees, having frequent communication, and so forth, leads to safety performance. The safety ensured in work leads to organizational identification. People tend to work in the organizations characterized by safety [61]. The hypothesis developed is:

Hypothesis 3. *There is a positive impact of a safety climate on safety performance.*

2.4. Safety Consciousness and Safety Performance

The employees' knowledge about safety standards encourages them to ensure safety performance. Worker engagement in safety may systematically act to reduce the probability of human errors from occurring by making workers more involved with and aware of their tasks/surroundings and associated risks, as well as the error traps that could be present. Thus, increased levels of worker engagement in safety activities could possibly be related to increased safety performance as measured by standard safety outcomes, i.e., accident rates [38].

Knowledge about safety standards and practices leads to enhanced levels of cognitive engagement [62]. The employees display focus, attention, and concentration on the safety aspects of the job. By displaying safety behavior, the employees working in the organization are known to be safety-minded people. Safety mindedness leads to leading others by example. They are the ones who are fond of continuous learning. They respond to feedback quickly and have strong communication skills. Safety-conscious people try not to harm others and make people learn safety practices by adopting safety organizational citizenship behaviors [63]. A positive safety climate is developed when the employees have a perception of management safety values and commitment to safety [48].

Safety consciousness refers to an "individual's own awareness of safety issues" [11]. This awareness works on both a cognitive and a behavioral level. Cognitively, safety consciousness means being mentally aware of safety in your work and knowing what behaviors foster operational safety. Behaviorally, safety consciousness enacts the behaviors that foster operational safety. Safety consciousness can be separated from the safety climate in a manner that safety consciousness is about the safety of oneself, whereas a safety climate is about the safety of the whole workplace in the organization. We argue that the extent to which the individuals are aware of the safety hazards and are aware of possibly avoiding them indicates whether they are in a better position to minimize the accidents, i.e., the safety performance. Safety performance is the extent to which companies are able to prevent accidents and errors.

Kelloway et al. [64] argued that if anything could reduce the chances of accidents, it would be employees' awareness of issues that threaten safety, their knowledge of how to prevent them, and their behaviors oriented toward preventing them (i.e., safety consciousness). Safety consciousness comes from the segments of the organization working together. Individuals, when seeing one another following the safety principles, tend to adopt safe work practices, which thus resembles the social systems theory. In light of the above arguments, the hypothesis developed is:

Hypothesis 4. *There is a positive impact of safety consciousness on safety performance.*

2.5. Responsible Leadership as Moderator for Safety Consciousness and Safety Performance

Clarke [60] noted that "there is very limited understanding of the impact of leadership styles on safety outcomes" (p. 1175). Except for a transformational leadership style, empowering leadership, and safety leadership, which drew more research attention, leadership styles have not been adequately investigated in this context [65–67]. Many argue that leaders are the prime drivers of high-reliability organizations (i.e., [68]). For example, top management is often responsible for the implementation of safety-enhancing systems and the development of a safety-oriented culture. When the responsible leaders weigh different stakeholder claims before deciding, it helps in building trust and people feel free to share their safety problems and seek solutions. This enhances safety consciousness and ensures safety performance. Rare evidence is available in the literature explaining responsible leadership with relation to safety outcomes. However, it is possible that when the leaders act as role models, as per social exchange theory, the people adopt the same behaviors as their role models [69]; this boosts safety compliance and performance.

Abbas et al. [70] argued that employees are the critical stakeholders of organizations and are responsible for protecting the organizational environment via their safety mindfulness and interpersonal interaction. The safety of mindfulness and interactions are shaped by the responsible leader's powerful forces of protection, acquisition, connection, and understanding [71]. In the presence of reinforcement from the responsible leaders, this mindfulness further leads to better safety performance.

Hypothesis 5. *Responsible leadership significantly moderates the relationship between safety consciousness and safety performance.*

2.6. Responsible Leadership as Moderator for Safety Climate and Safety Performance

Leaders demonstrate normatively appropriate conduct through personal actions and interpersonal relationships and promote such conduct to subordinates through two-way communication, reinforcement, and decision-making [72]. Rare evidence is available for responsible leaders influencing the safety outcomes. However, this mechanism can be explained as responsible leadership being characterized as involving stakeholders in decision-making and looking after their demands. Moreover, he has an idea of the consequences of his decisions on the stakeholders. This enables the employees to get involved in the safety procedures and they conduct periodic checks on the execution of the prevention plans. Furthermore, they participate in evaluating the risks. This premise is based on the social exchange theory. The positive exchanges taking place between the leader and the employees lead to compliance as a matter of showing gratitude. The hypothesis developed is:

Hypothesis 6. *Responsible leadership significantly moderates the relationship between safety climate and safety performance.*

3. Methodology

The population of the current study includes small and medium-sized pharmaceutical firms located in industrial zones of Lahore, Pakistan. A list of 100 small and medium-sized pharmaceutical firms operating in the industrial zone near Lahore, Pakistan was compiled. The criteria of the National SME Policy 2007 of Pakistan, "an enterprise with an employment size up to 250, capital of Rs. 25 million and annual sales up to Rs. 250 million", was used for defining an SME. Out of 100 firms, 37 agreed to participate in the study; hence, these 37 firms were contacted for data collection. CEO, plant manager, production manager, quality assurance manager, quality control manager, pharmacists, technical staff, and assistant managers were contacted via Google Forms, which was shared either through email or WhatsApp. A total of 209 fully completed self-report surveys were received and used for data analysis.

3.1. Data Collection

Self-administered survey forms were used for data collection. The purpose of the survey was to analyze the behavior of respondents toward the safety management practices, safety climate, level of safety consciousness, and safety performance of their firm and responsible leadership. A non-probability, convenience sampling technique was employed for respondent selection and data collection.

3.2. Instrumentation

For the measurement of safety management, an 18-item scale was adopted from Beatriz Fernández-Muñiz et al. [73]. The safety management scale has four subcategories, namely safety policy, training in safety, communication in prevention issues, and preventive planning. For the measurement of safety consciousness, a seven-item scale was adopted from Westaby and Lee [9]. Item samples are "I always take extra time to do things safely" and "People think of me as being an extremely safety-minded". A safety climate scale was adopted from Beatriz Fernández-Muñiz et al. [73] with seven items. Sample items are "Periodic checks conducted on execution of prevention plans and compliance level of regulations" and "Accidents and incidents reported, investigated, analyzed, and recorded". The variable safety performances were measured with the help of an eight-item scale developed and used by Beatriz Fernández-Muñiz et al. [74]. Similarly, a scale of responsible leadership with five items was adopted from Voegtlin [75]. Sample items are "My direct supervisor demonstrates awareness of the relevant stakeholder claims" and "My direct supervisor considers the consequences of decisions for the affected stakeholders". The survey instrument/questionnaire is attached in Appendix A.

4. Data Analysis

4.1. Descriptive Analysis

Majority of data collected were from males. Out of 209 responses, 128 were males, while the remaining 81 were females. Similarly, the majority of respondents were of the age group between 30–39 and were from lower- to middle-level management categories; 14% were holding undergraduate degrees, 67% had master's degrees, and the remaining 18% had higher-level degrees.

4.2. Common Method Variance

Self-reported data raise the issue of the potential effect of common method variance (CMV) [76]. Prior to hypothesis testing, CMV was tested using Harman's one-factor test by loading all items into a single factor. The results revealed that 33% of the variance is explained by the single factor that is below the recommended threshold value of 50%. The result revealed that the data are free from CMV.

4.3. Scale Validation

Confirmatory factor analysis (CFA), also known as the measurement model, was used as an analytical strategy for the validation of the scale. CFA was conducted using AMOS 17. SM 18, and SP 7 was removed at this stage as it was not successfully loaded into its latent construct. The results of CFA provided acceptable model-fit indices and are presented in Table 1.

Table 1. Results of confirmatory factor analysis (CFA).

Construct/Variable	βeta	Alpha	CR	AVE
Safety Management		0.973	0.975	0.740
SM1	0.775			
SM2	0.863			
SM3	0.866			
SM4	0.829			
SM5	0.831			
SM6	0.877			
SM7	0.833			
SM8	0.833			
SM9	0.778			
SM10	0.762			
SM11	0.787			
SM12	0.825			
SM13	0.853			
SM14	0.846			
SM15	0.862			
SM16	0.830			
SM17	0.780			
SM18				
Safety Consciousness		0.948	0.949	0.728
SC1	0.766			
SC2	0.843			
SC3	0.889			
SC4	0.858			
SC5	0.868			
SC6	0.895			
SC7	0.847			
Safety Climate		0.959	0.960	0.774
SCL1	0.830			
SCL2	0.867			
SCL3	0.889			
SCL4	0.889			
SCL5	0.906			
SCL6	0.897			
SCL7	0.880			
Responsible Leadership		0.903	0.907	0.662
RL1	0.744			
RL2	0.841			
RL3	0.886			
RL4	0.834			
RL5	0.753			
Safety Performance		0.948	0.949	0.728
SP1	0.848			
SP2	0.864			
SP3	0.862			
SP4	0.831			
SP5	0.859			
SP6	0.819			
SP8	0.887			
Goodness of fit indices				
$\chi^2 = 1482$; d.f. = 845; $\chi^2/\text{d.f.} = 1.75$; $p < 0.001$; CFI = 0.93; GFI = 0.76; AGFI = 0.73; RMR = 0.05; RMSEA = 0.06				

β: standardized coefficient; alpha: Cronbath's alpha; CR: composite reliability; AVE: average variance extracted.

4.4. Statistical Assumptions

The statistical assumptions including normality, reliability, and validity of the collected data were checked before hypothesis testing.

4.4.1. Normality Analysis

Univariate normality can be accessed through skewness and kurtosis indices, which should lie between the absolute value of 3 and 10, respectively [77]. The skewness values for the current data lies between −1.888 and 0.210, while kurtosis values were between −0.928 and 3.05, hence showing univariate normality in the dataset.

4.4.2. Reliability Analysis

Internal consistency and reliability of the dataset was checked using both Cronbatch's alpha values and composite reliability. The alpha values were calculated using SPSS 20, while composite reliability measures were obtained through CFA output. The overall scale provided the alpha of 0.911 while the alpha values were between 0.903 and 0.973 and composite reliability values were between 0.907–0.975 for each latent construct. The Cronbatch's alpha and composite reliability values for each latent construct presented in the model are given in Table 1.

4.4.3. Validity Analysis

Convergent validity can be achieved by getting the loadings of observed variables on their respective latent constructs significant ($p < 0.001$) and the squared multiple correlation value of each observed variable greater than 0.5. The validity analysis results indicated that the dataset was valid for further analysis. The values of squared multiple correlation are presented in Table 2.

Table 2. Descriptive statistics and correlations.

	Variable	No of Items	Mean	s.d.	SM	SC	SCL	RL	SP
1	SM	17	3.84	0.88	0.740				
2	SC	7	3.15	1.04	0.241 ** (0.058)	0.728			
3	SCL	7	3.44	1.06	0.159 * (0.025)	0.800 ** (0.640)	0.774		
4	RL	5	2.93	1.01	0.005 (0.0002)	0.233 ** (0.054)	0.181 ** (0.033)	0.662	
5	SP	7	3.91	0.89	0.024 (0.0005)	0.343 ** (0.1180)	0.431 ** (0.186)	−0.286 ** (0.082)	0.728

* correlation significant at 0.05. ** correlation significant at 0.01 shared variance are in parenthesis. AVE is on diagonal.

Similarly, the discriminant validity for the dataset was evaluated using the criteria presented by Fornell and Larker [78], where the shared variance of any construct should not be greater than the average variance extracted (AVE). The AVE value for every variable was greater than the shared variance of all variables, hence indicating a discriminant validity of the data.

4.5. Hypotheses Testing

All proposed hypotheses were tested using PROCESS Macro by Hayes [79]. PROCESS Macro was preferred over other analytical techniques because of its robustness and bootstrapping approach. The PROCESS Macro provides biased corrected 95% CI and can simultaneously analyze the moderation and mediation effect for complex models.

We have used an incremental approach to test our hypotheses, where at the first step we assessed two mediation models by taking safety consciousness and safety climate as mediators. After that, two moderation models taking safety consciousness and safety climate, respectively, were analyzed. Finally, the full mediation moderation model was assessed. In total, five models using PROCESS Macro have been analyzed.

4.6. Mediation Model

To test the first set of proposed hypotheses, PROCESS Macro (extension in SPSS) by Hayes [79] Model No. 4 was used. The results identified that SM has insignificant direct effect (B = −0.0641; $p > 0.10$) on SP. However, the indirect effect through SC is significant (B = 0.086; $p < 0.10$), hence identifying full mediation. Similarly, for safety climate as mediator, the SM has insignificant direct (B = −0.047; $p > 0.10$) and significant indirect effects (B = 0.069; $p < 0.10$) through safety climate, providing support for full mediation. The results of PROCESS Model 4 are presented in Tables 3 and 4.

Table 3. Five thousand bootstrap results for direct and indirect effects. PROCESS Model 4 (safety consciousness as mediator).

Path	Estimate	SE		
SM→SP (Direct Effect)	−0.0641	0.07		
SM→SC	0.285 *	0.08		
SC→SP	0.310 *	0.06		
Standardized Direct and Indirect Effects using 5000 Bootstrap 95% CI				
Path	Effect	SE	LL 95% CI	UL 95% CI
Direct Effect	−0.641	0.07	−0.199	0.071
Indirect Effect (SM→SC→SP)	0.086 *	0.04	0.025	0.164

SM: safety management; SP: safety performance: SC: safety consciousness; * $p < 0.10$.

Table 4. Five thousand bootstrap results for direct and indirect effects. PROCESS Model 4 (safety climate as mediator).

Path	Estimate	SE		
SM→SP (Direct Effect)	−0.047	0.06		
SM→SCL	0.192 *	0.08		
SCL→SP	0.371 *	0.05		
Standardized Direct and Indirect Effects using 5000 Bootstrap 95% CI				
Path	Effect	SE	LL 95% CI	UL 95% CI
Direct Effect	−0.047	0.06	−0.175	0.081
Indirect Effect (SM→SCL→SP)	0.069 *	0.04	0.066	0.144

SM: safety management; SP: safety performance: SCL: safety climate; * $p < 0.10$.

4.7. Moderation Analysis

PROCESS Macro (extension in SPSS) by Hayes [79] Model No. 1 was used to test the proposed moderation hypotheses for responsible leadership. PROCESS Macro by Hayes [79] was preferred over simple regression analysis using interaction term and structural equation modeling because of its robustness. PROCESS Macro uses a bootstrapping approach with biased corrected at 95% confidence intervals that calculates the Johnson-Neyman outputs for the interaction term. The variables that define product term were first mean centered. Conditioning values at mean and ±1SD and Johnson-Neyman outputs for the interaction graph were also calculated. We have used a separate PROCESS Model No. 1 for safety consciousness and safety climate. The result of PROCESS Model 1 are presented in Table 5.

Table 5. Five thousand bootstrap results for PROCESS Model No. 1, simple moderation analysis.

	DV: SP				DV: SP			
	Estimate	SE	LL 95% CI	UL 95% CI	Estimate	SE	LL 95% CI	UL 95% CI
SC	0.241 *	0.055	0.131	0.351				
RL	0.174 *	0.057	0.061	0.287				
SC*RL	−0.163 *	0.057	−0.265	−0.061				
SCL					0.302 *	0.053	0.196	0.407
RL					0.186 *	0.054	0.078	0.293
SCL*RL					−0.117 **	0.048	−0.212	−0.022
Model Fit								
F-value	17.22 *				23.02 *			
R2	0.20				0.25			
R2 Change	0.04 *				0.02 **			

SM: safety management; SP: safety performance: SCL: safety climate; SC: safety consciousness; RL: Responsible Leadership * $p < 0.01$, ** $p < 0.05$.

The results identified that the interaction terms for both SC (B = −0.163 *; $p < 0.01$) and SCL (B = −0.117 **; $p < 0.05$) were significant and there was no zero in the lower and upper bound of the 95% confidence interval. Interaction graphs for low and high (Mean ± SD) values of SC and RL and SCL and RL were plotted. The interaction graph of the SC and RL relationship (shown in Figure 2) suggests that RL significantly enhances the relationship between safety consciousness and safety performance when safety consciousness is low. The role of RL as moderator is significant at low levels of safety consciousness, and it becomes insignificant when safety consciousness is high. Similarly, for safety climate, in the interaction graph of the RL and SCL relationship (shown in Figure 3), RL is significant at low levels of safety climate. The slope test shows that the presence of RL enhances the positive relationship of SP and SC and SP and SCL when SC and SCL are low.

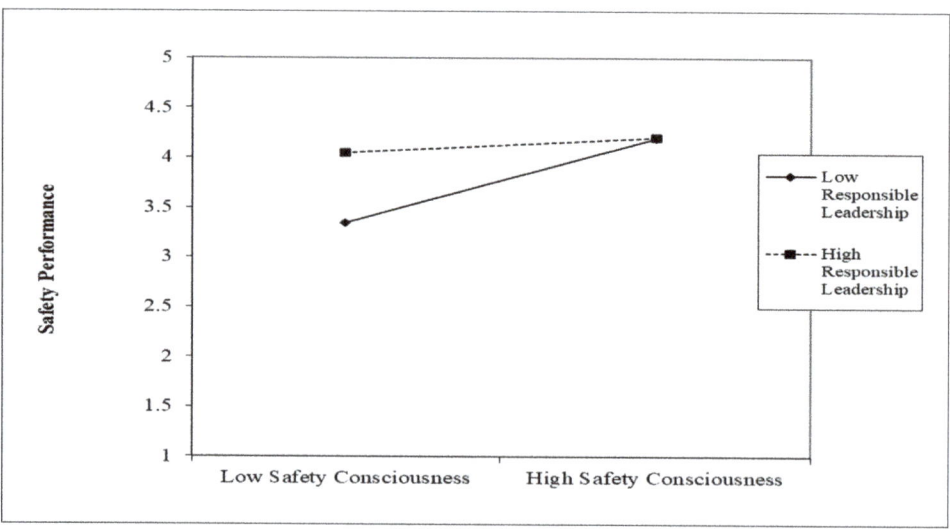

Figure 2. Interaction plot for responsible leadership and safety consciousness.

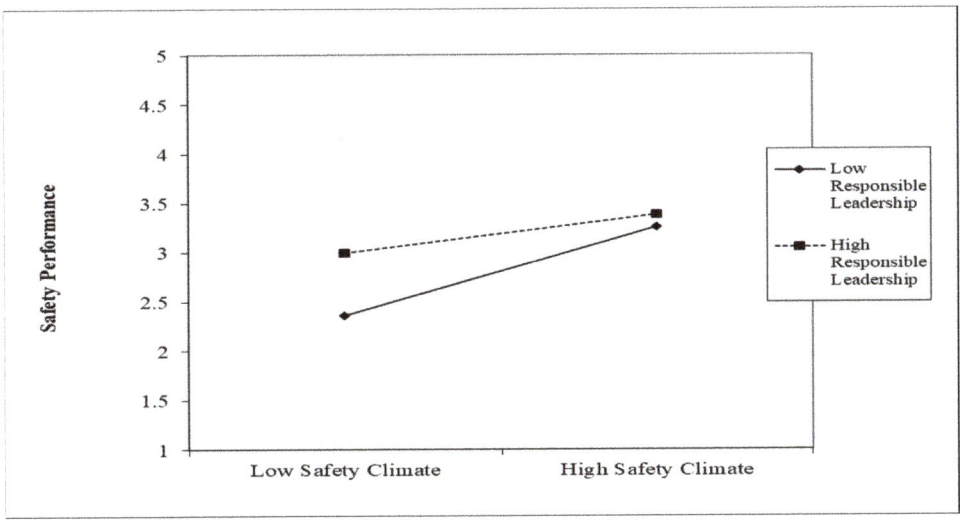

Figure 3. Interaction plot for responsible leadership and safety climate.

4.8. Mediated Moderation Analysis

Finally, to test mediation and moderation simultaneously, we have used PROCESS Macro Model No. 14 with 5000 bootstraps sampling and 95% biased corrected confidence intervals. We have run PROCESS Model No. 14 twice, one with safety consciousness as a mediator and one with safety climate as mediator. The results of moderated mediation analysis identified that there is a significant indirect effect of SM on SP through both SC and SCL. Out of the two proposed mediators, only safety consciousness has a significant index of mediated moderation (index = −0.457; LB: −0.1053; UB: −0.0069). Similarly, the conditional indirect effects (indirect effects in presence of moderators) of SM on SP were significant. The results of PROCESS Model No. 14 are presented in Table 6.

Table 6. Five thousand bootstrap results for PROCESS Model No. 14, mediated moderation analysis.

Path	Estimate	SE		
SM→SP (conditional direct Effect)	−0.025	0.06		
SM→SC	0.285 *	0.08		
SC→SP	0.247 *	0.06		
RL→SP	0.1730 *	0.06		
RL*SC→SP	−0.161 *	0.05		
SM→SP (conditional direct Effect)	−0.016	0.06		
SM→SCL	0.3045 *	0.05		
SCL→SP	0.192 **	0.08		
RL→SP	0.1856 *	0.05		
RL*SCL→SP	−0.167 **	0.07		
Conditional indirect effects of X on Y in presence of moderator using 5000 bootstrap 95% CI				
Path	Effect	SE	LL 95% CI	UL 95% CI
SA→SC→SP	0.4096 *	0.07	0.263	0.556
SA→SCL→SP	0.4214 *	0.06	0.296	0.547

SM: safety management; SP: safety performance: SCL: safety climate; SC: safety consciousness RL: Responsible Leadership, * $p < 0.01$, ** $p < 0.05$.

5. Discussion

Due to the considerable human and monetary costs associated with workplace accidents, it is important to study various factors that help reduce mishaps [80]. Various factors are examined to test the framework of this study. The results show a positive relationship between safety management and safety consciousness (Hypothesis 1) in the workplace. This study supports the findings of the earlier studies [81,82]. The employees are required to perform in a safer way that would not harm themselves and their co-workers [37]. This consciousness can be enhanced through developing a plan for work, reporting all the possible hazards, safety training, reporting all the hazards that actually occurred during the work, accepting the responsibility for any misconduct and taking measures to avoid them in the future, and teaching ourselves and our colleagues about preventing the accidents [38].

The safety standards and procedures enforced by the organization keep employees in touch with the use of safety procedures and can avoid dangerous situations [9]. Safety management can be made effective through safety policy, as a part of safety climate (Hypothesis 2). The policy helps coordinate the other HR policies to ensure employees well-being. The written policies show the management's concern for safety and this written document reminds the employees about the safety standards to be implemented while at work. The written documents also provide the procedures to follow to avoid any possible health hazards [13]. The policies available lead to continuous improvements in the workplace and save all from the dangers. Another important component of safety management is the priority of providing training to the employees to avoid any uneven situation at the workplace. The avoidance of dangerous situations and compelling others to be safe by themselves and keep others safe becomes mandatory while working, thus boosting safety consciousness [41].

The managers who provide safety training as a part of a safety climate, as a priority to learn safety measures, provide an opportunity to make a safe competitive environment that is safety performance (Hypothesis 3). People try to learn as much as they can to avoid accidents, thus adding to their safety consciousness [41]. The organizations must communicate about the risks associated with work. Frequent communications can help in two ways. First, the employees become aware of the hazards associated with their work, and, second, if anything goes wrong it will be well-communicated in time to reduce the damage as much as possible [45]. Better safety management frequently transmits the principles and rules of action. This makes people mindful of safety. Preventive planning is another way to add timely emergency plans that can reduce the possible level of danger at the workplace. Involving employees in making preventive plans can enable people to think of their safety, thus making people conscious of their safety. In short, policies, training, communication, and preventive planning collectively motivate employees to remain conscious of their workplace safety for positive outcomes [44] (Hypothesis 4).

The results of this study found a positive impact of safety management on the safety climate. Safety training, communication, preventive planning, and policy-making are important for developing a common sense of safety in the organization [41]. A written declaration available to and signed by all workers reflects management's concern for safety. This puts compulsion on the employees to develop a safe climate. Moreover, the safety policy puts emphasis on commitment to continuous improvement. This leads to conducting periodic checks on the execution of prevention plans [81].

The continuous and periodic training of employees enables them to apply their safety knowledge, skills, and abilities in a manner that saves themselves and their co-workers [9]. This also helps to keep procedures in place and to check the achievement of the objectives set. Similarly, the instruction manuals or work procedures elaborated can help employees prevent accidents. The frequent communication for transmitting the principles and rules of action leads to collective awareness [45]. Moreover, the written circulars and meetings inform workers about risks associated with their work and how to prevent possible accidents. Similarly, the written circulars and meetings force employees to conduct systematic inspections periodically. This ensures the effective functioning of the whole system.

Organizations that focus on emergency plans by practicing responsible leadership can protect employees from harm. Effective organizations always have emergency plans in place. The prevention plans are based on an assessment of the risk and employees are empowered to know the possible degree of risk. They keep themselves aware of the risks and try their best to be alert while assuming risky tasks [43] (Hypothesis 6).

The results show a positive impact of the safety climate on safety performance, i.e., consistent with the results [52,58,59]. The improvement in the safety climate means reducing potential safety threats. The employees conduct periodic checks as a result of the frequent communication and training provided to them. This enhances the compliance levels and ensures safety in the workplace [81]. The timetables available for the safety checks support compliance. The periodic checks of the procedures and equipment to use keep track of the personal protection equipment and keep the inventory up to date. That further strengthens the safety performance. The predetermined plans enable employees to improve working conditions by following the standard operating procedures and minimizing the errors involved. The minimized errors save time and other resources from wastage [47].

The results confirm the positivity in the relationship of these two variables, such as the findings of Lee et al. [82] and Wong et al. [81]. The higher the knowledge of the safety standards, the greater the application of the safety standards can be ensured. Moreover, one who is convinced about the use of safety procedures can compel himself and others to remain safety-minded [63]. At times it becomes difficult for the employees to use the safety equipment, but the policies and rules enforce the adoption of safety measures. The employees who remain involved in the evaluation of the safety risks tend to show discomfort when they see other people acting dangerously [44].

In the safety-enforced environment, the employees are compelled to make sure that other people do the things that are safe and healthy. Participation in setting the safety objectives and improving safety practices also gives a sense of ensuring collective safety at the workplace by inculcating safety-mindedness [52]. Compliance with the safety standards encourages employees to avoid dangerous situations. Participation of employees in the risk evaluations and safety inspections, and in making suggestions about improving the safety situation at the workplace, compel them to do the safest possible things as the best strategy [38].

Results found that responsible leadership is significant when the safety consciousness and safety performance relationship is low. The leaders play important roles in shaping safety behaviors (Hypothesis 5). As per the social exchange theory, socially responsible behaviors such as safety behaviors cannot be implemented without the influence of the leaders [30]. The leader's concern to take care of the stakeholders makes a stronger bond to keep closely in touch with the employees. The employees keep in touch with the leaders and share their concerns and problems about safety. The leader guides them and involves them in decision-making and setting the safety parameters. This involvement and the knowledge of the safety practices enhance the consciousness of employees and they become capable of avoiding accidents.

The results show that responsible leadership is a moderator for the safety climate and safety performance relationship (Hypothesis 6). The social exchange theory supports the leader's involvement in shaping the safety climate. The leaders who make people learn and develop a common sense of safety in the organization help people learn and retain the knowledge. This further leads to ensuring safety performance. Based on social identity theory and social exchange theory, this study aims to investigate the mechanisms underlying the responsible leadership, safety consciousness, and safety performance relationship.

Responsibility is one of the essential components of effective leadership in the field of organizational management [83]. Due to a lack of leadership accountability in today's accident-prone climate, businesses are experiencing a crisis of low trust. Lack of trust by employees make them pay less attention to the safety instructions given by their leaders, which leads to mishaps and a loss of health and safety. As a result, executives need to act more responsibly toward employees and other stakeholders. The socially responsible leaders are more effective and have greater impact on the organizations than other leadership styles [84]. As per social identity theory, the people are inclined to categorize themselves and others into social groups and establish a positive self-concept by identifying with groups that enhance their self-esteem.

Furthermore, individuals tend to boost their self-image by identifying with organizations recognized for their social engagement and responsibility [85], which subsequently motivates employees to strive for organizational safety objectives.

Additionally, people tend to feel better about themselves when they associate with organizations that are known for their social responsibility, such as with a safety climate [85]. This inspires employees to work toward the achievement of organizational safety objectives.

Furthermore, social exchange theory posits that individuals' voluntary actions are motivated by the returns they expect from others [25]; the responsible leaders take care of the stakeholders and in return the employees take care of the leaders and try to oblige them by following the safety standards, thus showing safety performance.

6. Conclusions

Three theories are supported through this examination: the social identity theory, the social systems theory, and the social exchange theory. Safety consciousness and safety climate are necessary for showing safety performance. Moreover, responsible leadership is the key to achieve better safety performance in the organization when the safety climate is weak or safety consciousness is low.

7. Implications

The following practical implications can be drawn from this investigation for the managers and policymakers. Prevention of accidents is only possible through inculcating safety consciousness, a safety climate, and safety performance in the organizations with responsible leaders who can enforce and implement safety standards in the organization through policy making, planning, training, and communication.

Safety management practices have a direct effect on the safety consciousness of the employees. Safety management can foster safety consciousness by means of policy-making, training, communication, and preventive planning that possibly protect the organizations from accidents and disasters. Employees with safety consciousness have a greater chance to avoid accidents and can remain healthy to perform without errors. The higher the level of consciousness, the greater will be the safety practices applied while doing work. Merely the presence of safety equipment or kits is not necessary, but the employees must have the tendency to remain safe and use the kits available to prevent dangers associated with their work.

The direct influence of management commitment on safety compliance can be considered as a result of the individual wisdom of the employees, earned from the overall interest shown by the management toward the safety of their employees, to protect themselves from accidents. Safety performance can become a priority for the employees by having the management's strong concern for safety. The role of responsible leadership is significant for developing safety consciousness, a safety climate, and safety performance of employees. The traits of responsible leadership should be developed in other top managers to prevent accidents.

8. Limitations

Like other research studies, this study has a few limitations. First, only a single sector/organization was selected for the study, which provided a limited sample size. Therefore, one should be cautious in generalizing the results of this study to other industries/sectors/organizations. Second, the companies with poor safety practices may have been reluctant to provide an original response to the questionnaire; therefore, there may be an influence from selection bias. Third, the survey itself was cross-sectional. A future longitudinal study could provide stronger support for causal relationships between safety climate and safety outcomes vis-a-vis the responsible leadership style used for the study.

Author Contributions: Conceptualization, F.S. and M.I.M.; methodology, F.S.; software, F.S.; validation, F.S. and M.I.M.; formal analysis, F.S.; investigation, F.S.; resources, F.S. and M.I.M.; data curation, F.S. and M.I.M.; writing—original draft preparation, F.S. and M.I.M.; writing—review and editing, M.I.M.; visualization, F.S. and M.I.M.; supervision, F.S. and M.I.M.; funding acquisition, F.S. All authors have read and agreed to the published version of the manuscript.

Funding: The APC was funded by Prince Sultan University, Riyadh, Saudi Arabia.

Informed Consent Statement: Informed consent was obtained from all subjects involved in the study.

Data Availability Statement: The data will be available on request from the corresponding author.

Acknowledgments: The authors would like to thank Prince Sultan University for providing APC for this article.

Conflicts of Interest: The authors declare no conflict of interest.

Appendix A. Survey Questionnaire

Safety consciousness adopted from and Westaby Lee [9]

1. I always take extra time to do things safely.
2. People think of me as being an extremely safety-minded person.
3. I always avoid dangerous situations.
4. I take a lot of extra time to do something safely even if it slows my performance.
5. I often find myself making sure that other people do things that are safe and healthy.
6. I get upset when I see other people acting dangerously.
7. Doing the safest possible thing is always the best thing.

Safety compliance and performance adopted from Beatriz Fernández-Muñiz et al. [74]

1. I always comply with the safety standards and procedures.
2. I am convinced about the importance of the safety procedures.
3. I use the personal protection equipment even if it is uncomfortable.
4. I participate in setting objectives and drawing up plans to improve safety.
5. I participate in evaluating risk.
6. I participate in the safety inspections.
7. I make suggestions about how to improve the working conditions.
8. I frequently discuss safety problems with their superiors.

Safety climate adopted from Beatriz Fernández-Muñiz et al. [73]

1. Periodic checks conducted on execution of prevention plans and compliance level of regulations.
2. Standards or pre-determined plans and actions are compared, evaluating implementation and efficacy in order to identify corrective action.
3. Procedures in place (reports, periodic statistics) to check achievement of objectives allocated to managers.
4. Systematic inspections conducted periodically to ensure effective functioning of whole system.
5. Accidents and incidents reported, investigated, analyzed, and recorded.
6. Firm's accident rates regularly compared with those of other organizations from same sector using similar production processes.
7. Firm's techniques and management practices regularly compared with those of other organizations from all sectors, to obtain new ideas about management of similar problems.

Safety management adopted from Beatriz Fernández-Muñiz et al. [73]

1. Safety policy:
    (1) Firm coordinates its health and safety policies with other HR policies to ensure commitment and well-being of workers.

(2) Written declaration is available to all workers reflecting management's concern for safety, principles of action and objectives to achieve.
(3) Safety policy contains commitment to continuous improvement, attempting to improve objectives already achieved.

2. Training in safety:
(1) Worker given sufficient training period when entering firm, changing jobs or using new technique.
(2) Training actions continuous and periodic, integrated in formally established training plan.
(3) Training plan decided jointly with workers or their representatives.
(4) Firm helps workers to train in-house (leave, grants).
(5) Instruction manuals or work procedures elaborated to aid in preventive action.

3. Communication in prevention issues:
(1) There is a fluent communication embodied in periodic and frequent meetings, campaigns or oral presentations to transmit principles and rules of action.
(2) Information systems made available to affected workers prior to modifications and changes in production processes, job positions or expected investments.
(3) Written circulars elaborated on and meetings organized to inform workers about risks associated with their work and how to prevent accidents.

4. Preventive planning:
(1) Prevention plans formulated setting measures to take on basis of information provided by risks assessment in all job positions.
(2) Standards of action or work procedures elaborated on basis of risk evaluation.
(3) Prevention plans circulated among all workers.
(4) Firm has elaborated emergency plan for serious risks or catastrophes.
(5) Firm has implemented its emergency plan.
(6) All workers informed about emergency plan.
(7) Periodic simulations carried out to check efficacy of emergency plan.

Responsible leadership adopted from Voegtlin (2011) [75]

1. My direct supervisor demonstrates awareness of the relevant stakeholder claims.
2. My direct supervisor considers the consequences of decisions for the affected stakeholders.
3. My direct supervisor involves the affected stakeholders in the decision-making process.
4. My direct supervisor weighs different stakeholder claims before making a decision.
5. My direct supervisor tries to achieve a consensus among the affected stakeholders.

References

1. Daito, A.; Riyanto, S.; Nusraningrum, D. Human Resource Management Strategy and Safety Culture as Competitive Advantages in Order to Improve Construction Company Performance. *Bus. Entrep. Rev.* **2020**, *20*, 123–140.
2. Majid, S.; Nugraha, A.; Sulistiyono, B.; Suryaningsih, L.; Widodo, S.; Kholdun, A.; Endri, E. The effect of safety risk management and airport personnel competency on aviation safety performance. *Uncertain Supply Chain Manag.* **2022**, *10*, 1509–1522. [CrossRef]
3. Zhang, S.; Hua, X.; Huang, G.; Shi, X. How Does Leadership in Safety Management Affect Employees' Safety Performance? A Case Study from Mining Enterprises in China. *Int. J. Environ. Res. Public Health* **2022**, *19*, 6187. [CrossRef]
4. Vinodkumar, M.N.; Bhasi, M. Safety management practices and safety behaviour: Assessing the mediating role of safety knowledge and motivation. *Accid. Anal. Prev.* **2010**, *42*, 2082–2093. [CrossRef]
5. Lan, T.; Goh, Y.M.; Jensen, O.; Asmore, A.S. The impact of climate change on workplace safety and health hazard in facilities management: An in-depth review. *Saf. Sci.* **2022**, *151*, 105745. [CrossRef]
6. Black, C.D.; Frost, D. *Health at Work—An Independent Review of Sickness Absence*; TSO: London, UK, 2011.
7. Intini, P.; Berloco, N.; Coropulis, S.; Gentile, R.; Ranieri, V. The use of macro-level safety performance functions for province-wide road safety management. *Sustainability* **2022**, *14*, 9245. [CrossRef]
8. Kirwan, B. Safety management assessment and task analysis—A missing link? In *Safety Management: The Challenge of Change*; Hale, A., Baram, M., Eds.; Elsevier: Oxford UK, 1998.
9. Westaby, J.D.; Lee, B.C. Antecedents of injury among youth in agricultural settings: A longitudinal examination of safety consciousness, dangerous risk taking, and safety knowledge. *J. Saf. Res.* **2003**, *34*, 227–240. [CrossRef]

10. Cheyne, A.; Cox, S.; Oliver, A.; Tomás, J.M. Modelling safety climate in the prediction of levels of safety activity. *Work Stress* **1998**, *12*, 255–271. [CrossRef]
11. Barling, J.; Loughlin, C.; Kelloway, E.K. Development and test of a model linking safety-specific transformational leadership and occupational safety. *J. Appl. Psychol.* **2002**, *87*, 488–496. [CrossRef]
12. Neal, A.; Griffin, M.A.; Hart, P.M. The impact of organizational climate on safety climate and individual behavior. *Saf. Sci.* **2000**, *34*, 99–109. [CrossRef]
13. De Koster, R.B.; Stam, D.; Balk, B.M. Accidents happen: The influence of safety-specific transformational leadership, safety consciousness, and hazard reducing systems on warehouse accidents. *J. Oper. Manag.* **2011**, *29*, 753–765. [CrossRef]
14. Skeepers, N.C.; Charles, M. A study on the leadership behaviour, safety leadership and safety performance in the construction industry in South Africa. *Proc. Manuf.* **2015**, *4*, 10–16. [CrossRef]
15. Posner, B.Z.; Schmidt, W.H. An updated look at the values and expectations of federal government executives. *Public Adm. Rev.* **1994**, *54*, 20–24. [CrossRef]
16. Hussain, S.; Nabeel, S. Tunneling: Evidence from family business groups of Pakistan. *Bus. Econ. Rev.* **2018**, *10*, 97–121. [CrossRef]
17. Sikandar, S.; Mahmood, W. Corporate governance and value of family-owned business: A case of emerging country. *Corp. Gov. Sustain. Rev.* **2018**, *2*, 6–12. [CrossRef]
18. State of SMEs in Pakistan. *Daily Pakistan*. 29 May 2021. Available online: https://dailytimes.com.pk/763512/state-of-smes-in-pakistan/ (accessed on 1 September 2022).
19. Khan, M. Scenario of manufacturing pharmaceutical small and medium enterprises (smes) in Pakistan. *Int. J. Bus. Manag. Econ. Stud.* **2015**, *1*, 14–20.
20. Jackson, M.C. Social systems theory and practice: The need for a critical approach. *Int. J. Gen. Syst.* **1985**, *10*, 135–151. [CrossRef]
21. Getzels, J.W.; Egon, G.G. Social behavior and the administrative process. *Sch. Rev.* **1957**, *65*, 423–441. [CrossRef]
22. Ornstein, A.C.; Hunkins, F.P. *Curriculum: Foundations, Principles and Issues*, 2nd ed.; Allyn and Bacon: Needham Heights, MA, USA, 1993.
23. Skyttner, L. *General Systems Theory: Problems, Perspectives, Practice*; World Scientific: Singapore, 2005.
24. Riehle, A.; Braun, B.I.; Hafiz, H. Improving patient and worker safety: Exploring opportunities for synergy. *J. Nurs. Care Qual.* **2013**, *28*, 99–102. [CrossRef]
25. Blau, P.M. Social exchange. *Int. Encycl. Soc. Sci.* **1968**, *7*, 452–457.
26. Törner, M. The "social-physiology" of safety. An integrative approach to understanding organisational psychological mechanisms behind safety performance. *Saf. Sci.* **2011**, *49*, 1262–1269. [CrossRef]
27. Ekeh, P. *Social Exchange Theory: The Two Traditions*; Harvard University Press: Cambridge, MA, USA, 1974.
28. Siegel, D.S. Responsible leadership. *Acad. Manag. Perspect.* **2014**, *28*, 221–223. [CrossRef]
29. De Cieri, H.; Shea, T.; Pettit, T.; Clarke, M. Measuring the Leading Indicators of Occupational Health and Safety: A Snapshot Review. Institute of Safety, Compensation and Recovery Research. 2012, pp. 5–30. Available online: https://workplacehealthsafetyresearch.files.wordpress.com/2014/11/measuring-the-leading-indicators-of-ohs-snapshot-review-2012.pdf (accessed on 1 September 2022).
30. Waldman, D.A.; Balven, R.M. Responsible leadership: Theoretical issues and research directions. *Acad. Manag. Perspect.* **2014**, *28*, 224–234. [CrossRef]
31. Hasan, O.; McColl, J.; Pfefferkorn, T.; Hamadneh, S.; Alshurideh, M.; Kurdi, B. Consumer attitudes towards the use of autonomous vehicles: Evidence from United Kingdom taxi services. *Int. J. Data Netw. Sci.* **2022**, *6*, 537–550. [CrossRef]
32. Khan, N.; Ahmad, I.; Ilyas, M. Impact of ethical leadership on organizational safety performance: The mediating role of safety culture and safety consciousness. *Ethics Behav.* **2018**, *28*, 628–643. [CrossRef]
33. Xi, Y.; Hu, S.; Yang, Z.; Fu, S.; Weng, J. Analysis of safety climate effect on individual safety consciousness creation and safety behaviour improvement in shipping operations. *Marit. Policy Manag.* **2022**, 1–16. [CrossRef]
34. Ajmal, M.; Isha, A.S.N.; Nordin, S.M.; Al-Mekhlafi, A.B.A. Safety-management practices and the occurrence of occupational accidents: Assessing the mediating role of safety compliance. *Sustainability* **2022**, *14*, 4569. [CrossRef]
35. Burke, R.J.; Clarke, S.; Cooper, C.L. (Eds.) *Occupational Health and Safety*; Gower Publishing, Ltd.: Aldershot, UK, 2011.
36. Nahrgang, J.D.; Morgeson, F.P.; Hofmann, D.A. Safety at work: A meta-analytic investigation of the link between job demands, job resources, burnout, engagement, and safety outcomes. *J. Appl. Psyc. Olog.* **2011**, *96*, 71–81. [CrossRef]
37. Klenke-Borgmann, L.; Digregorio, H.; Cantrell, M.A. Role clarity and interprofessional colleagues in psychological safety: A faculty reflection. *Simul. Healthc.* **2022**. [CrossRef]
38. Wachter, J.K.; Yorio, P.L. A system of safety management practices and worker engagement for reducing and preventing accidents: An empirical and theoretical investigation. *Accid. Anal. Prev.* **2014**, *68*, 117–130. [CrossRef]
39. Kiken, L.G.; Shook, N.J. Looking up: Mindfulness increases positive judgments and reduces negativity bias. *Soc. Psychol. Personal. Sci.* **2011**, *2*, 425–431. [CrossRef]
40. Zhang, J.; Wu, C. The influence of dispositional mindfulness on safety behaviors: A dual process perspective. *Acci. Anal. Prev.* **2014**, *70*, 24–32. [CrossRef] [PubMed]
41. Bahari, S.F. *An Investigation of Safety Training, Safety Climate and Safety Outcomes: A Longitudinal Study in a Malaysian Manufacturing Plant*; The University of Manchester: Manchester, UK, 2011.

42. Sawacha, E.; Naoum, S.; Fong, D. Factors affecting safety performance on construction sites. *Int. J. Proj. Manag.* **1999**, *17*, 309–315. [CrossRef]
43. Reason, J. *Managing the Risks of Organizational Accidents*; Routledge: London, UK, 2016.
44. García, M.G.; Cañamares, M.S.; Escribano, B.V.; Barriuso, A.R. Constructioń's health and safety Plan: The leading role of the main preventive management document on construction sites. *Saf. Sci.* **2021**, *143*, 105437. [CrossRef]
45. Pandit, B.; Albert, A.; Patil, Y.; Al-Bayati, A.J. Fostering safety communication among construction workers: Role of safety climate and crew-level cohesion. *Int. J. Environ. Res. Public Health* **2019**, *16*, 71. [CrossRef]
46. Flin, R. Measuring safety culture in healthcare: A case for accurate diagnosis. *Saf. Sci.* **2007**, *45*, 653–667. [CrossRef]
47. Singer, S.; Lin, S.; Falwell, A.; Gaba, D.; Baker, L. Relationship of safety climate and safety performance in hospitals. *Health Serv. Res.* **2009**, *44*, 399–421. [CrossRef]
48. Mearns, K.; Whitaker, S.M.; Flin, R. Safety climate, safety management practice and safety performance in offshore environments. *Saf. Sci.* **2003**, *41*, 641–680. [CrossRef]
49. Simard, M.; Marchand, A. The behaviour of first-line supervisors in accident prevention and effectiveness in occupational safety. *Saf. Sci.* **1994**, *17*, 169–185. [CrossRef]
50. Vinodkumar, M.N.; Bhasi, M. A study on the impact of management system certification on safety management. *Saf. Sci.* **2011**, *49*, 498–507. [CrossRef]
51. Guo, B.H.; Yiu, T.W.; González, V.A. Predicting safety behavior in the construction industry: Development and test of an integrative model. *Saf. Sci.* **2016**, *84*, 1–11. [CrossRef]
52. Borgheipour, H.; Eskandari, D.; Barkhordari, A.; Mavaji, M.; Tehrani, G.M. Predicting the relationship between safety climate and safety performance in cement industry. *Work* **2020**, *66*, 109–117. [CrossRef] [PubMed]
53. Cooper, M.D. Towards a model of safety culture. *Saf. Sci.* **2000**, *36*, 111–136. [CrossRef]
54. Griffin, M.A.; Neal, A. Perceptions of safety at work: A framework for linking safety climate to safety performance, knowledge, and motivation. *J. Occup. Health Psychol.* **2000**, *5*, 347–351. [CrossRef]
55. Hofmann, D.A.; Stetzer, A. A cross-level investigation of factors influencing unsafe behaviors and accidents. *Pers. Psychol.* **1996**, *49*, 307–339. [CrossRef]
56. Rebelo, M.F.; Santos, G.; Silva, R. A generic model for integration of quality, environment and safety management systems. *TQM J.* **2014**, *26*, 143–159. [CrossRef]
57. Shen, Y.; Tuuli, M.M.; Xia, B.; Koh, T.Y.; Rowlinson, S. Toward a model for forming psychological safety climate in construction project management. *Inter. J. Proj. Manag.* **2015**, *33*, 223–235. [CrossRef]
58. Jafari, M.J.; Eskandari, D.; Valipour, F.; Mehrabi, Y.; Charkhand, H.; Mirghotbi, M. Development and validation of a new safety climate scale for petrochemical industries. *Work* **2017**, *58*, 309–317. [CrossRef]
59. Eskandari, D.; Gharabagh, M.J.; Barkhordari, A.; Gharari, N.; Panahi, D.; Gholami, A.; Teimori-Boghsani, G. Development of a scale for assessing the organization's safety performance based fuzzy ANP. *J. Loss Prev. Process Ind.* **2021**, *69*, 104342. [CrossRef]
60. Clarke, S. The relationship between safety climate and safety performance: A meta-analytic review. *J. Occup. Health Psychol.* **2006**, *11*, 315–327. [CrossRef]
61. Imna, M.; Hassan, Z. Influence of human resource management practices on employee retention in Maldives retail industry. *Int. J. Account. Bus. Manag.* **2015**, *1*, 1–28. [CrossRef]
62. Rich, B.L.; Lepine, J.A.; Crawford, E.R. Job engagement: Antecedents and effects on job performance. *Acad. Manag. J.* **2010**, *53*, 617–635. [CrossRef]
63. Meng, X.; Zhai, H.; Chan, A.H. Development of scales to measure and analyse the relationship of safety consciousness and safety citizenship behaviour of construction workers: An empirical study in China. *Int. J. Environ. Res. Public Health* **2019**, *16*, 1411. [CrossRef]
64. Kelloway, E.K.; Mullen, J.; Francis, L. Divergent effects of transformational and passive leadership on employee safety. *J. Occup. Health Psychol.* **2006**, *11*, 76. [CrossRef] [PubMed]
65. Bavik, A.; Bavik, y.L.; Tang, P.M. Servant leadership, employee job crafting, and citizenship behaviors: A cross-level investigation. *Cornell Hosp. Q.* **2017**, *58*, 364–373. [CrossRef]
66. Chughtai, A.A. Creating safer workplaces: The role of ethical leadership. *Saf. Sci.* **2015**, *73*, 92–98. [CrossRef]
67. Martínez-Córcoles, M.; Gracia, F.; Tomás, I.; Peiró, J.M. Leadership and employees' perceived safety behaviours in a nuclear power plant: A structural equation model. *Saf. Sci.* **2011**, *49*, 1118–1129. [CrossRef]
68. McFadden, K.L.; Stock, G.N.; Gowen, C.R. Leadership, safety climate, and continuous quality improvement. *J. Nurs. Admi.* **2014**, *44*, S27–S37. [CrossRef]
69. Scarnati, J.T. Leaders as role models: 12 rules. *Care. Dev. Inter.* **2002**, *7*, 181–189. [CrossRef]
70. Abbas, A.; Chengang, Y.; Zhuo, S.; Manzoor, S.; Ullah, I.; Mughal, Y.H. Role of responsible leadership for organizational citizenship behavior for the environment in light of psychological ownership and employee environmental commitment: A moderated mediation model. *Front. Psychol.* **2021**, *12*, 756570. [CrossRef]
71. Afsar, B.; Maqsoom, A.; Shahjehan, A.; Afridi, S.A.; Nawaz, A.; Fazliani, H. Responsible leadership and employee's proenvironmental behavior: The role of organizational commitment, green shared vision, and internal environmental locus of control. *Corp. Soc. Responsib. Environ. Manag.* **2020**, *27*, 297–312. [CrossRef]

2. Brown, M.E.; Treviño, L.K.; Harrison, D.A. Ethical leadership: A social learning perspective for construct development and testing. *Organ. Behav. Hum. Decis. Process.* **2005**, *97*, 117–134. [CrossRef]
3. Fernández-Muñiz, B.; Montes-Peon, J.M.; Vazquez-Ordas, C.J. Safety management system: Development and validation of a multidimensional scale. *J. Loss Prev. Proc. Ind.* **2007**, *7*, 52–68. [CrossRef]
4. Fernández-Muñiz, B.; Montes-Peón, J.M.; Vázquez-Ordás, C.J. Safety leadership, risk management and safety performance in Spanish firms. *Saf. Sci.* **2014**, *70*, 295–307. [CrossRef]
5. Voegtlin, C. Development of a scale measuring discursive responsible leadership. In *Responsible Leadership*; Springer: Dordrecht, The Netherlands, 2011; pp. 57–73.
6. Podsakoff, N.P. Common method biases in behavioral research: A critical review of the literature and recommended remedies. *J. Appl. Psychol.* **2003**, *885*, 10–37. [CrossRef] [PubMed]
7. Kline, T. *Psychological Testing: A Practical Approach to Design and Evaluation*; Sage: Thousand Oaks, CA, USA; London, UK; New Delhi, India, 2005; pp. 1–10.
8. Fornell, C.; Larcker, D.F. Structural equation models with unobservable variables and measurement error: Algebra and statistics. *J. Mark. Res.* **1981**, *18*, 382–388. [CrossRef]
9. Hayes, A.F. *Introduction to Mediation, Moderation, and Conditional Process Analysis: A Regression-Based Approach*; The Guilford Press: New York, NY, USA, 2013.
10. Parboteeah, K.P.; Kapp, E.A. Ethical climates and workplace safety behaviors: An empirical investigation. *J. Bus. Ethics* **2008**, *80*, 515–529. [CrossRef]
11. Wong, T.K.M.; Man, S.S.; Chan, A.H.S. Exploring the acceptance of PPE by construction workers: An extension of the technology acceptance model with safety management practices and safety consciousness. *Saf. Sci.* **2021**, *139*, 105239. [CrossRef]
12. Lee, H.C.; Yeo, S.K.; Go, S.S. A study on the improving safety management by analyzing safety consciousness of construction labors. *J. Korea Inst. Build. Constr.* **2009**, *9*, 51–58. [CrossRef]
13. Dong, W.; Zhong, L. Responsible leadership fuels innovative behavior: The mediating roles of socially responsible human resource management and organizational pride. *Front. Psychol.* **2021**, *12*, 787833. [CrossRef]
14. Haque, A. The COVID-19 pandemic and the role of responsible leadership in health care: Thinking beyond employee well-being and organisational sustainability. *Leadersh. Health Serv.* **2021**, *34*, 52–68. [CrossRef] [PubMed]
15. Gond, J.P.; El-Akremi, A.; Igalens, J.; Swaen, V. Corporate social responsibility influence on employees. *Int. Cent. Corp. Soc. Responsib.* **2010**, *54*, 1–47.

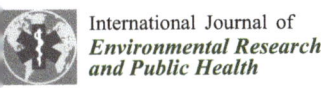

Article

Burnout and Quality of Work Life among Municipal Workers: Do Motivating and Economic Factors Play a Mediating Role?

Dina Pereira [1,2], João Leitão [1,2,3,4,*] and Ludovina Ramos [3]

[1] Centre for Management Studies of Instituto Superior Técnico (CEG-IST), University of Lisbon, 1049-001 Lisboa, Portugal
[2] Research Center in Business Sciences (NECE), University of Beira Interior, 6200-209 Covilhã, Portugal
[3] Faculty of Human and Social Sciences, University of Beira Interior, 6200-001 Covilhã, Portugal
[4] Instituto de Ciências Sociais (ICS), University of Lisbon, 1649-004 Lisboa, Portugal
* Correspondence: jleitao@ubi.pt

Abstract: This study analyzes the relationship between burnout and quality of work life among municipal workers subjected to higher levels of stress and emotional exhaustion, impacting their occupational health in the context of the COVID-19 pandemic. With a sample of 459 municipal workers, the relationship between burnout and quality of work life is tested by considering the isolated mediating effect of the feeling of contributing to productivity and the combined effects of two mediators representing the feeling of contributing to productivity and receiving an appropriate salary. The main findings include a negative association between the three dimensions of burnout: emotional exhaustion, feelings of cynicism, and a sense of being less effective, and the mediators: contribution to productivity and appropriate salary. Also detected was an important mediating role associated with the effects of not feeling contributive at work, as well as not being well paid, on the relation between the burnout syndrome dimension of low effectiveness and quality of work life. For future action by public authorities and public managers, the need is highlighted to create innovative human resource management frameworks and flexible work organization, with remuneration plans based on productivity goals and aimed at an improved balance between personal life and work.

Keywords: burnout; occupational health; public sector; quality of work life; well-being

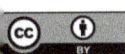

1. Background

The concepts of quality of work life (QWL) and job satisfaction are interrelated, when attempting to define a good work environment or a good and healthy life. Sirgy et al. [1] state that QWL relates to job satisfaction in the sense that job satisfaction is one of many outcomes of QWL. Job satisfaction is crucial because it influences job performance, customer satisfaction, employment retention, employee absenteeism, and organizational commitment [2]. Moreover, QWL does not only affect job satisfaction but also satisfaction in other life domains, such as family life, leisure life, social life, and financial life. In fact, women working from home during the COVID-19 lockdown experienced a set of negative effects from working remotely, namely the invasion of privacy, family time, the occurrence of distractions while working resulting in failures, and the increasing interference of work in private life [3]. Therefore, the focus of QWL goes beyond job satisfaction. It involves the effect of the workplace on satisfaction with the job; satisfaction in non-work life domains; and satisfaction with overall life, personal happiness, and subjective well-being [1].

Work occupies one's thoughts, determining decisions and thus contributing to one's social identity [4]. Such subjective and behavioral components of the QWL, namely supervisors' support, a good work environment, and collaborative support from co-workers, as well as the feeling of being respected professionally and personally, have an important influence on forming an employee's individual desire to contribute to the organization's productivity. This is also supported by the statement that QWL is associated with job satisfaction, motivation, productivity, health, job security, safety, and well-being, embracing four main axes: a safe work environment, occupational healthcare, appropriate working time, and an appropriate salary [5,6].

With the increasing workloads of the past decades, plus the COVID-19 pandemic, the number of employees experiencing psychological problems related to occupational stress has increased rapidly, raising costs in terms of absenteeism and loss of productivity and also increasing healthcare consumption and raising public health issues in the long term [7]. Conversely, not only at the employees' level, but also at the level of SME owners, who faced, during the COVID-19 crisis, high stress, mostly derived from the shortage of personnel, financial constraints, liquidities, repeated closures, and reopenings, as well as great difficulty in adapting to such a changing environment [8].

Added to the above, occupational stress and self-reported sleep quality are also strongly associated with both QWL and work ability, highlighting the urgent need for the screening and handling of these health issues [9]. Occupational stress leads to organizational burnout, whose effects were formerly analyzed as moderators of the relationship between employees' QWL and their perceptions of their contribution to the organization's productivity by integrating the QWL factors into the trichotomy of (de)motivators of productivity in the workplace [10]. Our previous findings suggest that QWL hygiene factors (e.g., safe work environment and occupational healthcare) have an important influence on productivity, and burnout de-motivator factors (that is, low effectiveness, cynicism, and emotional exhaustion) significantly moderate the relationship between QWL and the contribution to productivity.

The COVID-19 pandemic—which has been (and will continue to be) a key issue throughout and beyond the 2020s—had an effect on individual–organizational relations and consequently, on organizational performance [11]. This took a toll not only on frontline workers (physicians, nurses, and hospital workers) but also on other public servants, such as municipal workers, not studied so far, who were affected by the changing the location of their work, tasks, the demands at work, and the demands they face outside work, endangering the balance between professional and personal life [12,13].

Furthermore, the financial insecurity and financial stress that already interfered with work [14] increased unexpectedly as COVID-19 aggravated these concerns. Due to the COVID-19 pandemic, employees are generally more aware of financial security. According to Kulikowski and Sedlak (2020), studies on work engagement and job performance have shown that employees ranked financial security as a factor of the highest significance [15]. These concerns could trigger stress, impacting employees' health and leading to mental illnesses such as post-traumatic stress disorder (PTSD) [13] but also high rates of tension, anger, anxiety, depressed mood, mental fatigue, and sleep disturbances. Such problems, usually referred to overall as distress, are often classified as neurasthenia, adjustment disorders, or burnout [7,16]. Focusing on younger, unmarried female healthcare workers with low monthly incomes who were studied in Jordan during the pandemic, they revealed high anxiety symptoms, which were exacerbated one year after the beginning of COVID-19, particularly for the physicians, with intense schedules, and those who were infected [17]. This situation is intensified in the public healthcare system, during pandemics, as it is characterized by a scarcity of resources and reduced accountability, thus increasing the lack of trustworthiness in the health system [18]. Strategies to improve healthcare systems' efficiency, physicians' motivation, management routines, patient flows, and information are a need during extreme crises, such as COVID-19. These strategies were implemented in a nodal-designated COVID-19 center in Qatar and proved to be effective, lowering mortality and increasing efficacy, capabilities, and patient satisfaction [19].

Furthermore, employees' mental health has a positive relationship with job performance, although this same relationship is mediated by innovative behavior and work engagement, which are also positively associated with job performance [20].

Knowledge on the influencers of QWL has remained relatively limited. In order to forecast and make possible an anticipated action on the part of responsible managers, it is essential to assess hypothetical unexplored effects associated with other mediating factors of the core relationship between burnout and QWL [21].

Set against this background, a relevant research question arises concerning the need to advance the still limited knowledge about other types of motivating and economic mediators affecting municipal workers' QWL, especially in terms of disorders associated with burnout, in the context of the COVID-19 pandemic. An effective response to the COVID-19 pandemic required effective administration, which in turn depended on the effort and capacity of millions of public sector workers from the front line to central administration. Added to the above, for many public servants, COVID-19 has fundamentally changed not only where and how they work but also the increasing demands of their jobs and day-to-day life [12].

2. Burnout during COVID-19 for Public Servants

When the World Health Organization (WHO) declared the outbreak of a new coronavirus disease (COVID-19) and then characterized it as a pandemic, all working people were affected. Not only because of their (or their relatives') health, but also due to the implications for the workplace. Here, we can identify three main groups of people who could be affected by burnout, namely: (a) people who kept their jobs and continued to work in the same location, (b) people who kept their jobs but started to work from home, and (c) people who lost their jobs.

The term "burnout" was first used by Freudenberger (1974), who described his own experience as "a combination of feelings, exhaustion and fatigue, a lingering cold, headache and gastrointestinal disturbances, sleeplessness and shortness of breath" [22]. The discussion on burnout has grown since then, being continuously updated in terms of symptoms but also in terms of consequences, not only for the employee, but also for the employer.

The multidimensional theory of burnout [23–25] defines burnout as being grounded in three core components: (i) emotional exhaustion, as the individual stress dimension of burnout, refers to energy depletion or the draining of emotional resources; (ii) depersonalization, which represents the interpersonal dimension, refers to the development of negative, cynical attitudes towards the recipients of one's service or care; and (iii) reduced or lack of personal accomplishment, which refers to a decline in one's feeling of competence and successful achievement in one's career; this is the self-evaluation dimension of burnout. Furthermore, burnout is characterized by: (a) loss of enthusiasm for work; (b) psychological exhaustion; (c) indolence, and the appearance of negative attitudes and behaviors towards patients and the organization; and (d) the appearance, in some cases, of feelings of guilt [26].

Globally, burnout entails a state of physical, emotional, and mental exhaustion resulting from a long period of involvement in highly emotional demanding work situations [27]. Burnout is a psychological syndrome of exhaustion, cynicism, and inefficacy in the workplace. It is also considered to be an individual stress experience embedded in a context of complex social relationships, involving a person's perception of both the self and others on the job [28,29], associated with limited resources, low abilities, and low energies and interest in long-term work [30]. This condition involves emotional exhaustion, depersonalization, and a lack of personal accomplishment. Burnout can arise through stress disorders triggered by stress on the job and is also often defined as an emotional-exhaustion experience by employees [15,31]. Theoretical frameworks such as the JD-R model claim that high, unfavorable job demands are consistently related to burnout [32–36]. Moreover, the combination of those high demands with low job resources can lead to some kind of long-lasting burnout and employee disengagement.

As a phenomenon that is context-specific, it is worthwhile to try to deepen the still-scarce knowledge about the impact of pandemic circumstances on occupational health, insofar as it has influenced working conditions, involvement, QWL, and burnout levels, bearing in mind the limited knowledge about the situation for public servants, including municipal workers. According to Meyer et al. (2021, p. 1) [37], " (. . .) the COVID-19 pandemic poses new challenges for employees' psychological health that go beyond previous findings in the area of demands and resources (e.g., [35,38]).

The spread of COVID-19, followed by swift responses by companies and government created many new challenges that have brought about profound changes and affected the normal health routines and lifestyles of people of all ages, restricting outdoor or physical activity, increasing sedentary time, and consequently, disrupting sleep [39]. Nevertheless, the same authors outline that the isolation of workers at home had mixed effects on adult health behaviors in China, stressing that those workers focused more on their eating quality and patterns, which had a positive influence on their quality of life. The biggest change for most workers was the remote work experience. Prior to COVID-19, most workers had little remote working experience, nor were they or their organizations prepared to adopt this practice. Now, the unprecedented pandemic has required millions of people across the world to become remote workers, inadvertently leading to a de facto global experiment on remote working [40,41]. According to a study by Moretti et al. (2001) of the home-working population, home workers perceived themselves to be less productive compared to their office working period and less satisfied due to isolation [42].

In this respect, COVID-19 highlights employees' and employers' vulnerability. As many businesses around the world will be restructured or disappear due to the pandemic, workers will be retrained or laid off and the economic, social–psychological, and health costs of these actions are likely to be immense. Indeed, the impacts of the pandemic affect some groups of workers more than others, for example, based on their age, race and ethnicity, gender, or personality [41]. These impacts were affirmed by Wang et al. (2021), who stated that, as schools in China shut down during the COVID-19 outbreak, working parents faced a challenge in balancing work and family roles and time, creating higher levels of exhaustion, depression, and burnout [40].

Blake at al. (2020) conducted a survey of frontline/healthcare workers to understand the psychological impacts on employees and how these translated into negative consequences for organizations [43]. They found that the extreme pressure experienced by workers during the COVID-19 pandemic might increase their risk of burnout, which has adverse outcomes, not only for their individual well-being, but also for patient care and for the healthcare system. In addition, fear of exposure to COVID-19 or even due to the scarcity of personal protective equipment (PPE), allocation of resources, accountability, and the efficient management of patient flows, as well as a lack of or a reduction in training on practical skills to deal with emergency situations and critical care, can put even more pressure on frontline/health professionals [18,44]. There is also the fear of taking the disease home or even being responsible for bringing it to the workplace, infecting other patients. All this combined with the normal challenges of supporting a family, changes in workload and schedules, and facing new or unknown clinical situations may substantially increase levels of anxiety, emotional strain, and physical exhaustion.

At the coalface of the pandemic, healthcare workers and public service providers have jobs and occupations that have proven to be associated with increased mental health problems during pandemic crises and high personal and work-related burnout [13].

A survey applied to Portuguese healthcare workers during the COVID-19 pandemic wherein frontline working positions were associated with higher levels of stress and depression, showed a significant association with increased burnout levels. In this survey higher levels of satisfaction with life and resilience were highly associated with lower levels of burnout [45]. This is also supported in the research developed by Hofmam and Hubie (2020), wherein surveys conducted among frontline workers from two health units in Cascavel-PR (Brazil) identified that all participants obtained higher than expected burnout scores, emotional exhaustion, and a feeling of low professional achievement [46].

Pandemics bring new ways of performing jobs in several sectors of activity, including among public servants not directly working in health-related areas, as happens with municipal workers. The institutionalization of remote working and the rapid, sometimes reckless, digitalization by companies and public organizations has increased the frequency of workers' burnout with consequences for families' personal life and budget [47].

During the COVID-19 pandemic, municipal workers working in sectors closer to citizens were forced to work remotely, which has caused unique supervisory demands for human resources managers [12], as well as exacerbated burnout caused by self-isolation policies, which can increase social isolation and relationship difficulties [48].

Other public sector activities and their workers, for instance, those connected with education, were also put under pressure by the effects of pandemics. Marelli et al. (2021) showed a high percentage of both students and university administration staff workers denoting symptoms of depression or anxiety [49], and Evanoff et al. (2020) pointed out the important prevalence of stress, anxiety, depression, work exhaustion, burnout, and worsened well-being among university employees [50]. Another study on insomnia among employees in occupations critical to the functioning of society (e.g., health, education, welfare, and emergency services) during the COVID-19 pandemic also found that employees reported higher levels of insomnia symptoms compared to normative data collected before the pandemic [51]. These findings only highlight the associations of health and well-being with additional personal and work factors beyond the COVID-19 pandemic, without addressing the role played by motivating and economic mediators of the relationship between burnout and QWL.

A study of social workers in the United States during the COVID-19 pandemic, showed a high level of PTSD and burnout symptoms among the participants enrolled in frontline jobs dealing directly with the risk of contagion [52]. Bapuji et al. (2020) stated that organizational and societal inequalities feed into each other, giving rise to concerns that growing inequality after COVID-19 will also contribute to a downward spiral of negative trends in the workplace in the form of decreased work centrality and increased burnout, absenteeism, deviant behaviors, bullying, and higher job rotation [53].

3. Methods

3.1. Research Question and Model Design

The aim of this study is to address the following core research question: Does the feeling of contributing to productivity and receiving an appropriate salary mediate the relationship between the burnout condition and the QWL of municipal workers in the context of the COVID-19 pandemic?

To address this research question, the model specification presented in Figure 1 below intends to evaluate the relationship between three burnout dimensions and QWL, mediated by motivating and economic factors, including both the feeling of contributing to productivity and receiving an appropriate salary, regarding municipal workers.

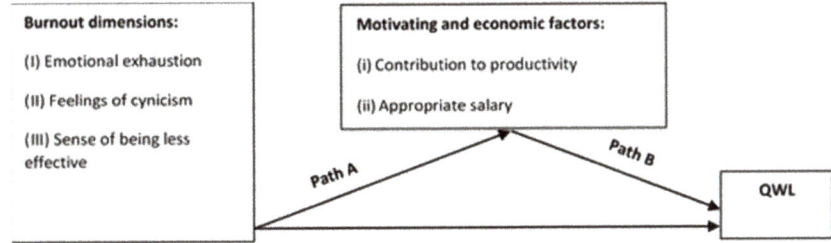

Figure 1. Mediators of burnout and QWL: Model design.

3.2. Study Design and Participants

This cross-sectional quantitative study examined municipal workers in Portugal. The survey was administered by emailing the questionnaire to Portuguese municipalities, from December 2020 to April 2021, with 459 responses being received from municipal workers developing professional activities during the COVID-19 pandemic, with a diversified set of socio-economic characteristics and professional profiles, in municipal institutions with different sizes, as presented below in Table 1.

Table 1. Socio-economic characteristics, professional profiles, and the size of the institutions of the municipal workers.

	Socio-Economic Characteristics	
Gender	Female	67.00%
	Male	33.00%
Age	20–25 years	0.60%
	26–35 years	8.00%
	36–45 years	34.00%
	46–55 years	38.00%
	>55 years	19.40%
Age	Single	19.00%
	Married	67.00%
	Other	14.00%
	Professional profiles	
Insitutional role	Leadership positions	25.60%
	Qualified workers	66.40%
	Non-qualified workers	8.00%
Education	Post-graduate	24.00%
	College	48.00%
	Secondary school	28.00%
Contract	Permanent	50.00%
	Open	40.00%
	Fixed period	5.00%
	Temporary	5.00%
	Municipal Institutions	
Size	<50 employees	5.00%
	[50; 249] employees	10.00%
	[250; 999] employees	36.00%
	≥1000 employees	49.00%

3.3. Survey Procedures

The research methodology was developed using different surveys, which were designed taking a set of eleven international benchmarks into consideration, namely: (i) health and well-being at work: a survey of employees, 2014, UK, Department for Work and Pensions [54]; (ii) ACT Online Employee Health and Wellbeing Survey 2016, Australian Capital Territory Government [55]; (iii) British Heart Foundation 2012, employee survey [56]; (iv) British Heart Foundation 2017, staff health and wellbeing template survey [57]; (v) Rand Europe (2015), Health, wellbeing and productivity in the workplace—Britain's Healthiest Organization summary report [58]; (vi) South Australia Health, Government of South Australia staff needs assessment, staff health and wellbeing survey; (vii) Southern Cross Health Society and Business NZ, Wellness in the Workplace Survey 2017 [59]; (viii) State Government Victoria, Workplace Health & Wellbeing needs survey; (ix) East Midlands Public Health Observatory, Workplace Health Needs Assessment for Employers, February 2012 [60]; (x) Tool for Observing Worksite Environments (TOWE). U.S. Department of Health & Human Services [1]; and (xi) Measure of QWL, as originally proposed in [61].

With the motivation of accomplishing the objectives, this study was analytical and correlational, because it sought to explore the variables and the relationships between them, and it was cross-sectional because the sample was collected in a single period. The purpose of the study was descriptive because it aimed to analyze the relationship between burnout and quality of work life among municipal workers subjected to higher levels of stress and emotional exhaustion, interacting with their occupational health in the context of the COVID 19 pandemic. Through a quantitative, objectivist, and, therefore, deductive approach, this research was supported by models built on results and previous research, with quantitative indicators collected through a survey.

The survey includes four sections: (i) health, (ii) well-being, (iii) QWL, and (iv) sample characterization (gender, age, marital status, role in the organization, type of employee contract, academic qualifications, size of the organization). In the first three sections, Likert scales were used (ranging from 1 to 7), in order to evaluate the level of agreement with a set of affirmations, which were used to assess the level of agreement with a set of sentences in each sub-section. These scales had been transformed into binary considering the variables under analysis. In the fourth section, levels of answers were used, considering values ranging from 1 to 4 equaling 0 and values 5, 6, and 7 equal to 1.

The study period included a declaration of national calamity twice and two subsequent stages of easing lockdown measures following the states of national emergency (between 19 March and 4 May 2020 and between 15 January and 15 March 2021). A questionnaire built in the Google platform was provided to participants via a link shared through direct e-mail to municipalities' contacts.

3.4. Measures and Covariates

Socio-demographic and other mental health related data were collected through a self-administered survey. The variables used in to measure burnout were: emotional exhaustion, cynicism, and low effectiveness [8]. All items were scored on a 7-point Likert scale. The variables used to measure QWL were: supervisor support, co-worker support, good work environment, professional respect, work–life balance, and skills development [4]. QWL was then generated as a new variable, computed by using the six prior variables, attributing the value 1 if the levels of agreement were positive and 0 otherwise. Regarding the mediators, the variables of contribution to productivity and appropriate salary were used. The former was scored on a 7-point Likert scale, ranging from 1 if the worker felt they contribute to the organization's productivity, 0 otherwise, while the latter ranged from 1 to 7, 1 being if the workers did not agree and 7 if they totally agreed.

3.5. Data Analysis

The data collected from Google® Forms were exported to an Excel spreadsheet, and all statistical analyses were carried out using STATA Statistics (version 14.1). Variable characterization was performed by means of absolute and relative frequencies, means and standard deviations (SDs).

Two mediation analyses were performed using two models. Model 1 used the intermedate variable (contribution to productivity), and Model 2 used two intermediate variables (contribution to productivity and appropriate salary). These mediators intend to explain how or why a set of independent variables influences an outcome (here the QWL). To do so, structural equation modeling (SEM) was used, as it is a powerful multivariate technique, which makes use of a conceptual model, path diagram, and system of linked regression-style equations in order to capture complex and dynamic relationships within an agglomerate of both observed and unobserved variables. This technique allows a reciprocal role played by a variable and enables the inference of causal relationships. According to Gunzler et al. (2013), the option for the SEM framework in a mediation analysis is advantageous when the model comprises latent variables such as quality of life or stress, as it will make interpretation and estimation easier [61]. As SEM was created partly to test complex mediation models in a single analysis, this technique simplifies the testing of mediation hypotheses. Moreover, the option here is also justified as this work extends the mediation process to multiple independent variables.

4. Findings and Discussion

4.1. Sample Profile

The selection of this population was justified as it ensured a diversified sample with the representation of distinct municipal workers with distinct socio-economic characteristics, professional roles, education, contracts, and working in different sized municipal institutions. Due to limitations, in terms of data access, the convenience sample procedure tried to incorporate the maximum number of institutions, for a total number of 308 municipalities in Portugal, in order to ensure the total geographical coverage of Portugal, including five regions of continental Portugal: north, center, metropolitan area of Lisbon, Alentejo, and Algarve, and also two autonomous regions: Madeira and Azores. Based on the complete survey responses from 459 respondents, the convenience sample was generated. Previously, we described the socio-economic characteristics, professional profiles, and the size of the municipal employees' institutions (see Table 1).

A total of 89.98% of participants reported a feeling of contributing to productivity, with 69.28% stating that they felt they were experiencing a good QWL. Nevertheless, only 27.67% of workers considered their salary appropriate. Taking as reference the three dimensions of assessing burnout, i.e., emotional exhaustion, cynicism, and low effectiveness, 44.23% agreed they experienced emotional exhaustion and feelings of high levels of stress/anxiety in the workplace; 28.54% expressed feelings of cynicism, stating they had become more critical at work, both of colleagues and working conditions; and 30.06% felt low effectiveness at work, lacking satisfaction in job achievements. Table 2, presented below, summarizes this descriptive information.

Table 2. Sample characteristics (n = 459).

Characteristics	n	%
Contribution to productivity	413	89.98
QWL	318	69.28
Appropriate salary	127	27.67
Emotional exhaustion	203	44.23
Cynicism	131	28.54
Low effectiveness	138	30.06

4.2. Burnout and QWL: Contribution to Productivity as Mediator (Model 1)

Concerning model 1, the direct effects (Table 3), indirect effects (Table 4), and total effects (Table 5) were assessed using one mediator variable, i.e., contribution to productivity. The level of z (and/or p) considered to be significant for the statistical analyses was 0.05. Regarding the first dimension of burnout, i.e., emotional exhaustion, the total effect is -0.8160712, which is the effect found if there is no mediator in the model. It is significant with a z of -4.79. The direct effect of emotional exhaustion is -0.8076825, which, while still significant ($z = -4.74$), is smaller than the total effect. The indirect effect of emotional exhaustion that passes through the contribution to productivity is -0.008388 and is not significant.

The proportion of the total mediated effect is $-0.008388/-0.8160712$, resulting in -0.8263497. The ratio of the indirect to direct effect is $-0.008388/-0.8076825$, equaling -0.0103852. The ratio of the total to direct effect corresponds to $-0.8160712/-0.8076825$, equaling -1.0103861. The proportion of the total effect that is mediated is almost -0.83, which is a respectable amount. The ratio of the indirect effect to the direct effect is about -0.010, and the total effect is about -1.010 times the direct effect.

Table 3. Model 1: Direct effects.

OIM	Coef.	Std.Err.	z	P > z	[95%	Conf.Int]
Structural						
contribution to productivity						
QWL	0.0744012	0.099308	0.75	0.454	−0.1202389	0.2690412
Burnout Dimension I						
Emotional-exhaustion	<-					
contribution to productivity	−0.1127498	0.0799756	−1.41	0.159	−0.2694992	0.0439995
QWL	−0.8076825 ***	0.1702603	−4.74	0.000	−1.141387	−0.4739784
Burnout Dimension II						
Cynicism	<-					
contribution to productivity	−0.1562514 *	0.0802144	−1.95	0.051	−0.3134687	0.000966
QWL	−0.8447911 ***	0.1707687	−4.95	0.000	−1.179492	−0.5100907
Burnout Dimension III						
Low-effectiveness	<-					
contribution to productivity	−0.2946748 ***	0.0829586	−3.55	0.000	−0.4572706	−0.1320789
QWL	−1.732726 ***	0.1766108	−9.81	0.000	−2.078877	−1.386575

Legend: *** 1% statistical significance; and * 10% statistical significance.

Table 4. Model 1: Indirect effects.

OIM	Coef.	Std.Err.	z	P > z	[95%	Conf.Int]
Structural						
contribution to productivity						
QWL	0	(no	path)			
Burnout Dimension I						
Emotional-exhaustion	<-					
contribution to productivity	0	(no	path)			
QWL	−0.0083887	0.0126798	−0.66	0.508	−0.0332407	0.0164633
Burnout Dimension II						
Cynicism	<-					
contribution to productivity	0	(no	path)			
QWL	−0.0116253	0.0166251	−0.70	0.484	−0.0442099	0.0209594
Burnout Dimension III						
Low-effectiveness	<-					
contribution to productivity	0	(no	path)			
QWL	−0.0219241	0.0299074	−0.73	0.464	−0.0805416	0.0366933

Table 5. Model 1: Total effects.

OIM	Coef.	Std.Err.	z	P > z	[95%	Conf.Int]
Structural						
contribution to productivity						
QWL	0.0744012	0.099308	0.75	0.454	−0.1202389	0.2690412
Burnout Dimension I						
Emotional-exhaustion	<-					
contribution to productivity	−0.1127498	0.0799756	−1.41	0.159	−0.2694992	0.0439995
QWL	−0.8160712 ***	0.1705243	−4.79	0.000	−1.150293	−0.4818497
Burnout Dimension II						
Cynicism	<-					
contribution to productivity	−0.1562514 *	0.0802144	−1.95	0.051	−0.3134687	0.000966
QWL	−0.8564164 ***	0.1713683	−5.00	0.000	−1.192292	−0.5205407
Burnout Dimension III						
Low-effectiveness	<-					
contribution to productivity	−0.2946748 ***	0.0829586	−3.55	0.000	−0.4572706	−0.1320789
QWL	−1.75465 ***	0.1789124	−9.81	0.000	−2.105312	−1.403988

Legend: *** 1% statistical significance; and * 10% statistical significance.

Concerning the second dimension of burnout, i.e., cynicism, its total effect is −0.8564164, which is the effect found if there is no mediator in the model. It is significant, with a z of −5.00. The direct effect of cynicism is −0.1562514, which, while still significant (z = −1.95), is smaller than the total effect. The indirect effect of cynicism that passes through the contribution to productivity is −0.0116253 and is also not significant.

The proportion of the total effect mediated is −0.0116253/−0.8564164, resulting in −0.0135743. The ratio of the indirect to direct effect is −0.0116253/−0.8447911, equaling −0.0137611. The ratio of the total to direct effect corresponds to −0.8564164/−0.8447911, equaling −1.0137611. The proportion of the total effect that is mediated is almost −0.014, which is a small amount. The ratio of the indirect effect to the direct effect is about −0.014, and the total effect is about −1.014 times the direct effect.

Concerning the third dimension assessed for burnout, i.e., the feeling of low effectiveness, its total effect is −1.75465, which is the effect found if there is no mediator in the model. It is significant, with a z of −9.81. The direct effect of low effectiveness is −0.2946748, which, while still significant (z = −3.55), is smaller than the total effect. The indirect effect of low effectiveness that passes through the contribution to productivity is −0.0219241, and it is also not significant.

The proportion of the total effect mediated is −0.0219241/−1.75465, resulting in −0.0124948. The ratio of the indirect to direct effect is −0.0219241/−1.732726, equaling −0.0126529. The ratio of the total to direct effect corresponds to −1.75465/−1.732726, equaling −1.0126528. The proportion of the total effect that is mediated is almost -0.013, which is a small amount. The ratio of the indirect effect to the direct effect is about -0.013, and the total effect is about −1.013 times the direct effect.

4.3. Burnout and QWL: Contribution to Productivity and Appropriate Salary as Mediators (Model 2)

Considering model 2, the same set of effects are analyzed (cf. Tables 6–8), evaluating two mediators (i.e., contribution to productivity and appropriate salary). For the first dimension of burnout, i.e., emotional exhaustion, the total effect is −1.054325, which is the effect found if there are no mediators in the model. It is significant, with a z of −6.64. The direct effect for emotional exhaustion is -1.019637, which is still quite significant (z = −5.99), although slightly smaller than the total effect. The indirect effect of emotional exhaustion that passes through the contribution to productivity and appropriate salary is −0.0346888 and is not significant.

The proportion of the total effect mediated is −0.0346888/−1.054325, resulting in −0.0329014. The ratio of the indirect to direct effect is −0.0346888/−1.019637, equaling −0.0340207. The ratio of the total to direct effect corresponds to −1.054325/−1.019637, equaling −1.0340199. The proportion of the total effect that is mediated is almost −0.33, which is a respectable amount. The ratio of the indirect effect to direct effect is about −0.03, and the total effect is about −1.034 times the direct effect.

Concerning the second dimension of burnout, i.e., cynicism, its total effect is -1.011313, which is the effect found if there are no mediators in the model. It is significant, with a z of −6.30. The direct effect for cynicism is −0.9078191, which, while still significant (z = −5.29), is smaller than the total effect. The indirect effect of cynicism that passes through the contribution to productivity is −0.01034937 and is also not significant.

The proportion of the total effect mediated is −0.01034937/−1.011313, resulting in −0.0102335. The ratio of the indirect to direct effect is −0.01034937/−0.9078191, equaling −0.0114001. The ratio of the total to direct effect corresponds to −1.011313/−0.9078191, equaling −1.1140027. The proportion of the total effect that is mediated is almost −0.010, which is a small amount. The ratio of the indirect effect to direct effect is about -0.011, and the total effect is about −1.114 times the direct effect.

Table 6. Model 2: Direct effects.

OIM	Coef.	Std.Err.	z	P > z	[95%	Conf.Int]
Structural contribution to productivity						
QWL	0.2031458 **	0.0940108	2.16	0.031	0.018888	0.3874035
Appropriate salary	<-					
QWL	1.210284 ***	0.1492337	8.11	0.000	0.9177917	1.502777
Burnout dimension I Emotional-exhaustion	<-					
contribution to productivity	−0.0748569	0.0787106	−0.95	0.342	−0.2291269	0.0794131
Appropriate salary	−0.016097	0.0495843	−0.32	0.745	−0.1132804	0.0810865
QWL	−1.019637 ***	0.1703282	−5.99	0.000	−1.353474	−0.6857996
Burnout dimension II Cynicism	<-					
contribution to productivity	−0.1226739	0.0793634	−1.55	0.122	−0.2782234	0.0328755
Appropriate salary	−0.0649211	0.0499955	−1.30	0.194	−0.1629105	0.0330683
QWL	−0.9078191 ***	0.1717408	−5.29	0.000	−1.244425	−0.5712133
Burnout Dimension III Low-effectiveness	<-					
contribution to productivity	−0.2445894 ***	0.0820851	−2.98	0.003	−0.4054733	−0.0837055
Appropriate salary	−0.1833378 ***	0.0517101	−3.55	0.000	−0.2846877	−0.0819878
QWL	−1.444998 ***	0.1776306	−8.13	0.000	−1.793147	−1.096848

Legend: *** 1% statistical significance; and ** 5% statistical significance.

Table 7. Model 2: Indirect effects.

OIM	Coef.	Std.Err.	z	P > z	[95%	Conf.Int]
Structural contribution to productivity						
QWL	0	(no	path)			
Appropriate salary	<-					
QWL	0	(no	path)			
Burnout dimension I Emotional-exhaustion	<-					
contribution to productivity	0	(no	path)			
Appropriate salary	0	(no	path)			
QWL	−0.0346888	0.0627665	−0.55	0.580	−0.1577088	0.0883312
Burnout dimension II Cynicism	<-					
contribution to productivity	0	(no	path)			
Appropriate salary	0	(no	path)			
QWL	−0.1034937	0.0646212	−1.60	0.109	−0.2301489	0.0231615
Burnout Dimension III Low-effectiveness	<-					
contribution to productivity	0	(no	path)			
Appropriate salary	0	(no	path)			
QWL	−0.2715781 ***	0.0741744	−3.66	0.000	−0.4169573	−0.126199

Legend: *** 1% statistical significance.

Regarding the third dimension of burnout, i.e., the feeling of low effectiveness, its total effect is −1.716576, which is the effect found if there are no mediators in the model. It is significant, with a z of −10.15. The direct effect for low effectiveness is −1.444998, which, while still significant (z = −8.13), is smaller than the total effect. The indirect effect of low effectiveness that passes through the contribution to productivity is −0.2715781, and it is also highly significant.

Table 8. Model 2: Total effects.

OIM	Coef.	Std.Err.	z	P > z	[95%	Conf.Int]
Structural						
contribution to productivity						
QWL	0.2031458 **	0.0940108	2.16	0.031	0.018888	0.3874035
Appropriate salary	<-					
QWL	1.210284 ***	0.1492337	8.11	0.000	0.9177917	1.502777
Burnout dimension I						
Emotional-exhaustion	<-					
contribution to productivity	−0.0748569	0.0787106	−0.95	0.342	−0.2291269	0.0794131
Appropriate salary	−0.016097	0.0495843	−0.32	0.745	−0.1132804	0.0810865
QWL	−1.054325 ***	0.1586904	−6.64	0.000	−1.365353	−0.743298
Burnout dimension II						
Cynicism	<-					
contribution to productivity	−0.1226739	0.0793634	−1.55	0.122	−0.2782234	0.0328755
Appropriate salary	−0.0649211	0.0499955	−1.30	0.194	−0.1629105	0.0330683
QWL	−1.011313 ***	0.1605389	−6.30	0.000	−1.325963	−0.6966623
Burnout Dimension III						
Low-effectiveness	<-					
contribution to productivity	−0.2445894 ***	0.0820851	−2.98	0.003	−0.4054733	−0.0837055
Appropriate salary	−0.1833378 ***	0.0517101	−3.55	0.000	−0.2846877	−0.0819878
QWL	−1.716576 ***	0.1691313	−10.15	0.000	−2.048067	−1.385085

Legend: *** 1% statistical significance; and ** 5% statistical significance.

The proportion of the total effect mediated is −0.2715781/−1.716576, resulting in −0.1582091. The ratio of the indirect to direct effect is −0.2715781/−1.444998, equaling −0.1879435. The ratio of the total to direct effect corresponds to −1.716576/−1.444998, equaling −1.1879435. The proportion of the total effect that is mediated is almost −0.16, which is quite an important amount. The ratio of the indirect effect to direct effect is about −0.19, and the total effect is about −1.19 times the direct effect.

4.4. Discussion

The COVID-19 pandemic showed an increase of stress levels and emotional-exhaustion experiences related to employees' occupational health, with higher absenteeism rates, loss of productivity, and increased healthcare consumption [7]. In fact, such impacts showed an important correlation with the loss of QWL and work ability [9].

The findings from this study show that, concerning the three dimensions of burnout assessment, i.e., emotional exhaustion, cynicism, and low effectiveness, approximately 44% answered that they were experiencing a condition of emotional exhaustion, feeling high stress/anxiety levels in the workplace. Almost 29% expressed feelings of cynicism, stating they had become more critical at work, both of colleagues and working conditions. For 30% of workers, feelings of being less effective at work and lacking satisfaction in job achievements occurred often.

Aligned with the results of prior research, COVID-19 not only impacted negatively on stress levels and QWL among frontline workers in the healthcare sector (physicians, nurses, and hospital workers) but also on other public servants [12,13]. Public servants closer to citizens, such as municipal workers, were suddenly forced to work remotely, changing public-sector work environments, raising contingent supervisory demands [12], and acting as a major stressor, increasing chronic anxiety, social isolation, and relationship difficulties [48].

The findings presented here confirm the burnout syndrome as a multidimensional phenomenon whose dimensions affect QWL in different ways. To understand how much of the measured effect of the independent variable (burnout dimensions) on the dependent variable (QWL) is attributable to motivating and economic mediator variables: contribution to productivity (in model 1) and satisfaction with salary (in model 2), we used mediation analysis. In model 1 (cf. Tables 2–4), the total effect comprises a direct effect pathway of the independent variables on the dependent variable (path C) and an indirect pathway of the independent variables on the dependent variable through the mediator (path A and path B). The first model analyzed the mediator effect of the contribution to productivity on the relation between the first dimension analyzed for burnout, i.e., emotional exhaustion, on QWL. Our results revealed a significant direct effect but found no significance in the mediating role of the worker feeling productive between this dimension of burnout and QWL. This mediating role had no significant effect concerning the second dimension, cynicism, or the third dimension, the feeling of low effectiveness, only showing important direct effects.

In contrast, model 2, assessing the mediation role of workers' contribution to productivity if associated with lower satisfaction with salary in the relation between municipal workers' burnout and decreased QWL (cf. Tables 5–7), our findings confirm the significant direct effects, for the first two dimensions of burnout on QWL but, as in model 1, found no significance in the mediating role of the worker feeling productive and satisfied with salary between this dimension of burnout and QWL. Nevertheless, and contrasting with the first dimensions of the burnout syndrome, the third one, i.e., the sense of low effectiveness, revealed not only important direct effects but highly significant indirect effects, which are in line with prior research highlighting the multidimensionality of burnout and the diverse effects on QWL.

The results of the present study are aligned with the literature on the determinants of QWL, which highlights the association between altered work conditions, including for public servants not directly working in health-related areas, and increased worker burnout exacerbated by the consequences for families' personal life and budget [47].

5. Conclusions

This study contributes to the literature on occupational health, with an application for the public sector, especially the situation of municipal workers developing professional activities during the COVID-19 pandemic. It addressed the relationship between the multidimensional construct of burnout and QWL, by innovating in empirical assessment, considering both the isolated mediator of contribution to productivity and the joint mediator of the contribution to productivity and an appropriate salary.

In fact, the set of evidence presented outlines an important mediating role of not feeling contributive at work, as well as not being well paid, in the link between the burnout syndrome dimension of low effectiveness and QWL. These findings shed new light on the need for public managers in leading roles, as well as human resource departments in the public sector, to design innovative incentives, appropriate measures, and work schedules to counterbalance such tendencies.

Regarding implications for public authorities, and based on our previous direct contacts and auscultation in the context of online training delivered to municipal workers, in order to address the negative association between the three burnout dimensions: emotional exhaustion, feelings of cynicism, and feeling less effective, and the motivating and economic mediators: contribution to productivity and appropriate salary; progressive remuneration mechanisms should be created, including a (fixed) basic salary and a (variable) supplementary salary indexed to productivity goals, and aligned with a new production and evaluation framework, to be implemented in public administration. Also taking into consideration the results of brainstorming, co-creation, and open innovation groups dynamics promoted in the previously referred online training delivered to municipal workers, further action is required to promote occupational health, QWL, and gender equality in public administration, aiming to diminish income inequality and foster the work–life balance of both female and male public servants.

Adding to the above, and considering the previous experience and project-based and organization innovation views of the authors collected in the previous exercise of public administration roles, it is suggested that public managers adopt innovative organizational practices, including flexible work schedules; project management practices; work innovation labs; mindfulness programs; hybrid work formats; and special incentives for workers with families, including children at school and older people with special needs, in order to tackle the negative associations and mediating effects found in the current study.

Despite the important set of discoveries made in the course of the current study, it is not free of limitations that should be considered in future research. Firstly, this study uses a cross-sectional online survey, which might have limited access by municipal workers who are less familiar with the internet or less likely to use it, for instance, manual workers rather than office workers. The convenience sampling procedure was obtained by direct contact with chief positions (middle managers) in the municipalities during online training courses, something that could bias access by some groups or individuals. This is a non-probability sampling method wherein units are selected for inclusion in the sample because they are the easiest for the researcher to access. The use of this non-random sampling can be due to availability at a given time or willingness to participate in the research, as occurred in the context of the previously referred online training.

One limitation associated with the empirical test of the convenience sample is that mixing functions and qualifications of municipal workers could bias the results, making it impossible to focus on one category of municipal workers. Nevertheless, bearing in mind the sample's dimension and the observed diversified set of institutional roles, it was found to be advantageous to consider municipal workers with leadership roles, as well as qualified and non-qualified workers.

It is also worthwhile to outline that the limited sample size was confined to Portuguese municipalities and, therefore, these results cannot be generalized to municipalities in other countries. Another aspect associated with the representativeness is the fact that the sample is related only to public municipalities, excluding from the study other public municipal firms. Therefore, representativeness is limited, and the results of the study cannot be generalized to the entire Portuguese municipal system, including the entrepreneurial units with the participation of municipal bodies.

The study was carried out during a five-month period, during a pandemic, which corresponded to one lockdown and then the relaxation of some lockdown measures. Furthermore, the inexistence of data gathered before the pandemic means comparisons cannot be made. Future studies could focus on participants who already felt burnout symptoms before the COVID-19 pandemic, to examine the increase, maintenance, or decrease of symptoms during the pandemic. When gathering information through a questionnaire, bias can appear linked to the tendency to present a favorable image of oneself. This tendency could be increased as sending the invitations to the leading positions inside the institutions can also produce a biased collection. In the sample used, 26% have leadership positions and 65% were qualified workers, while only 8% were non-qualified workers.

Future research endeavors on the relationship between burnout and QWL should perform a comparative analysis of different hierarchical positions, for different activities in the public sector, in order to assess the mediating effects of the contribution to productivity and appropriate salary, considering different cohorts of remuneration, education, and age.

Author Contributions: Conceptualization, D.P., J.L. and L.R.; validation, J.L.; estimation, D.P. and J.L.; data curation, D.P.; writing—original draft preparation, D.P.; writing—review and editing, D.P., J.L. and L.R; supervision, J.L. All authors have read and agreed to the published version of the manuscript.

Funding: The Portuguese Foundation for Science and Technology (Grants and NECE- UIDB/04630/2020) provided financial support for this study.

Institutional Review Board Statement: Ethical review and approval were waived for the study on human participants in accordance with the European legislation and institutional requirements applicable in this study, which was not conducted in our own higher education institution. The study was funded in the scope of the R.E.NewAL. SKILLS project (Project Number: 591861-EPP-1-2017-1-IT-EPPKA2-SSA) and the board governance structure of this project established a quality assurance, evaluation, and monitoring framework, through which the R.E.NewAL. SKILLS Contents Quality Plan (REC-QP) was created to ensure defined and shared quality standards for the contents production, including the questionnaires for gathering data, as well as identifying key roles among partner representatives and scores to be achieved by the contents produced. This plan created a set of committees to ensure ethical procedures, quality control, efficiency, and monitoring: a General Assembly, the ultimate decision-making body of the consortium and supervisory body for the execution of the project, coordinated by a representative of the Lead Partner (Coordinator of the General Assembly) acting as chairperson; and a Curriculum Committee (CC) made of RENewAL Contents Quality Managers (CQMs), selected by partner organizations among their staff, responsible for the quality control of R.E.NewAL. SKILLS contents, such as the survey questionnaire. The design of the questionnaire and methodology used to collect data was approved by the General Assembly, the partners, and the CC, assuring that the methods of data collection, the conformity of the questionnaires, and the subsequent anonymized treatment complied with ethical and quality standards, with published results not containing any entity-identifying information. Finally, the Education, Audio visual and Culture Executive Agency (EACEA) approved the outputs of the R.E.NewAL. SKILLS and closed the project with success.

Informed Consent Statement: Informed written consent was obtained from all subjects involved in the study.

Data Availability Statement: The data presented in this study are available on request from the corresponding author.

Acknowledgments: All the authors acknowledge the highly valuable comments and suggestions provided by the editors and reviewers, which contributed to improving the clarity, focus, contribution, and scientific soundness of the current study. The study was conducted with the support of FEFAL-Portuguese Foundation for the Studies and Training of Municipalities, which made possible the administration of the survey in a sample of 459 municipal workers.

Conflicts of Interest: The authors declare no conflict of interest.

References

1. Sirgy, M.; Efraty, D.; Siegel, P.; Lee, D. A new measure of quality of work life (QWL) based on need satisfaction and spillover theories. *Soc. Indic. Res.* **2001**, *55*, 241–302. [CrossRef]
2. Kooli, C. Challenges of working from home during the COVID-19 pandemic for women in the UAE. *J. Public Aff.* **2022**, e2829. [CrossRef] [PubMed]
3. Raub, S.; Blunschi, S. The Power of Meaningful Work: How Awareness of CSR Initiatives Fosters Task Significance and Positive Work Outcomes in Service Employees. *Cornell Hosp. Q.* **2014**, *55*, 10–18. [CrossRef]
4. Martel, J.P.; Dupuis, G. Quality of work life: Theoretical and methodological problems, and presentation of a new model and measuring instrument. *Soc. Indic. Res.* **2006**, *77*, 333–368. [CrossRef]
5. Leitão, J.; Pereira, D.; Gonçalves, Â. Quality of Work Life and Organizational Performance: Workers' Feelings of Contributing, or Not, to the Organization's Productivity. *Int. J. Environ. Res. Public Health* **2019**, *16*, 3803. [CrossRef]
6. Pandey, M.K.; Tripathi, P. Examine the relationship between level of aspiration, believes in just world, psychological well-being and quality of work-life. *Indian J. Health Well-Being* **2018**, *9*, 53–59.
7. Van der Klink, J.J.L.; Blonk, R.W.B.; Schene, A.H.; Van Dijk, F.J.H. The benefits of interventions for work-related stress. *Am. J. Public Health* **2001**, *91*, 270–276. [PubMed]
8. Messabia, N.; Fomi, P.R.; Kooli, C. Managing restaurants during the COVID-19 crisis: Innovating to survive and prosper. *J. Innov. Knowl.* **2022**, *7*, 100234. [CrossRef]
9. Bergman, E.; Löyttyniemi, E.; Myllyntausta, S.; Rautava, P.; Korhonen, P.E. Factors associated with quality of life and work ability among Finnish municipal employees: A cross-sectional study. *BMJ Open* **2020**, *10*, e035544. [CrossRef]
10. Leitão, J.; Pereira, D.; Gonçalves, Â. Quality of work life and contribution to productivity: Assessing the moderator effects of burnout syndrome. *Int. J. Environ. Res. Public Health* **2021**, *18*, 2425. [CrossRef] [PubMed]
11. Rasdi, R.M.; Zaremohzzabieh, Z.; Ahrari, S. Financial Insecurity During the COVID-19 Pandemic: Spillover Effects on Burnout–Disengagement Relationships and Performance of Employees Who Moonlight. *Front. Psychol.* **2021**, *12*, 610138. [CrossRef]

12. Schuster, C.; Weitzman, L.; Mikkelsen, K.S.; Meyer-Sahling, J.; Bersch, K.; Fukuyama, F.; Paskov, P.; Rogger, D.; Mistree, D.; Kay, K. Responding to COVID-19 through Surveys of Public Servants. *Public Adm. Rev.* **2020**, *80*, 792–796. [CrossRef]
13. Johnson, S.U.; Ebrahimi, O.V.; Hoffart, A. PTSD symptoms among health workers and public service providers during the COVID-19 outbreak. *PLoS ONE* **2020**, *15*, e0241032. [CrossRef]
14. Kim, J.; Garman, E.T. Financial Stress, Pay Satisfaction and Workplace Performance. *Compens. Benefits Rev.* **2004**, *36*, 69–76. [CrossRef]
15. Kulikowski, K.; Sedlak, P. Can you buy work engagement? The relationship between pay, fringe benefits, financial bonuses and work engagement. *Curr. Psychol.* **2020**, *39*, 343–353. [CrossRef]
16. Ceschi, A.; Costantini, A.; Dickert, S.; Sartori, R. The impact of occupational rewards on risk taking among managers. *J. Pers. Psychol.* **2017**, *16*, 104–111. [CrossRef]
17. Yassin, A.; Al-Mistarehi, A.H.; El-Salem, K.; Karasneh, R.A.; Al-Azzam, S.; Qarqash, A.A.; Khasawneh, A.G.; Alaabdin, A.M.Z.; Soudah, O. Prevalence Estimates and Risk Factors of Anxiety among Healthcare Workers in Jordan over One Year of the COVID-19 Pandemic: A Cross-Sectional Study. *Int. J. Environ. Res. Public Health* **2022**, *19*, 2615. [CrossRef]
18. Kooli, C. COVID-19: Public health issues and ethical dilemmas. *Ethics Med. Public Health* **2021**, *17*, 100635. [CrossRef]
19. Barman, M.; Hussain, T.; Abuswiril, H.; Illahi, M.N.; Sharif, M.; Saman, H.T.; Hassan, M.; Gaafar, M.; Abu, J.; Ahmad, M.K.K.; et al. Embracing Healthcare Delivery Challenges during a Pandemic. Review from a nodal designated COVID-19 center in Qatar. *Avicenna* **2021**, *2021*, 8. [CrossRef]
20. Lu, X.; Yu, H.; Shan, B. Relationship between Employee Mental Health and Job Performance: Mediation Role of Innovative Behavior and Work Engagement. *Int. J. Environ. Res. Public Health* **2022**, *19*, 6599. [CrossRef]
21. Ramos, D.; Cotrim, T.; Arezes, P.; Baptista, J.; Rodrigues, M.; Leitão, J. Frontiers in Occupational Health and Safety Management. *Int. J. Environ. Res. Public Health* **2022**, *19*, 10759. [CrossRef]
22. Freudenberger, H.J. Staff Burn-Out. *J. Soc. Issues* **1974**, *30*, 159–165. [CrossRef]
23. Leiter, M.P.; Maslach, C. The impact of interpersonal environment on burnout and organizational commitment. *J. Organ. Behav.* **1988**, *9*, 297–308. [CrossRef]
24. Maslach, C.; Jackson, S.E. The measurement of experienced burnout. *J. Organ. Behav.* **1981**, *2*, 99–113. [CrossRef]
25. Maslach, C.; Leiter, M.P. *Burnout: What It Is and How to Measure It*; Harvard Business Review Press: Boston, MA, USA, 2021; pp. 211–221.
26. Gil-Monte, P.R. *El síndrome de quemarse por el trabajo (burnout). Una enfermedad laboral en la sociedad del bienestar [The Syndrome of Being Burned by Work (Burnout). An Occupational Disease in the Welfare Society]*; Pirámide: Portonovo, Spain, 2005.
27. Schaufeli, W.B.; Greenglass, E.R. Introduction to special issue on burnout and health. *Psychol. Health* **2001**, *16*, 501–510. [CrossRef]
28. Maslach, C.; Leiter, M.P. Burnout. In *Encyclopedia of Stress*, 2nd ed.; Fink, G., Ed.; Elsevier: Amsterdam, The Netherlands, 2007; pp. 358–362.
29. Demerouti, E.; Mostert, K.; Bakker, A.B. Burnout and Work Engagement: A Thorough Investigation of the Independency of Both Constructs. *J. Occup. Health Psychol.* **2010**, *15*, 209–222. [CrossRef] [PubMed]
30. West, C.P.; Dyrbye, L.N.; Shanafelt, T.D. Physician burnout: Contributors, consequences and solutions. *J. Intern. Med.* **2018**, *283*, 516–529. [CrossRef]
31. Srivastava, S.; Misra, R.; Madan, P. 'The Saviors Are Also Humans': Understanding the Role of Quality of Work Life on Job Burnout and Job Satisfaction Relationship of Indian Doctors. *J. Health Manag.* **2019**, *21*, 210–229. [CrossRef]
32. Bakker, A.B.; de Vries, J.D. Job Demands–Resources theory and self-regulation: New explanations and remedies for job burnout. *Anxiety Stress Coping* **2021**, *34*, 1–21. [CrossRef]
33. Bakker, A.B.; Demerouti, E. Job demands-resources theory: Taking stock and looking forward. *J. Occup. Health Psychol.* **2017**, *22*, 273–285. [CrossRef]
34. Bakker, A.; Demerouti, E. The job demands-resources model: State of the art. *J. Manag. Psychol.* **2007**, *22*, 309–328. [CrossRef]
35. Bakker, A.B.; Shimazu, A.; Demerouti, E.; Shimada, K.; Kawakami, N. Work engagement versus workaholism: A test of the spillover-crossover model. *J. Manag. Psychol.* **2014**, *29*, 63–80. [CrossRef]
36. Demerouti, E.; Nachreiner, F.; Bakker, A.B.; Schaufeli, W.B. The job demands-resources model of burnout. *J. Appl. Psychol.* **2001**, *86*, 499–512. [CrossRef] [PubMed]
37. Meyer, B.; Zill, A.; Dilba, D.; Gerlach, R.; Schumann, S. Employee psychological well-being during the COVID-19 pandemic in Germany: A longitudinal study of demands, resources, and exhaustion. *Int. J. Psychol.* **2021**, *56*, 532–550. [CrossRef]
38. Sonnentag, S. Wellbeing and burnout in the workplace: Organizational causes and consequences. In *International Encyclopedia of the Social & Behavioral Sciences*, 2nd ed.; Elsevier: Amsterdam, The Netherlands, 2015; Volume 25, pp. 537–540.
39. Wang, X.; Lei, S.M.; Le, S.; Yang, Y.; Zhang, B.; Yao, W.; Gao, Z.; Cheng, S. Bidirectional influence of the COVID-19 pandemic lockdowns on health behaviors and quality of life among Chinese adults. *Int. J. Environ. Res. Public Health* **2020**, *17*, 5575. [CrossRef]
40. Wang, B.; Liu, Y.; Qian, J.; Parker, S.K. Achieving Effective Remote Working During the COVID-19 Pandemic: A Work Design Perspective. *Appl. Psychol.* **2021**, *70*, 16–59. [CrossRef]
41. Kniffin, K.M.; Narayanan, J.; Anseel, F.; Antonakis, J.; Ashford, S.P.; Bakker, A.B.; Bamberger, P.; Bapuji, H.; Bhave, D.P.; Choi, V.K.; et al. COVID-19 and the workplace: Implications, issues, and insights for future research and action. *Am. Psychol.* **2021**, *76*, 63–77. [CrossRef]

42. Moretti, A.; Menna, F.; Aulicino, M.; Paoletta, M.; Liguori, S.; Iolascon, G. Characterization of home working population during COVID-19 emergency: A cross-sectional analysis. *Int. J. Environ. Res. Public Health* **2020**, *17*, 6284. [CrossRef]
43. Blake, H.; Bermingham, F.; Johnson, G.; Tabner, A. Mitigating the psychological impact of COVID-19 on healthcare workers: A digital learning package. *Int. J. Environ. Res. Public Health* **2020**, *17*, 2997. [CrossRef]
44. Helmi, M.; Sari, D.; Sulistyowati, Y.; Meliala, A.; Trisnantoro, L.; Nurrobi, T.; Ratmono, T. The challenge of education and training in the COVID-19 National Emergency Hospital Wisma Atlet Kemayoran in Jakarta. *Avicenna* **2021**, *2021*, 10. [CrossRef]
45. Duarte, I.; Teixeira, A.; Castro, L.; Marina, S.; Ribeiro, C.; Jácome, C.; Martins, V.; Ribeiro-Vaz, I.; Pinheiro, H.C.; Silva, A.R.; et al. Burnout among portuguese healthcare workers during the COVID-19 pandemic. *BMC Public Health* **2020**, *20*, 1885. [CrossRef]
46. Hofmam, A.C.; Hubie, A.P.S. Burnout syndrome in employees of two health units in a city in the west of Paraná. *FAG J. Health* **2020**, *4*, 429–433. [CrossRef]
47. Charbonneau, É.; Doberstein, C. An Empirical Assessment of the Intrusiveness and Reasonableness of Emerging Work Surveillance Technologies in the Public Sector. *Public Adm. Rev.* **2020**, *80*, 780–791. [CrossRef]
48. Bavel, J.J.V.; Baicker, K.; Boggio, P.S.; Capraro, V.; Cichocka, A.; Cikara, M.; Crockett, M.J.; Crum, A.J.; Douglas, K.M.; Druckman, J.N.; et al. Using social and behavioural science to support COVID-19 pandemic response. *Nat. Hum. Behav.* **2020**, *4*, 460–471. [CrossRef]
49. Marelli, S.; Castelnuovo, A.; Somma, A.; Castronovo, V.; Mombelli, S.; Bottoni, D.; Leitner, C.; Fossati, A.; Ferini-Strambi, L. Impact of COVID-19 lockdown on sleep quality in university students and administration staff. *J. Neurol.* **2021**, *268*, 8–15. [CrossRef] [PubMed]
50. Evanoff, B.A.; Strickland, J.R.; Dale, A.M.; Hayibor, L.; Page, E.; Duncan, J.G.; Kannampallil, T.; Gray, D.L. Work-related and personal factors associated with mental well-being during the COVID-19 response: Survey of health care and other workers. *J. Med. Internet Res.* **2020**, *22*, e21366. [CrossRef] [PubMed]
51. Sørengaard, T.A.; Saksvik-Lehouillier, I. Insomnia among employees in occupations with critical societal functions during the COVID-19 pandemic. *Sleep Med.* **2022**, *91*, 185–188. [CrossRef]
52. Holmes, M.R.; Rentrope, C.R.; Korsch-Williams, A.; King, J.A. Impact of COVID-19 Pandemic on Posttraumatic Stress, Grief, Burnout, and Secondary Trauma of Social Workers in the United States. *Clin. Soc. Work J.* **2021**, *49*, 495–504. [CrossRef] [PubMed]
53. Bapuji, H.; Ertug, G.; Shaw, J.D. Organizations and societal economic inequality: A review and way forward. *Acad. Manag. Ann.* **2020**, *14*, 60–91. [CrossRef]
54. Steadman, K.; Wood, M.; Silvester, H. *Health and Wellbeing at Work: A Survey of Employees*; Department for Work and Pensions: London, UK, 2014.
55. ACT Government. *ACT Online Employee Health and Wellbeing Survey*; ACT Government: Canberra, Australia, 2015.
56. British Heart Foundation. Health at Work Employee Survey. 2012. Available online: https://www.bhf.org.uk/informationsupport/publications/health-at-work/health-at-work-employee-survey (accessed on 26 May 2021).
57. Hafner, M.; Van Stolk, C.; Saunders, C.; Krapels, J.; Baruch, B. *Health, Wellbeing and Productivity in the Workplace: A Britain's Healthiest Company Summary Report*; RAND Corporation: Santa Monica, CA, USA, 2015.
58. Southern Cross Health Society & BusinessNZ. Wellness in the Workplace. The Personnel Administrator. New Zealand. 2017. Available online: https://www.southerncross.co.nz/-/media/Southern-Cross-Health-Society/Health-insurance/Sales-collateral/Employer/Wellness-in-the-Workplace-Survey-2017.pdf?la=en (accessed on 26 May 2021).
59. Staff Health and Wellbeing Survey. Available online: https://www.sahealth.sa.gov.au/wps/wcm/connect/public+content/sa+health+internet/resources/staff+needs+assessment+tool+healthy+workers+healthy+futures (accessed on 26 May 2021).
60. RTI. Tool for Observing Worksite Environments (TOWE). Available online: https://www.cdc.gov/workplacehealthpromotion/pdf/TOWE-508.pdf (accessed on 26 May 2021).
61. Gunzler, D.; Chen, T.; Wu, P.; Zhang, H. Introduction to mediation analysis with structural equation modeling. *Shanghai Arch Psychiatry* **2013**, *25*, 390–394.

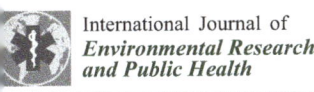

Article

Relationship between Employee Mental Health and Job Performance: Mediation Role of Innovative Behavior and Work Engagement

Xifeng Lu [1], Haijing Yu [2,*] and Biaoan Shan [2]

[1] College of Accounting, Jilin University of Finance and Economics, Changchun 130117, China; luxifeng621@163.com
[2] School of Business and Management, Jilin University, Changchun 130012, China; shanbiaoan@jlu.edu.cn
* Correspondence: yuhj101@163.com

Abstract: The relationship between employee mental health and job performance has been one of the key concerns in workplace. However, extant studies suffer from incomplete results due to their focus on developed economies' contexts and the unclear path of employee mental health's impact on performance. In this paper, we investigate the mechanism of employee mental health influencing job performance. We use the data of Chinese firms to test these hypotheses. Drawing on a sample of 239 firms from China, we find that employee mental health positively impacts job performance, and such relationship is mediated by innovative behavior and work engagement. The findings not only enrich the discipline's knowledge on mental health in an emerging economy setting but also extend the implications of mental health, innovative behavior, and work engagement to job performance.

Keywords: mental health; job performance; innovative behavior; work engagement; emerging economy

1. Introduction

Employee mental health has long been a topic of concern for researchers and practitioners alike [1]. One reason for this interest is that employee mental health is increasingly prominent within workplaces, which leads to significant costs including absenteeism, burnout, employee compensation claims, work–family conflict and low productivity [2,3]. In particular, with the outbreak of COVID-19, the uncertainties and fears associated with the virus outbreak, along with survival crisis of enterprises, lead to increases in employees' mental disorders [4–6]. For example, Xiong et al. [7] found that people in China, Spain, Italy and five other countries had higher levels of symptoms of anxiety, depression, traumatic stress disorder and other mental health problems during the COVID-19 pandemic. Bufquin et al. [8] showed that since the outbreak, employees in the restaurant industry experienced higher levels of psychological distress and drug and alcohol use than furloughed employees. In this regard, it is timely to examine the influence of the mental health of employees on outcomes.

Recent studies have shown the relationship between employee mental health and different organizational outcomes, including employee emotional expression, job satisfaction, daily work behavior, job performance and firm performance [6,9–12]. Among these, the relationship between employee mental health and job performance has been an important research topic and has received more and more attention. Scholars suggested that employees with good mental health will show a positive working state and devote themselves to work tasks with more enthusiasm [13], whereas poor mental health may lead to inactivity at work and degradations in interpersonal relationships, which, in turn, negatively impacts employees' work performance [14–17].

Although the relationship between mental health and job performance has been well-documented, there still remain some insufficiencies in the previous research. As a result, our extant knowledge on how employee mental health shapes job performance has remained fragmented and limited. First, the path of how employee mental health affects job performance is still unclear. The psychological characteristic–behavior–outcome framework indicates that although a strong individual attribute is important for an outcome, it does not automatically yield that outcome; instead, it influences outcome via appropriate behaviors. Second, such studies have been primarily conducted in Western economic contexts, whereas examinations in Eastern cultures such as China are lacking, which impedes upon the field's global relevance. Studies have shown that culture, such as individualism and collectivism, will affect individuals' mental health [18,19]. Therefore, the impact of mental health on performance may be different under different cultural backgrounds.

With the goal of addressing this gap of the unclear path of employee mental health-job performance in the literature, we consider the mediating role of employee innovation behavior and work engagement on this relationship. It additionally aims to identify the antecedents of job performance. Because research on the employee mental health–job performance relationship in emerging economies is lacking, we also aim to analyze the role of employee mental health in job performance in China. To achieve the goals adopted in the study, we examine the employee mental health–job performance relationship, innovation behavior, the work engagement–job performance relationship, and the mediating role of innovation behavior and work engagement in the mental health–job performance relationship using data from Chinese firms. Our results show that employee mental health is positively associated with job performance, and that these effects are mediated by employee innovative behavior and work engagement.

The present paper contributes to the literature in several ways. First, complementing previous research investigating the role of employee mental health in job performance in developed economies, we examine employee mental health's impact on job performance in China. Second, we contribute to the research on job performance by analyzing the role of innovative behavior and work engagement in job performance. Although prior research has provided insightful understanding of the drivers of job performance, knowledge on job performance could benefit from identifying further drivers that explain this important concept. Third, we explored the pathways of employee mental health affecting job performance ignored by extant research, thus extending the relationship between employee mental health and job performance.

The rest of the article is structured as follows. Firstly, the literature on employee mental health is reviewed, and the corresponding theoretical hypotheses are put forward. Second, this study proposes the methods and results. Then, we conclude by discussing our results and their implications for theory and practice and suggesting future research directions. Finally, we draw a conclusion of this study.

2. Literature Review and Hypothesis Development

2.1. Employee Mental Health

The World Health Organization [20] defines mental health as "a state of well-being in which the individual realizes his or her own abilities, can cope with the normal stresses of life, can work productively and fruitfully, and is able to make a contribution to his or her community". Over the years, researchers have developed a variety of operational definitions. For example, Ford et al. [13] suggest that mental health refers to an individual's affective experiences and behavior. Montano et al. [16] define mental health as a continuum of neurophysiological and cognitive states related to thinking, mood and emotion, and behavior including negative and positive mental health states. Sharma et al. [21] show that mental health is a positive expression, which is the absence of anxiety, social dysfunction and the presence of condition. Based on these definitions, scholars have developed a variety of measurement instruments that include both positive and negative terms in order to describe mental health more accurately [22]. Although definitions and measurements differ among scholars, it is widely accepted that positive affective states are often described as 'good' mental health, while a state of emotional suffering such as depression and anxiety is often used to refer to 'poor' mental health [8,23].

2.2. Employee Mental Health and Job Performance

The relationships between mental health and job performance have received increased attention in the organizational literature. We propose that employee mental health is positively correlated with job performance. This view is consistent with the happy–productive worker hypothesis that suggests that mental health is positively related to job performance [24,25]. Specifically, mentally healthy employees with positive affective states can improve cognitive flexibility and find more solutions to problems in work tasks [26]. Thus, employees with good mental health perform better on work tasks than those with poor mental health. Moreover, positive affective states are associated with individuals building good interpersonal relationships [27], which enable them to receive help from their leaders and colleagues at work. Studies also showed that good social relationships are an important source of job-related information and knowledge [28]. Finally, many studies also support this hypothesis. For example, in a meta-analytic study from 111 independent samples obtained from a search of the literature, Ford et al. [13] indicated that psychological health was a moderate-to-strong correlate of work performance. Similarly, Zacher, Jimmieson and Winter [25] showed that employees' mental health had a positive effect on work performance in the sample of 165 employees providing in-home eldercare, as well as one colleague and one family member of each employee. At the same time, several meta-analytical findings indicate that poor mental health such as anxiety, depressive symptoms and job stress has a negative impact on job performance [16]. Hence, we expect:

Hypothesis 1. *Employee mental health is positively related to job performance.*

2.3. Work Engagement, Innovative Behavior and Job Performance

Work engagement is defined as an active state of work characterized by vigor, dedication, and absorption [29,30]. Engaged employees are energetic and passionate about their work and are often fully immersed in their work [31,32]. In this regard, by investing their cognitive, emotional and social resources into their work, employees can enhance their responsibilities and emotional connection to work, and put more effort and more time into work, which is conducive to achieving high work performance [33]. At the same time, employees with high work engagement have a strong work identity and expect to achieve good results such as high performance through work [34]. Indeed, several studies have shown that work engagement is positively related to job performance [35–37].

We further propose that employee innovative behavior has a positive effect on job performance. Innovative behavior is a process of going beyond given paradigms and routines and generating new ideas and implementing them through experimentation [38]. In this process, employees can access a broad range of information to generate creative and new ideas, which facilitate a more detailed understanding of existing problems and alternative solutions through experimentation [39,40]. Moreover, experimentation and trial and error in innovation behavior produce a larger and more elaborate pool of knowledge and involve the recombination or creation of resources [41,42]. This again will facilitate learning and develop capacity [42,43], which in turn improve work performance. Hence, we expect:

Hypothesis 2a. *Employee work engagement is positively related to job performance.*

Hypothesis 2b. *Employee innovative behavior is positively related to job performance.*

2.4. Work Engagement and Innovative Behavior as Mediators

Finally, we propose that mental health has an effect on work engagement and innovative behavior, which, in turn, is positively related to work performance. In other words, we argue that work engagement and innovative behavior mediate the relationship between mental health and work performance. Specifically, according to the broaden-and-build theory of positive emotions, positive emotions expand people's thought–action repertoires and build their enduring personal resources including self-efficacy and resilience [26,44]. Studies have shown that such personal resources have a strong motivational potential and are vital antecedents of work engagement [45–48]. In addition, positive mental health leads to higher work motivation [13]. Employees with positive affect will set high goals for work and expect that engaging in work generates positive outcomes [49]. Finally, positive affect also leads to a heuristic and global information processing pattern that allows employees to concentrate on an ongoing activity, which is an important aspect of work engagement. In contrast, poor mental health such as depression and anxiety is associated with overestimations of risk and underestimations of self-worth, which may lead to lower effort when working [13].

At the same time, the broaden-and-build theory of positive emotions also indicates that positive emotions broaden the array of individual's existing cognitive frameworks [26], which increases individual cognitive flexibility and the cognitive resources available for recognizing the potential connections between things [44]; this, in turn, helps individuals generate novel ideas not previously available [27,50]. Moreover, some theories propose that affect provides information about the world around us [51–53]. A positive emotional state signals that everything is going well and the current situation poses no serious threat [27,50,54,55]. These reactions, in turn, encourage employees to engage in active efforts to try novel things such as innovation [54]. In addition, innovative behavior is a multi-stage process from idea generation to implementation of new and useful ideas within an organization [56–58], which is filled with high uncertainty and risks [42,59]. Employees with good mental health have confidence to overcome obstacles in innovation processes and persist longer in efforts to develop and implement innovative ideas [60,61].

In sum, we suggest that the better one's mental health, the higher their work engagement and innovative behavior. Moreover, work engagement and innovative behavior are shown to be direct antecedents of work performance. Hence, we expect:

Hypothesis 3a. *Work engagement mediates the relationship between mental health and job performance.*

Hypothesis 3b. *Innovative behavior mediates the relationship between mental health and job performance.*

3. Methodology

3.1. Data Collection and Samples Characteristics

Considering the impacts of COVID-19, an online survey was conducted to test the hypotheses in this study. In order to let participants fully understand the purpose of this survey, we provided important information about the online questionnaire on the first page. In addition, we provided an informed consent at the front of the questionnaire. Additionally, all subjects were required to give their informed consent for inclusion before they started the survey. The questionnaires were from employees' self-reports. Participants were anonymous and they could quit at any time during the survey. Therefore, this study did not collect any data without consent.

According to the study of Shan et al. [62], the process of developing the questionnaire is shown as follows: First, several employees from different companies were interviewed. This step let us understand more about the core concepts of this study, including job performance and employees' mental health. Then, we developed a draft questionnaire based on the interviews and previous studies. Finally, we conducted a pilot study to test the preliminary questionnaire. Based on a small-scale survey, we revised the questionnaire and a formal questionnaire for this study was generated. The process could ensure the accuracy of the questionnaire.

Based on the above, this study carried out a formal survey in China. The survey was conducted from October to December, 2021. Participants came from different companies in several provinces, such as Jilin Province, Shandong Province, and Yunnan Province. These companies were located in different regions in China. Our team members sent the questionnaires or links by WeChat, email and other ways. Participants were employees in different positions, such as managers (e.g., middle-level managers) and technical engineers (e.g., employees in production line). About 500 questionnaires or links were sent out to the target employees. We confirmed the samples and eliminated the samples for which the completion rate was low (less than 75%).

Finally, we collected 239 valid samples. These samples came from different industries, including manufacturing industry, construction industry, and service industries. Additionally, the samples were distributed in different regions, such as Northeast, East coast and Southwest China. The characteristics of the samples are as follows. Most participants (73%) are grass-roots employees, and 27% of participants are middle-level or above. 69.2% participants have received a Bachelor's degree, Master's degree, or Ph.D., while 30.8% of participants' education level is low, including Junior college, High school or below. Most participants (66.7%) have worked for less than eight years. Most participants (62.3%) are from mature companies (created more than 10 years ago).

3.2. Measurement

We utilized a seven-point Likert scale to measure the core variables in this study. All scales of the related variables have been tested in other studies.

Dependent variable: job performance. Based on the research of Williams and Anderson [63], we utilized four items to measure the variable of job performance. Example items include "I am satisfied with my job performance", "I could adequately complete assigned duties" and ""I try to work as hard as possible" (Cronbach's α = 0.858).

Independent variable: Employee mental health. Employee mental health used nine items, mainly from the study of Kashyap and Singh [64]. Example items include "I am always very nervous and feel stressed", "I always feel unhappy or depressed" and "I always could not concentrate when I do something" (Cronbach's α = 0.952).

Mediating variables: Work engagement and employee innovative behavior. First, we used four items to measure work engagement based on the study of Suárez-Albanchez et al. [65]. Example items include "I am passionate about my work", "I feel full of energy when I am working" and "Time flies when I'm working" (Cronbach's α = 0.849). Second, according to the research of Scott and Bruce [66], we used eight items to measure the variable of employee innovative behavior. Example items include "Always search for ideas for new technologies, processes, and/or products", "Always generate creative ideas" and "Always promote and support ideas to others" (Cronbach's α = 0.958).

Control variables: The selection of control variables is important for the results. In this study, firm age, the number of firm employees (firm size), the educational background of employees, and the work experience of employees were set as control variables. Firm age is calculated by the years since the firm was created (1–5 years, 1; 6–10 years, 2; 11–15 years, 3; more than 15 years, 4). Firm size is determined by the number of employees (more than 200 employees, 4; 51–200 employees, 3; 21–50 employees, 2; 20 or fewer employees, 1). Employees' educational background reflects the levels of employees' education (high school degree or below, 1; junior college education, 2; Bachelor's degree, 3; Master's degree, Ph.D., 4). Work experience refers to the year(s) an employee has worked in the company.

3.3. Validity and Common Method Bias

Firstly, we test the possible problem of common method bias. According to a study of Podsakoff and Organ [67], Harman's one-factor test could be utilized. This method has been widely used in previous studies. The results show that there is no significant problem of common method bias because the largest factor in this study only explained 38.121% of the entire variance. Secondly, the validity of the samples is conducted. The results show that all factor loadings are greater than 0.7 and none were below 0.6. Thus, the validity of the samples is very high in this study.

4. Data Analysis and Results

SPSS (IBM, Armonk, NY, USA) was used in this study. First, we calculate the correlations among core variables of this study. The results are shown in Table 1. The coefficients are not high. Second, the descriptive statistics are calculated. We can see that there is no significant problem with the mean and S.D. (standard deviation) of the core variable. All the correlation coefficients do not exceed 0.7. Third, the multicollinearity issue may impact the results. Consequently, we calculate the coefficients of variance inflation factors (VIFs). The results show that there is no VIF that exceeds 10. This indicates that there is no significant multicollinearity based on the view of Hair et al. [68].

Table 1. The results of the correlation matrix and descriptive statistics.

	1	2	3	4	5	6	7	Mean	S.D.
Firm age	1							2.978	1.064
Number of employees	0.676 ***	1						3.830	1.420
Education background	0.162 *	0.359 ***	1					2.760	0.790
Work experience	0.202 *	0.186 *	−0.074	1				5.800	4.214
Employee mental health	−0,015	−0.041	−0.056	0.135	1			4.657	1.458
work engagement	0,060	−0.11	−0.073	0.095	0.235 ***	1		4.873	1.288
innovative behavior	−0.036	−0.122	−0.042	0.069	0.382 ***	0.572 ***	1	5.188	1.210
job performance	0.027	−0.031	−0.049	0.162	0.292 ***	0.524 ***	0.609 ***	5.219	1.170

Note: *** $p < 0.001$; * $p < 0.05$.

Fourth, we apply hierarchical linear analysis (HLA) to test the hypotheses proposed in this study. Seven models are created and the results are shown in Tables 2 and 3. We control the firm age, the number of firm employees, the educational background of employees, and the work experience of employees. Model 1 showed the results of the impact of three control variables on job performance. The results of model 1 verified that the influence of control variables is not significant. Then, the results of model 2 indicated that H1 was verified. The coefficient for employee mental health is 0.256, which is significant at $p < 0.01$. (Model 2). Therefore, the influence of employee mental health is positive. Model 3 was built to test H2a and H2b. From the results of model 3, both coefficients for work engagement and employee innovative behavior were positive and significant. The results show that work engagement and innovative behavior are positively related to job performance.

Table 2. The results of regression analysis (models 1–3).

Variables	Dependent Variable: Job Performance		
	Model 1	Model 2	Model 3
Control variables			
Firm age	0.078	0.080	−0.008
Number of employees	−0.070	−0.045	0.019
Education background	0.004	0.032	−0.003
Work experience	0.164	0.126	0.113
Independent variable			
Employee mental health		0.256 **	
Mediating variables			
Work engagement			0.309 **
Innovative behavior			0.295 ***
R^2	0.031	0.094	0.313
Adj-R^2	0.001	0.058	0.280
F-value	1.038	2.642 *	9.628 ***

Note: *** $p < 0.001$; ** $p < 0.01$; * $p < 0.05$.

Table 3. The results of regression analysis (models 4–7).

Variables	Job Performance		Work Engagement	Innovative Behavior
	Model 4	Model 5	Model 6	Model 7
Control variables				
Firm age	0.008	0.023	0.161	0.129
Number of employees	−0.035	0.051	−0.023	−0.217
Education background	0.034	−0.012	−0.005	0.098
Work experience	0.113	0.105	0.030	0.048
Independent variable				
Employee mental health	0.129	0.108	0.284 ***	0.335 ***
Mediating variables				
Work engagement	0.447 ***			
Innovative behavior		0.444 ***		
R^2	0.273	0.262	0.103	0.142
Adj-R^2	0.239	0.227	0.068	0.109
F-value	7.949 ***	7.524 ***	2.949 **	4.252 ***

Note: *** $p < 0.001$; ** $p < 0.01$.

In order to test H3a and H3b, we built models 6 and 7 (Table 3). The results show that the impact of employee mental health on work engagement is positive (Model 6: β = 0.284; $p < 0.001$). Additionally, the impact of employee mental health on innovative behavior is positive (Model 7: β = 0.335; $p < 0.001$). The results indicated that both H3a and H3b were verified by the samples.

Model 4 was built based on model 2, which was applied to test the mediating role of work engagement. The results of model 4 indicated that the coefficient for work engagement is significant (model 4, β = 0.447; $p < 0.001$). However, the coefficient for employee mental health was not significant (model 4, β = 0.129; ns). From the results of model 2, model 4 and model 6, we could see that the positive mediating effect of work engagement on the relationship between employee mental health and job performance is significant. Therefore, hypothesis 4a is supported by the samples.

Model 5 was built based on model 2, which was applied to test the mediating role of innovative behavior. The results of model 5 indicated that the coefficient for innovative behavior was significant (model 5, β = 0.444; $p < 0.001$). However, the coefficient for employee mental health is also not significant (model 5, β = 0.108; ns). From the results of model 2, model 5 and model 7, we could see that the positive mediating effect of innovative behavior is significant. Therefore, hypothesis 4b is supported by the samples.

The endogeneity problem may be driven by some unobservable characteristics of the firm and employee [69]. Therefore, we consider several control variables in the model. We control the firm age, the number of firm employees, the educational background of employees, and the work experience of employees. Moreover, job satisfaction is considered as a proxy variable of employee mental health. We conduct the hierarchical linear analysis (HLA) and find that Hypotheses 1–3 are supported by data. Therefore, the results show there is not a significant endogeneity problem.

5. Discussion

The present study pursued three goals in extending the extant knowledge on the relationship between employee mental health and job performance. First, we set out to investigate how employee' mental health influences job performance in an emerging economy context. In line with previous theories and research in developed economies [25], we predicted and found that employee mental health also exerts a positive influence on job performance in China. This finding indicates that the mental health of employees is an important factor to predict job performance. Moreover, the result that employee mental health positively affects job performance is robust and valid.

Second, to enrich our insights into the antecedents of job performance, we predicted and found that employee innovation behavior and work engagement positively affect job performance. It is plausible that job performance is enhanced because employees who are more dedicated to work and exhibit more innovative behavior are more effective in meeting the demands of firms, thereby leads to better development of the firm. Importantly, this result extends the findings on factors that promote job performance.

Third, we found that employee mental health is indirectly associated with job performance via innovative behavior and work engagement, which addresses tasks associated with work effectiveness. The positive affect state inherent to mental health is conveyed through innovative behavior and work engagement that are important for work demands. In turn, these two behaviors are positively associated with job performance. These results concerning indirect effects suggest an important nomological chain that begins with the mental health of the employee, which is positively connected with investing more energy and resources via innovative behavior and work engagement to create positive, productive work conditions, leading to better job performance. This indirect connection leads to useful insights into the mental health–job performance relationship.

5.1. Theoretical Implications

There are several theoretical implications. Firstly, this study explores the relationship between employee mental health and job performance and tests it in a Chinese context. The important role of employees' mental health in an organization is a concern for existing scholars. More and more studies observe that mental health strongly influences the individual performance and organizational performance. However, previous studies examine the mental health-job performance relationship in developed countries. Few studies test the relationship in emerging economies such as China. Using the samples from China, we find a positive relationship. By doing so, the findings of this study contribute to the literature on the roles of employees' mental health in an emerging economy.

Secondly, we identify two types of employee behaviors and analyze their impacts on job performance. Work engagement and innovative behavior are important behaviors that may influence individual work efficiency. In this study, we explore the impacts of work engagement and innovative behavior on job performance. By doing so, the findings extend the antecedents of job performance.

Thirdly, this study reveals the paths of how employee mental health affects job performance, and find that employees' work engagement and innovative behavior play a positive mediating role in the relationship between employee mental health and job performance. Existing studies have ignored the impact mechanism of employee mental health on job performance. What remains unknown is how employee mental health influences individual performance. Based on the framework of individual characteristics–behaviors–outcome, we view employees' work engagement and innovative behavior as two salient types of behavior that are affected by mental health. This study examines and finds that employees' work engagement and innovative behavior mediate the mental health–job performance relationship. These findings further extend the relationship between employee mental health and job performance.

5.2. Managerial Implications

The managerial implications of this study are reflected in the following aspects. Firstly, employees (or managers) should pay attention to mental health problem and make necessary adjustments. Poor mental health may lead to absenteeism and low productivity [2]. For employees in a highly competitive environment, the mental health problem is becoming a big challenge for them to improve job performance. Especially under the context of the outbreak of COVID-19, many employees are suffering from mental health problems. It is important for them to maintain their mental health. This requires them to adjust their mental state. Secondly, top managers or leaders in different organizFations could stimulate employees' work engagement and encourage them to engage in innovative behavior. Especially for employees with good mental health, their intention to work and innovation is strong. How to utilize their passion is important for organization. Hence, managers should observe employees and apply their healthy mentality to improve their job performance. Thirdly, we suggest companies (or organizations) care about employees' mental health and foster an atmosphere to improve it. Employees are the core capital of companies. Employees with good mental health support enterprises to achieve high organizational performance. Therefore, companies should be concerned about their employees' mental health and foster a healthy mentality for them.

5.3. Limitations and Future Research

There are still some limitations which should be taken into account in future studies. Firstly, the data and samples of this study were collected in China. There are many other emerging economies, such as India and Brazil. In the future, more samples from other emerging economies could be considered to test the model. Additionally, future studies could compare the results of different countries or regions. Secondly, we identify work engagement and innovative behaviors as the mediating variables of the impact of employee mental health on job performance. Are there any other more important mediating variables to be considered? This question should be addressed by future research. Thirdly, we do not consider contextual factor(s) in this study. The relationship between employee mental health and job performance may be influenced by some contextual factors, such as perceived environment, individual personality, and so on. Therefore, future studies could identify certain moderating variables to further explore the relationship between employee mental health and job performance. Finally, this study does not consider the impact of different industries. In different industries, the situation of employees' mental health may be different, such as the IT industry, manufacturing industry, etc. Hence, future studies could consider the results of different industries, as well as test the model in them.

6. Conclusions

Based on existing research gaps, this study explores the impact of employee mental health on job performance. Considering that few studies in the literature focus on the context of China, an emerging economy, this study uses samples in China and finds that employee mental health plays an important role in improving job performance. Chinese organizations should try to maintain employee mental health to achieve high job performance. Furthermore, we discuss the employee mental health–job performance relationship. The paths of how employee mental health influence job performance are revealed in this study. The results show that work engagement and innovative behaviors play positive mediating roles in the relationship between employee mental health and job performance. These findings reveal the relationship between employee mental health and job performance and further enrich the literature on employee behaviors. Furthermore, this study extends the research of employees' characteristics and their influences on job performance.

Author Contributions: Conceptualization, X.L., H.Y. and B.S.; methodology, X.L. and B.S.; formal analysis, H.Y. and B.S.; investigation, X.L., H.Y. and B.S.; writing—original draft preparation, X.L., H.Y. and B.S.; writing—review and editing, X.L. and H.Y.; supervision, B.S.; project administration, X.L. and B.S. All authors have read and agreed to the published version of the manuscript.

Funding: This research received no external funding.

Institutional Review Board Statement: Not applicable.

Informed Consent Statement: Informed consent was obtained from all participants involved in the study.

Data Availability Statement: The data presented in this study are available upon request from the corresponding author.

Conflicts of Interest: The authors declare no conflict of interest.

References

1. Robbins, J.M.; Ford, M.T.; Tetrick, L.E. Perceived unfairness and employee health: A meta-analytic integration. *J. Appl. Psychol.* **2012**, *97*, 235–272. [CrossRef] [PubMed]
2. Dimoff, J.K.; Kelloway, E.K. With a little help from my boss: The impact of workplace mental health training on leader behaviors and employee resource utilization. *J. Occup. Health Psychol.* **2019**, *24*, 4–19. [CrossRef] [PubMed]
3. Van Gordon, W.; Shonin, E.; Zangeneh, M.; Griffiths, M.D. Work-related mental health and job performance: Can mindfulness help? *Int. J. Ment. Health Addict.* **2014**, *12*, 129–137. [CrossRef]
4. Liu, W.; Xu, Y.; Ma, D. Work-Related Mental Health under COVID-19 Restrictions: A Mini Literature Review. *Front. Public Health* **2021**, *9*, 788370. [CrossRef]
5. Usher, K.; Durkin, J.; Bhullar, N. The COVID-19 pandemic and mental health impacts. *Int. J. Ment. Health Nurs.* **2020**, *29*, 315. [CrossRef]
6. Yu, J.; Park, J.; Hyun, S.S. Impacts of the COVID-19 pandemic on employees' work stress, well-being, mental health, organizational citizenship behavior, and employee-customer identification. *J. Hosp. Mark. Manag.* **2021**, *30*, 529–548. [CrossRef]
7. Xiong, J.; Lipsitz, O.; Nasri, F.; Lui, L.M.; Gill, H.; Phan, L.; Chen-Li, D.; Iacobucci, M.; Ho, R.; Majeed, A.; et al. Impact of COVID-19 pandemic on mental health in the general population: A systematic review. *J. Affect. Disord.* **2020**, *277*, 55–64. [CrossRef]
8. Bufquin, D.; Park, J.Y.; Back, R.M.; de Souza Meira, J.V.; Hight, S.K. Employee work status, mental health, substance use, and career turnover intentions: An examination of restaurant employees during COVID-19. *Int. J. Hosp. Manag.* **2021**, *93*, 102764. [CrossRef]
9. Cao, X.; Zhang, H.; Li, P.; Huang, X. The Influence of Mental Health on Job Satisfaction: Mediating Effect of Psychological Capital and Social Capital. *Front. Public Health* **2022**, *10*, 797274. [CrossRef]
10. Ipsen, C.; Karanika-Murray, M.; Nardelli, G. Addressing mental health and organisational performance in tandem: A challenge and an opportunity for bringing together what belongs together. *Work Stress* **2020**, *34*, 1–4. [CrossRef]
11. Lee, M.S.M.; Lee, M.B.; Liao, S.C.; Chiang, F.T. Relationship between mental health and job satisfaction among employees in a medical center department of laboratory medicine. *J. Formos. Med. Assoc.* **2009**, *108*, 146–154. [CrossRef]
12. Stephan, U. Entrepreneurs' mental health and well-being: A review and research agenda. *Acad. Manag. Perspect.* **2018**, *32*, 290–322. [CrossRef]
13. Ford, M.T.; Cerasoli, C.P.; Higgins, J.A.; Decesare, A.L. Relationships between psychological, physical, and behavioural health and work performance: A review and meta-analysis. *Work Stress* **2011**, *25*, 185–204. [CrossRef]
14. Caveen, M.; Dewa, C.S.; Goering, P. The influence of organizational factors on return-to-work outcomes. *Can. J. Community Ment. Health* **2007**, *25*, 121–142. [CrossRef]
15. Kircanski, K.; Joormann, J.; Gotlib, I.H. Cognitive aspects of depression. *Wiley Interdiscip. Rev. Cogn. Sci.* **2012**, *3*, 301–313. [CrossRef] [PubMed]
16. Montano, D.; Reeske, A.; Franke, F.; Hüffmeier, J. Leadership, followers' mental health and job performance in organizations: A comprehensive meta-analysis from an occupational health perspective. *J. Organ. Behav.* **2017**, *38*, 327–350. [CrossRef]
17. Shain, M.; Arnold, I.; GermAnn, K. The road to psychological safety: Legal, scientific, and social foundations for a Canadian National Standard on Psychological Safety in the Workplace. *Bull. Sci. Technol. Soc.* **2012**, *32*, 142–162. [CrossRef]
18. Haar, J.M.; Russo, M.; Sune, A.; Ollier-Malaterre, A. Outcomes of work-life balance on job satisfaction, life satisfaction and mental health: A study across seven cultures. *J. Vocat. Behav.* **2014**, *85*, 361–373. [CrossRef]
19. Scott, G.; Ciarrochi, J.; Deane, F.P. Disadvantages of being an individualist in an individualistic culture: Idiocentrism, emotional competence, stress, and mental health. *Aust. Psychol.* **2004**, *39*, 143–153. [CrossRef]
20. World Health Organization. *Promoting Mental Health: Concepts, Emerging Evidence, Practice: Summary Report*; World Health Organization: Geneva, Switzerland, 2004.
21. Sharma, P.K.; Kumra, R. Relationship between workplace spirituality, organizational justice and mental health: Mediation role of employee engagement. *J. Adv. Manag. Res.* **2020**, *17*, 627–650. [CrossRef]
22. Winefield, H.R.; Gill, T.K.; Taylor, A.W.; Pilkington, R.M. Psychological well-being and psychological distress: Is it necessary to measure both? *Psychol. Well-Being Theory Res. Pract.* **2012**, *2*, 3. [CrossRef]
23. Jiang, S. Psychological well-being and distress in adolescents: An investigation into associations with poverty, peer victimization, and self-esteem. *Child. Youth Serv. Rev.* **2020**, *111*, 104824. [CrossRef]
24. Luthans, F.; Avolio, B.J.; Avey, J.B.; Norman, S.M. Positive psychological capital: Measurement and relationship with performance and satisfaction. *Pers. Psychol.* **2007**, *60*, 541–572. [CrossRef]
25. Zacher, H.; Jimmieson, N.L.; Winter, G. Eldercare demands, mental health, and work performance: The moderating role of satisfaction with eldercare tasks. *J. Occup. Health Psychol.* **2012**, *17*, 52–64. [CrossRef]
26. Fredrickson, B.L. The role of positive emotions in positive psychology: The broaden-and-build theory of positive emotions. *Am. Psychol.* **2001**, *56*, 218–226. [CrossRef]
27. Baron, R.A. The role of affect in the entrepreneurial process. *Acad. Manag. Rev.* **2008**, *33*, 328–340. [CrossRef]
28. Shan, B.; Lu, X. Founder's social ties, learning and entrepreneurial knowledge acquisition in China. *Asia Pac. Bus. Rev.* **2020**, *26*, 209–229. [CrossRef]

29. Bakker, A.B.; Demerouti, E.; Lieke, L. Work engagement, performance, and active learning: The role of conscientiousness. *J. Vocat. Behav.* **2012**, *80*, 555–564. [CrossRef]
30. Schaufeli, W.B.; Bakker, A.B.; Salanova, M. The measurement of work engagement with a short questionnaire: A cross-national study. *Educ. Psychol. Meas.* **2006**, *66*, 701–716. [CrossRef]
31. Ozturk, A.; Karatepe, O.M.; Okumus, F. The effect of servant leadership on hotel employees' behavioral consequences: Work engagement versus job satisfaction. *Int. J. Hosp. Manag.* **2021**, *97*, 102994. [CrossRef]
32. Xanthopoulou, D.; Bakker, A.B.; Fischbach, A. Work engagement among employees facing emotional demands. *J. Pers. Psychol.* **2013**, *12*, 74–84. [CrossRef]
33. Rich, B.L.; Lepine, J.A.; Crawford, E.R. Job engagement: Antecedents and effects on job performance. *Acad. Manag. J.* **2010**, *53*, 617–635. [CrossRef]
34. Xanthopoulou, D.; Bakker, A.B.; Demerouti, E.; Schaufeli, W.B. Work engagement and financial returns: A diary study on the role of job and personal resources. *J. Occup. Organ. Psychol.* **2009**, *82*, 183–200. [CrossRef]
35. Bakker, A.B.; Bal, M.P. Weekly work engagement and performance: A study among starting teachers. *J. Occup. Organ. Psychol.* **2010**, *83*, 189–206. [CrossRef]
36. Şahin, S.; Yozgat, U. Work–family conflict and job performance: Mediating role of work engagement in healthcare employees. *J. Manag. Organ.* **2021**, 1–20. [CrossRef]
37. Shimazu, A.; Schaufeli, W.B.; Kubota, K.; Kawakami, N. Do workaholism and work engagement predict employee well-being and performance in opposite directions? *Ind. Health* **2012**, *50*, 316–321. [CrossRef]
38. Utsch, A.; Rauch, A.; Rothfufs, R.; Frese, M. Who becomes a small scale entrepreneur in a post-socialist environment: On the differences between entrepreneurs and managers in East Germany. *J. Small Bus. Manag.* **1999**, *37*, 31.
39. Kim, M.S.; Koo, D.W. Linking LMX, engagement, innovative behavior, and job performance in hotel employees. *Int. J. Contemp. Hosp. Manag.* **2017**, *29*, 3044–3062. [CrossRef]
40. Van Zyl, L.E.; Van Oort, A.; Rispens, S.; Olckers, C. Work engagement and task performance within a global Dutch ICT-consulting firm: The mediating role of innovative work behaviors. *Curr. Psychol.* **2021**, *40*, 4012–4023. [CrossRef]
41. Kollmann, T.; Stöckmann, C.; Meves, Y.; Kensbock, J.M. When members of entrepreneurial teams differ: Linking diversity in individual-level entrepreneurial orientation to team performance. *Small Bus. Econ.* **2017**, *48*, 843–859. [CrossRef]
42. Rosenbusch, N.; Brinckmann, J.; Bausch, A. Is innovation always beneficial? A meta-analysis of the relationship between innovation and performance in SMEs. *J. Bus. Ventur.* **2011**, *26*, 441–457. [CrossRef]
43. Van de Ven, A.H.; Polley, D. Learning while innovating. *Organ. Sci.* **1992**, *3*, 92–116. [CrossRef]
44. Fredrickson, B.L. What good are positive emotions? *Rev. Gen. Psychol.* **1998**, *2*, 300–319. [CrossRef] [PubMed]
45. Bakker, A.B.; Demerouti, E. Towards a model of work engagement. *Career Dev. Int.* **2008**, *13*, 209–223. [CrossRef]
46. Burić, I.; Macuka, I. Self-efficacy, emotions and work engagement among teachers: A two wave cross-lagged analysis. *J. Happiness Stud.* **2018**, *19*, 1917–1933. [CrossRef]
47. Kim, K.S. The influence of hotels high-commitment hrm on job engagement of employees: Mediating effects of workplace happiness and mental health. *Appl. Res. Qual. Life* **2019**, *14*, 507–525. [CrossRef]
48. Schleupner, R.; Kühnel, J. Fueling Work Engagement: The Role of Sleep, Health, and Overtime. *Front. Public Health* **2021**, *9*, 619. [CrossRef]
49. Hakanen, J.J.; Bakker, A.B.; Schaufeli, W.B. Burnout and work engagement among teachers. *J. Sch. Psychol.* **2006**, *43*, 495–513. [CrossRef]
50. Binnewies, C.; Wörnlein, S.C. What makes a creative day? A diary study on the interplay between affect, job stressors, and job control. *J. Organ. Behav.* **2011**, *32*, 589–607. [CrossRef]
51. Schwarz, N.; Clore, G.L. Mood as information: 20 years later. *Psychol. Inq.* **2003**, *14*, 296–303. [CrossRef]
52. Schwarz, N.; Clore, G.L. Mood, misattribution, and judgments of well-being: Informative and directive functions of affective states. *J. Personal. Soc. Psychol.* **1983**, *45*, 513. [CrossRef]
53. Sirén, C.; He, V.F.; Wesemann, H.; Jonassen, Z.; Grichnik, D.; von Krogh, G. Leader emergence in nascent venture teams: The critical roles of individual emotion regulation and team emotions. *J. Manag. Stud.* **2020**, *57*, 931–961. [CrossRef]
54. Foo, M.D. Emotions and entrepreneurial opportunity evaluation. *Entrep. Theory Pract.* **2011**, *35*, 375–393. [CrossRef]
55. Forgas, J.P. Mood and judgment: The affect infusion model (AIM). *Psychol. Bull.* **1995**, *117*, 39. [CrossRef]
56. Janssen, O. Innovative behaviour and job involvement at the price of conflict and less satisfactory relations with co-workers. *J. Occup. Organ. Psychol.* **2003**, *76*, 347–364. [CrossRef]
57. Krause, D.E. Influence-based leadership as a determinant of the inclination to innovate and of innovation-related behaviors: An empirical investigation. *Leadersh. Q.* **2004**, *15*, 79–102. [CrossRef]
58. Pieterse, A.N.; Van Knippenberg, D.; Schippers, M.; Stam, D. Transformational and transactional leadership and innovative behavior: The moderating role of psychological empowerment. *J. Organ. Behav.* **2010**, *31*, 609–623. [CrossRef]
59. Eisenhardt, K.M.; Martin, J.A. Dynamic capabilities: What are they? *Strateg. Manag. J.* **2000**, *21*, 1105–1121. [CrossRef]
60. Sy, T.; Côté, S.; Saavedra, R. The contagious leader: Impact of the leader's mood on the mood of group members, group affective tone, and group processes. *J. Appl. Psychol.* **2005**, *90*, 295–305. [CrossRef]
61. Wu, T.J.; Wu, Y.J. Innovative work behaviors, employee engagement, and surface acting: A delineation of supervisor-employee emotional contagion effects. *Manag. Decis.* **2019**, *57*, 3200–3216. [CrossRef]

62. Shan, B.; Liu, X.; Gu, A.; Zhao, R. The effect of occupational health risk perception on job satisfaction. *Int. J. Environ. Res. Public Health* **2022**, *19*, 2111. [CrossRef] [PubMed]
63. Williams, L.J.; Anderson, S.E. Job satisfaction and organizational commitment as predictors of organizational citizenship and in-role behaviors. *J. Manag.* **1991**, *17*, 601–617. [CrossRef]
64. Kashyap, G.C.; Singh, S.K. Reliability and validity of general health questionnaire (GHQ-12) for male tannery workers: A study carried out in Kanpur, India. *BMC Psychiatry* **2017**, *17*, 102. [CrossRef] [PubMed]
65. Suárez-Albanchez, J.; Blazquez-Resino, J.J.; Gutierrez-Broncano, S.; Jimenez-Estevez, P. Occupational health and safety, organisational commitment, and turnover intention in the Spanish IT consultancy sector. *Int. J. Environ. Res. Public Health* **2021**, *18*, 5658. [CrossRef] [PubMed]
66. Scott, S.G.; Bruce, R.A.; Bruce, R.A. Determinants of Innovative Behavior: A Path Model of Individual Innovation in the Workplace. *Acad. Manag. J.* **1994**, *37*, 580–607.
67. Podsakoff, P.M.; Organ, D.W. Self-reports in organizational research: Problems and prospects. *J. Manag.* **1986**, *12*, 531–544. [CrossRef]
68. Hair, J.R.; Anderson, R.E.; Tatham, R.L.; Black, W.C. *Multivariate Data Analysis*, 5th ed.; Prentice Hall: Englewood Cliffs, NJ, USA, 1998.
69. Coles, J.L.; Li, Z.F. *An Empirical Assessment of Empirical Corporate Finance*; Social Science Electronic Publishing: Waltham, MA, USA, 2019. [CrossRef]

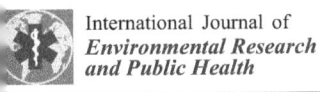

Review

Knowledge of Medical Imaging Professionals on Healthcare-Associated Infections: A Systematic Review and Meta-Analysis

Suresh Sukumar [1], Shovan Saha [2], Winniecia Dkhar [1], Nitika C. Panakkal [1], Visakh Thrivikraman Nair [1], Tulasiram Bommasamudram [3], K Vaishali [4], Ravishankar Nagaraja [5], Sneha Ravichandran [1] and Rajagopal Kadavigere [6,*]

1. Department of Medical Imaging Technology, Manipal College of Health Professions (MCHP), Manipal Academy of Higher Education (MAHE), Manipal 576104, India
2. Department of Occupational Therapy, Manipal College of Health Professions (MCHP), Manipal Academy of Higher Education (MAHE), Manipal 576104, India
3. Department of Exercise and Sports Sciences, Manipal College of Health Professions (MCHP), Manipal Academy of Higher Education (MAHE), Manipal 576104, India
4. Department of Physiotherapy, Manipal College of Health Professions (MCHP), Manipal Academy of Higher Education (MAHE), Manipal 576104, India
5. Department of Biostatistics, Vallabhbhai Patel Chest Institute, University of Delhi, Delhi 110021, India
6. Department of Radiodiagnosis and Imaging, Kasturba Medical College (KMC), Manipal Academy of Higher Education (MAHE), Manipal 576104, India
* Correspondence: rajagopal.kv@manipal.edu; Tel.: +91-9448158901

Abstract: Healthcare-associated infections (HCAIs) are a significant concern for both healthcare professionals and patients. With recent advances in imaging modalities, there is an increase in patients visiting the radiology department for diagnosis and therapeutic examination. The equipment used for the investigator is contaminated, which may result in HCAIs to the patients and healthcare professionals. Medical imaging professionals (MIPs) should have adequate knowledge to overcome the spread of infection in the radiology department. This systematic review aimed to examine the literature on the knowledge and precaution standard of MIPs on HCIAs. This study was performed with a relative keyword using PRISMA guidelines. The articles were retrieved from 2000 to 2022 using Scopus, PubMed, and ProQuest databases. The NICE public health guidance manual was used to assess the quality of the full-length article. The search yielded 262 articles, of which Scopus published 13 articles, PubMed published 179 articles, and ProQuest published 55 articles. In the present review, out of 262 articles, only 5 fulfilled the criteria that reported MIPs' knowledge of Jordan, Egypt, Sri Lanka, France, and Malawi populations. The present review reported that MIPs have moderate knowledge and precautionary standards regarding HCIAs in the radiology department. However, due to the limited studies published in the literature, the current review limits the application of the outcome in the vast MIPs population. This review recommended further studies to be conducted among the MIPs worldwide to know the actual knowledge and precaution standards regarding HCIAs.

Keywords: knowledge; attitude; healthcare-associated infection; medical imaging professionals; occupational health; risk assessment

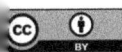

1. Introduction

Medical imaging professionals, such as radiologists, radiologic technologists, and other imaging specialists, may have some knowledge of healthcare-associated infections (HAIs). However, their level of knowledge may vary depending on their specific area of expertise and their exposure to patients with HAIs. HAIs are infections that patients acquire while receiving medical care, and they can occur in any healthcare setting, including hospitals, outpatient clinics, and long-term care facilities. HAIs are a significant public health concern, and healthcare professionals across all specialties are responsible for preventing and controlling these infections. Medical imaging professionals may have some knowledge of HAIs because they work closely with patients and often come into contact with contaminated equipment and surfaces. They may be trained in infection control measures, such as proper hand hygiene, cleaning and disinfection of equipment, and the use of personal protective equipment (PPE) to reduce the risk of transmission. In addition, medical imaging professionals may be involved in the diagnosis and treatment of patients with HAIs, particularly those that affect the respiratory system, such as tuberculosis or pneumonia. They may use imaging techniques such as chest X-rays, computed tomography (CT), or magnetic resonance imaging (MRI) to detect and monitor the progression of these infections. Overall, medical imaging professionals are an essential part of the healthcare team and play a critical role in preventing and controlling HAIs. While their specific knowledge of HAIs may vary, they should receive ongoing education and training on infection control measures to ensure the safety of both patients and healthcare workers.

The pandemic outbreak of Zoonotic viral diseases such as Corona, Nipah, and Ebola has resulted in a public health emergency with months of lockdown and financial loss to major tax-collecting departments such as tourism, aviation, and import–export. Further, the Zoonotic viral diseases have threatened the world economy with the loss of manpower, funds rerouting to the healthcare sector and vaccine research, and the health of human beings, leading to mass deaths and hospitalizations [1]

The World Health Organization (WHO) notified COVID-19 as a pandemic disease on 11 March 2020, and the global containment and quarantine efforts contamination incidents continue to increase post-haste. In developing countries such as India, there is a noticeable increase in the in-flow of infected patients to the hospital due to the recent and past outbreaks of pandemic Zoonotic viral diseases. The chances of cross infections increase with more immunocompromised patients visiting the hospital for other underlying cases. Still, they become infected with nosocomial infections, creating the need to assess cross-infection locations.

The infected patients with Zoonotic viral diseases primarily presented with dyspnoea, fever, and dry cough [2]. Further, these patients are highly contagious, and the infection is transmitted between people through droplets, close contact, and fomite [3,4]. The virus-like COVID-19 remains viable for 72 h on plastic and stainless steel and up to 3 h in aerosols [5]. The estimated half-life of the virus in the aerosol ranged from 1.1 to 2.1 h. Metals such as stainless steel have a half-life of 5.5 h, and the half-life of the plastic is 6.8 h [6]. The presence of bioaerosol in the surrounding air has profoundly influenced the health of humans, animals, and plant life. Further, both the viable and nonviable pathogens such as bacteria, fungi, and viruses present in the surrounding environmental air may also influence health [7,8].

Colonized and highly contagious infected patients visiting the hospital for different treatments may increase the chance of HCAI for patients and healthcare workers. Developing countries have a much higher risk of HCAI, with a radio of 20:1 as compared to developed countries [9]. In the past, HCAI was limited to inpatients. However, the recent pandemic virus outbreak resulted in increased HCAI in outpatients. Since the Department of Radiodiagnosis and Imaging plays a significant role in diagnosing different infectious diseases, there is a high probability of HCAI among radiology staff and patients [10]. Equipment such as radiography, magnetic resonance imaging, computed tomography, fluoroscopy, ultrasound, echocardiography and positron emission tomography used for diagnostic and therapeutic examinations were more prone to infection, resulting in healthcare-associated infections (HCAI). The other infected equipment in the Radiology Department (RD) including the imaging tables, keyboard, touchscreen, computer mouse, lead apron, radiographic markers, and transferring table are also more prone to the HCAIs [11–18].

However, despite the improvement in the practices, HCAI is still prevalent in the healthcare facilities affecting patients worldwide each year. In the recent outbreak, HCAI has reported that 3.8% of the total infections are related to COVID-19 [19]. To overcome the challenges of HCAIs, the knowledge and precautionary standards regarding HCPs must improve [20]. The HCPs such as Medical Imaging Professionals (MIP) working in the radiology equipment should know standardized operating protocols to minimize the spread of HCAIs via the radiology equipment [21,22].

Since there is limited research regarding the knowledge of the HCAI among the HCPs reported in the literature, the awareness of MIPs on the HCAI has also been underexplored.

The purpose of this study is to interpret research reports pertaining to knowledge and precaution standards among MIPs.

2. Materials and Methods

This systematic review was performed to identify MIPs' knowledge and precautionary standards regarding HCAIs in the radiology department. PRISMA-reporting guidelines were followed in this study [23].

2.1. Search Strategy

The electronic databases PubMed, Scopus, and ProQuest were considered to retrieve the studies reported from 2000 to 2022. The literature search was performed from 1 June 2022 to 30 June 2022 and restricted to studies published in English. The keywords and search strategy used are presented in Table 1. A manual search was also performed to identify the relevant articles using the included studies' citations.

Table 1. Keywords Strategy.

Sl. No.	Search
1	"(nosocomial infections or hospital-acquired infections or healthcare-associated infections)"
2	"(knowledge or education or understanding or awareness)"
3	" (radiographer or radiologist technologist)."
	1 AND 3
	1 AND 2 AND 3
4	" (nosocomial Infections)"
5	"(knowledge) "
6	" (radiographer)"
	4 AND 5 AND 6

2.2. Selection Criteria

Research papers focused on the "knowledge", or "education", or "understanding", or "awareness" of the HCAI among the MIPs were included. Articles published in the English language were considered for this study. The full-length research papers were independently reviewed by the two reviewers and then shortlisted. The disagreement between the reviewers over eligibility were resolved through discussion and concession with the third reviewer.

2.2.1. Selection of the Studies

The title and abstract of the articles were appraised for relevance to the aim of the present review. The articles that were not relevant were eliminated. The full text of the remaining article fulfilled the objective of the evaluation and was acquired to assess further relevance based on the inclusion and exclusion criteria. The full-length research papers were independently reviewed by the two reviewers and then shortlisted. The third reviewer verified shortlisted articles based on the review criteria. The disagreement between the reviewers over eligibility was resolved through discussion and concession with the third reviewer.

2.2.2. Data Extraction

The data of the included full-length articles were extracted into the Microsoft Excel sheet. The year, country, samples, study design, number of items present, validation of the questionnaires, ethical approval of the studies, and mode of data collection were considered during the data extraction.

2.2.3. Risk of Bias

The NICE public health guidance manual was used to assess the risk of bias for the included studies [21,22] (Table 2). Two reviewers performed the assessments independently, and the correlation was determined.

Table 2. Criteria to assess the risk of bias.

Criteria's	Score
Clarity of the questioners	+/−
Details of the study methodology	+/−
Details of data collection	+/−
Research content	+/−
Data analysis	+/−
Result revenant to the study's objective	+/−
Ethics approval	+/−
Overall	++/+/−

++ must meet at least six criteria indicated above. + must meet at least four criteria mentioned above. ++ denotes the low level of bias; + means the moderate level of bias; and − indicates a poor level of bias.

2.2.4. Criteria for Inclusion and Exclusion

Exclusion: focus on HCP, not focus on medical imaging, other language.
Inclusion: focus on the medical imaging, published in English.

2.2.5. Data Analysis

The Kappa test was performed to determine the two reviewers' agreement using SPSS 16. A meta-analysis was used to obtain the pooled estimate. The random-effects model was used for the meta-analysis. Chi-square statistics and I-square statistics were used to report heterogeneity. A meta-analysis was performed using STATA software version 13.1.

3. Results

The magnitude of the publication related to the knowledge and standard precautions of HCAIs among the MIPs was initially unknown. Therefore, the present research question was focused on MIPS. The literature searches across the three electronic databases resulted in 247 articles in the current review. The additional 14 articles were obtained by the manual search based on the references. Once the duplicate papers were eliminated, the study number was reduced to 238 articles. A total of 221 articles that were not focused on the MIPs were removed. The full text of the remaining 11 articles [24–34] was collected and screened for the inclusion and exclusion criteria, out of which only 5 articles are eligible for review and evaluation [24,25,29,30,32]. The PRISMA is presented in Figure 1 [23].

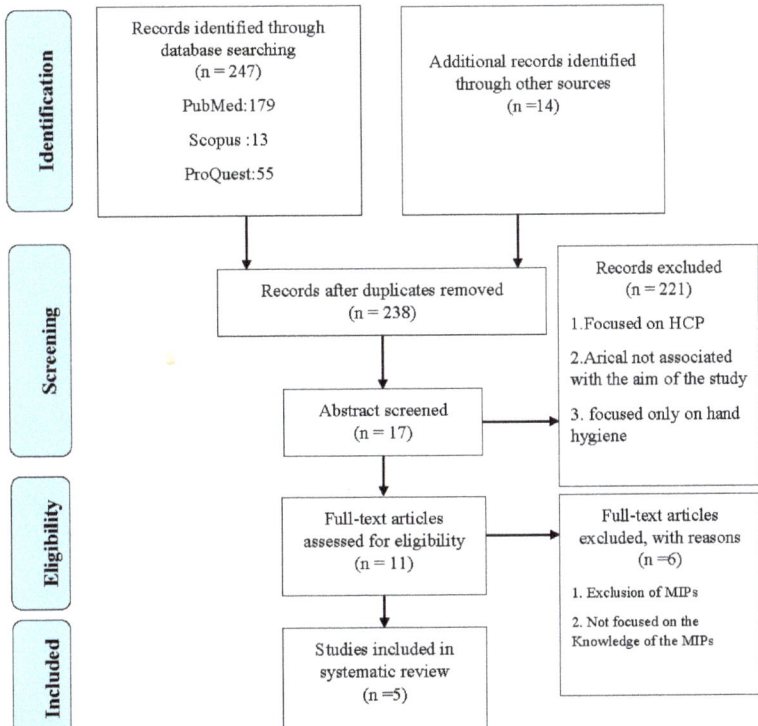

Figure 1. Flow diagram of the article selection process.

3.1. Characteristics of the Included Studies

A total of five articles published from Jordan, Egypt, Sri Lanka, France, and Malawi were considered for the present review [24,25,29,30,32]. All the articles were published between 2008 and 2018 (Table 3). Out of five studies, only two studies reported the questionnaire specific to the MIPs' knowledge of infection control practices specific to the RD. However, all the items included in the questionnaire were validated before the data collection. The questionnaire used in the studies to evaluate the knowledge and precautionary standards varied from 18 to 50 items. All the included studies reported that ethical approval was obtained to collect the data via a self-administered survey.

Table 3. Characteristics of the included studies.

	Author				
	M.A. Abdelrahman et al. [25]	El-Gilany et al. [24]	Jayasinghe et al. [29]	Marie-Pierre et al. [32]	Nyirenda, D. et al. [30]
Year	2017	2012	2014	2008	2018
Country	Jordan	Egypt	Sri Lanka	France	Malawi
Samples	128	14	213	94	62
Study design	CS	CS	CS	CS	CS
No of items	41	50	18	25	36
Ethical approval	Yes	Yes	Yes	Yes	Yes

Table 3. *Cont.*

	Author				
	M.A. Abdelrahman et al. [25]	El-Gilany et al. [24]	Jayasinghe et al. [29]	Marie-Pierre et al. [32]	Nyirenda, D. et al. [30]
Mode of data collection	SA	SA	SA	SA	SA
Validation	Yes	Yes	Yes	Yes	Yes
Items specific to radiology	Yes	No	No	No	No
Environment and HCAIs	Poor	*	Poor	poor	Good
Intervention and HCAIs	Good	*	Moderate	Good	*
Standard precaution and HCAIs	Good	Moderate	Good	Good	Moderate
Gloves recommend and HCAIs	Poor	*	Poor	Moderate	*

* indicates Not reported, and CS indicates a Cross-sectional study, SA—Self Administered.

3.2. Methodological Quality

The quality of the selected articles has been summarized in Table 4. All five studies were found to be of quality ++. A moderate agreement was reported between the two reviewers, with a kappa value of 0.545.

Table 4. Quality of the articles.

Study	Items							
	1	2	3	4	5	6	7	Overall
M.A. Abdelrahman et al. [25]	+	+	+	+	+	+	+	++
El-Gilany et al. [24]	+	+	+	+	+	+	+	++
Jayasinghe et al. [29]	+	+	+	+	-	+	+	++
Marie-Pierre et al. [32]	+	+	+	+	+	+	+	++
Nyirenda, D. et al. [30]	+	+	+	+	-	+	+	++

1—Clarity of the questioners, 2—Details of the study methodology, 3—Details of the data collection, 4—Research content, 5—Data analysis, 6—Result relevant to the study's objective, 7—Ethics approval. ++ denotes the low level of bias; + means the moderate level of bias; and − indicates a poor level of bias.

3.3. Meta-Analysis

In the present review, out of five included studies, only three studies [25,29,32] were considered for the meta-analysis. The pooled effect of the outcome measures related to the "Environment as a major source of infection," "Invasive procedures increase the risk of nosocomial infection," "Gloves recommendation" and "Precaution standards during the procedure" is reported in Table 5. The studies which did not report the specific outcome measures were excluded from the meta-analysis [24,30].

Table 5. The effect size of the outcome measures.

Outcome Measure	Effect Size (95% CI)
"The environment (air, water, inert surfaces) is the major source of bacteria responsible for nosocomial infection."	0.18 (0.08, 0.28)
"Invasive procedures increase the risk of nosocomial infection."	0.76 (0.44, 1.07)
"Medical Imaging Professionals knowledge on standard precautions recommend the use of gloves."	0.41 (0.17, 0.65)
"Precaution standards to protect the patients and the healthcare workers."	0.87 (0.77, 0.97)

3.4. Environment and HCIAs

The MIPs show poor knowledge with a pooled effect size of 0.18 (0.08, 0.28). Considerable heterogeneity is present among the studies, with I² of 85.39% and $p \leq 0.001$ (Figure 2).

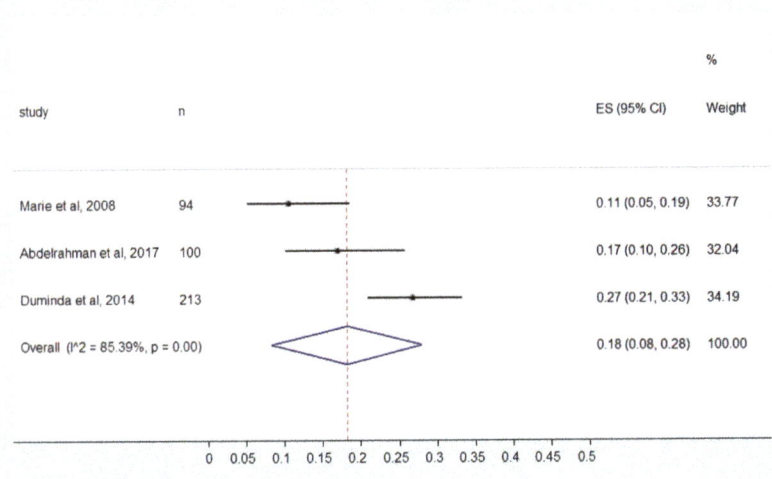

Figure 2. MIPs' knowledge of "The environment (air, water, inert surfaces) is the major source of bacteria responsible for nosocomial infection". (Marie et al., 2008 [32], Abdelrahman et al., 2017 [25], Duminda et al., 2014 [29]).

3.5. Gloves Recommendation during the Procedure

The MIPs reported poor knowledge with a pooled effect size of 0.41 (0.17, 0.65). Considerable heterogeneity is present among the studies included, with I² of 96.25% and $p \leq 0.001$ (Figure 3).

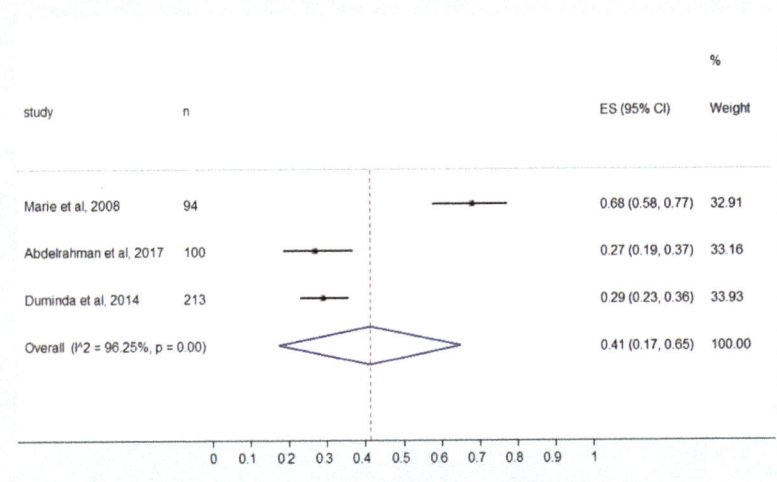

Figure 3. MIPs knowledge on "Gloves recommendation during the procedure." (Marie et al., 2008 [32], Abdelrahman et al., 2017 [25], Duminda et al., 2014 [29]).

3.6. Precaution Standards

The MIPs possess excellent knowledge with a pooled effect size of 0.87 (0.77, 0.97). Considerable heterogeneity is present among the studies included, with I^2 of 96.96% and $p \leq 0.001$ (Figure 4).

In the present review, the medical imaging professional shows good knowledge, with a pooled effect size of 0.76 (0.44, 1.07). Considerable heterogeneity is present among the studies included, with I^2 of 98.91% and $p \leq 0.001$ (Figure 5).

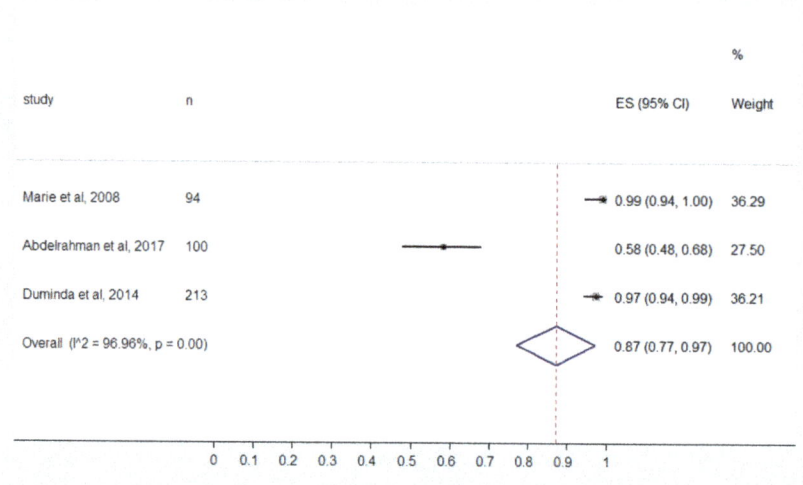

Figure 4. MIPs' knowledge of "Precaution standards to protect the patients and the HCPs". (Marie et al., 2008 [32], Abdelrahman et al., 2017 [25], Duminda et al., 2014 [29]).

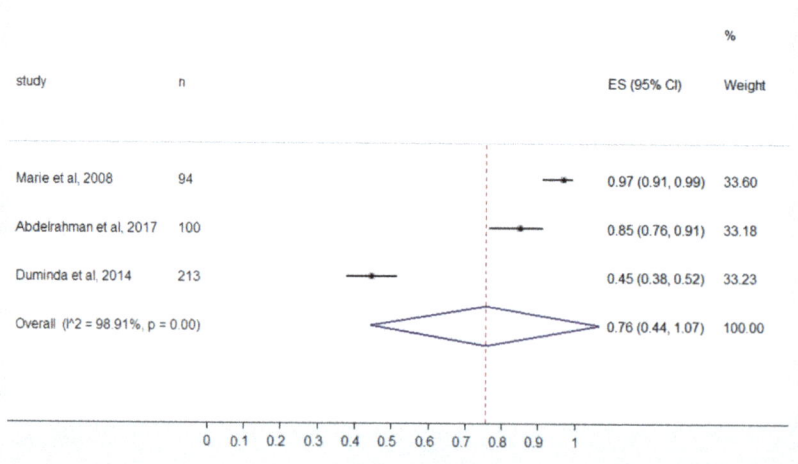

Figure 5. MIPs' knowledge of "Invasive procedures increase the risk of HCAIs". (Marie et al., 2008 [32], Abdelrahman et al., 2017 [25], Duminda et al., 2014 [29]).

4. Discussion

This systematic review was aimed at investigating the knowledge of the MIPs on the HCAIs. The literature search resulted in five articles, of which three articles were considered for the meta-analysis.

4.1. The Spread of Infection

The RD plays a vital role in the diagnosis and treating of the patient's disease using X-ray, CT scanner, MRI Scanner, interventional radiology, and ultrasound (USG). The probability of the HCAIs may increase due to the colonized and infected patients waiting for the diagnostic procedure [13]. Further, the contaminated hand is considered to be one of the primary sources of transferring the HCAIs. The contaminated hand of the MIPs and the other HCPs, including nurses, practitioners, and attendees, can lead to the transfer of the infection pathogens from one person to another person, adjacent surface, and equipment [35]. Nyirenda et al. reported that 98% of Malawi MIPs have good knowledge about the primary source and spread of infection [30]. However, in the present review, the MIPs reported that the environment was a major source of multi-resistant bacterial transmission, with a pooled effect size of 0.18 (0.08, 0.28). Giacometti et al. reported that 41.7% of the X-ray tube, 91.7% of control panels and imaging plates, and 8% of the X-ray cassettes were contaminated, which may transmit the HCAIs [36]. Therefore, faculty working in the RD should have updated knowledge and standard operating procedure to reduce the HCAIs spread via radiology equipment or the HCP in the RD.

4.2. Knowledge of Hand and Machine Hygiene in RD

Olu O. et al. [37] reported 95% of healthcare professionals acquired the HCAI during the outbreak of Ebola in 2014. Therefore, the HCAI in the Healthcare Professional (HCP) may accelerate the transmission and result in mortality [5]. However, if healthcare professionals adhere to the guidelines and protocol of disinfection and isolation, the risk of HCAI may drop to 10.7% [37]. The HCAI can be overcome by hand hygiene and sanitation practices, which may lower the incidence of the disease, as opposed to treating the disease [38].

The microbial growth on an MIP's hand can be effectively overcome by sterilization of the hand. The alcohol-based hand sanitisers were most commonly used for the sterilization of hand fields [13]. Further, proper sterilization of the imaging equipment can prevent one-third of the HCIAs [36]. Carling et al. reported that 88% of MIPs were aware that the primary reason for the contamination of the radiology equipment is due to the inadequate disinfection procedures followed in the department [39]. Cleaning the equipment and cassette between the patient's examinations using the alcohol wipe and chlorhexidine-based detergents is effective, and they are recommended as compared to soap and water [40,41]. The alcohol gel, disinfecting wipes, and the standard hand wash are recommended to disinfect the radiographer's markers during the procedure [40]. However, special consideration is required for the ribbon markers [42].

The American Institute of USG in medicine recommended using water and soap or quaternary ammonium disinfectant spray for the USG [40]. The MRI machine's disinfection is difficult compared to the other imaging equipment in the RD [41]. However, it is recommended to use the solution of 1000 parts of hypochlorite with a million parts of chloride to disinfect the MRI machine [11]. Abdel-Hady El-Gilany et al. reported that the MIPs have inadequate knowledge about sanitation practices as compared to the other HCPs [24].

During the portable examination of the infected patients, especially EBOLA and COVID-19 patients, specific emphasis on hand hygiene is necessary [35]. Further, additional precaution measures include the proper use of gloves while performing and handling high-risk patients. The gloves are also recommended when there is a risk of MIPs in contact with blood during the procedure [11]. However, it is not recommended to use gloves for every radiological procedure [25]. In the present review, the MIPs show poor knowledge of the glove's recommendation, with a pooled effect size of 0.41 (0.17, 0.65).

4.3. Recommendations of Precaution Standards to Protect the Patients and HCP

The MIPs can break the chain of HCAIs from other HCPs through proper education, hand hygiene surveillance, vaccination against preventable disease, and prevention of needle-struck injury. Abdel-Hady El-Gilany et al. reported that the MIPs have inadequate knowledge about needle-struck injury as compared to the other HCPs [24].

Training the MIPs with high-quality education can break the spread of the HCAIs in the radiology department [22]. Bello et al. reported that only half of the MIPs have intermediate knowledge of infection control measures [43]. However, in the present study, the MIPs show poor knowledge about the "Precaution standards recommendations to protect the patients and the healthcare workers" with a pooled effect size of 0.87 (0.77, 0.97).

4.4. Invasive Procedures and HCIAs

Interventional radiology is considered a high-risk area for imparting HCAIs [36,44]. The radiation protective equipment used during the intervention procedure has also been observed to be more prone to HCAIs [45]. The reduction in infection in interventional radiology requires the identification of the risk, the appropriate use of antibiotic prophylaxis, and appropriate patient care [46]. In the present review, the medical imaging professional shows good knowledge about invasive procedures that increase the risk of HCAIs, with a pooled effect size of 0.76 (0.44, 1.07).

Overall, the discrepancy in the result is present among the studies included in the current review. The MIPs have poor knowledge of the spread of HCIAs infection and the gloves recommendation. However, MIPs reported good knowledge of precaution standards to protect the patients and healthcare workers.

4.5. Limitations of the Included Studies

According to the hierarchy of evidence, the cross-section and observational study design ranked low as compared to the randomized control trials [42]. All five studies included in this review are of the cross-section study design that typically lacks the adequate methodology rigour that minimizes the effect of bias. However, applying a rigid design hierarchy to this research is potentially less significant than evaluating the precision of the study methodology [47]. Of the five systematic review studies, one used a sample of fewer than fifty subjects. However, no studies justified the sample size. The small sample size may result in the probability of non-significant results [48]. Out of five studies, only one was reported using random sampling techniques. This further limits the further the ability to find the wider population. Of the rest of the studies, one used convenience sampling, and four did not state the sampling procedure. The ability to extrapolate the survey to the other MIPs is difficult due to the limited number of studies. Variable types of items in the questionnaire were used in the surveys. In the current review, three out of five studies used similar questions, of which only one study reported specific to the MIPs.

4.6. Limitation of the Present Review

In the present review, the literature search was performed based on only three electronic databases (PubMed, Scopus, and ProQuest). Further, the systematic review was limited to the articles published between 2000 to 2022 and restricted to studies published in English. Due to the limited number of papers published and the diversity in the items present in the questionnaire, a meta-analysis for the present study was performed with three articles with similar items. However, the outcome of the current review on MIPs' knowledge and precautionary standards regarding HCAIs may limit the application of the result to the vast population.

4.7. Future Recommendations from the Present Review

Based on the current review, several research gaps have been identified. A minimal study was undertaken and published worldwide. Further research can be performed to develop a valid tool for understanding the MIPs' knowledge specific to the radiology department in preventing the HCAIs. All the studies included in this review are questionnaire-based quantitative studies. There was no study reported in the qualitative research methodology. Conducting the focus group discussion may result in a better understanding of the knowledge of MIPs on HCAIs. The present review has not focused on other allied health professionals. A systematic review needs to be undertaken among all the allied health professionals. Further, a study on infection control with proper guidelines and the HCP's compliance in involving these measures may be imperative in reducing the HCAIs, thereby reducing the burden and improving both HCP and patient outcomes [15].

4.8. Future Scopes

The qualitative and quantitative study on the awareness of the spread of infection among MIPs may provide better knowledge and understanding among imaging professionals. Diversity in the items in the questionnaire was observed; therefore, a standardized questionnaire must be developed to assess knowledge, awareness, and practice of handling infectious diseases in the Radiology Department. Further reviews have to be conducted on MIPs' understanding of the HCAI and the application of modern imaging techniques during the outbreak of infectious disease to reduce the risk of HCAI to MIPs.

5. Conclusions

The current review aimed to understand MIPs' knowledge and the precaution standards regarding the HCAIs in the RD. The present study resulted in five articles which fulfilled the inclusion criteria. Of these, only three used similar items related to the spread of infection, knowledge of precaution standards and hygiene, and risk of disease in invasive procedures. The present study reported that MIPs have moderate knowledge and precautionary standards toward the HCIAs in the RD. However, due to the limited studies published in the literature, the outcome of the current review may limit the application of the outcome results in the vast MIPs population worldwide. This review recommended further qualitative and quantitative studies to be conducted among imaging professionals worldwide to discern the actual knowledge and precaution standards regarding HCIAs.

Author Contributions: Conceptualization: S.S. (Suresh Sukumar), R.K. and K.V.; methodology, R.K., W.D. and S.S. (Suresh Sukumar); software, N.C.P., V.T.N. and T.B.; validation, R.N.; formal analysis R.K., W.D. and S.S. (Shovan Saha); writing original draft—R.K. and S.S. (Suresh Sukumar), writing review—R.K., W.D. and S.R.; supervision R.K. All authors have read and agreed to the published version of the manuscript.

Funding: This research did not receive any specific grant from funding agencies in the public, commercial, or not-for-profit sectors.

Data Availability Statement: The data for this review is available in "Sukumar, Suresh, 2022, Knowledge of Medical Imaging Professionals on Healthcare-Associated Infections: A systematic review and meta-analysis, https://doi.org/10.7910/DVN/OTG4YZ".

Acknowledgments: We would like to thank the following people for their assistance in the production of this report: Hari Prakash. P., Department of Speech and Hearing Manipal College of Health Professionals, Manipal Academy of Higher Education, Manipal 576 104, Karnataka, India for his assistance in data extraction. Baskaran Chandrasekaran, HOD-In charge, Department of Exercise and Sports Sciences and Coordinator, Center for Sports Science, Medicine and Research Manipal College of Health Professions Manipal Academy of Higher Education, Manipal 576104, Karnataka for his for their help in the search for files. Poovitha Shruthi P., Division of Yoga Center for Integrative Medicine and Research, Manipal Academy of Higher Education Manipal, Karnataka 576104 for their comments on the final draft. Abhimanyu Pradhan, Radiological Safety Officer, Department of Medical Imaging Technology, Manipal College of Health Professions (MCHP) at Manipal Academy of Higher Education (MAHE), Manipal 576 104, Karnataka, India for the comments and inputs. Nagarajan. T, PhD Scholar Visual Neurosciences, Department of Optometry, Manipal College of Health Professions (MCHP) at Manipal Academy of Higher Education (MAHE)), Manipal 576 104, Karnataka, India for his comments on the final draft. Guruprasad V, Department of Occupational Therapy, Department of Optometry, Manipal College of Health Professions (MCHP) at Manipal

Academy of Higher Education (MAHE)), Manipal 576 104, Karnataka, India for his assistance in data extraction and comments on the final draft. Pradeep Yuvaraj, Department of Speech Pathology and Audiology G14, OPD Block, National Institute of Mental Health and Neuro Sciences (NIMHANS), Hosur Road/Marigowda Road, (Lakkasandra, Wilson Garden), Bangalore 560029, Karnataka, India for his assistance in the data extraction, valuable inputs and motivation during the review process.

Conflicts of Interest: The authors have no conflict of interest to declare. All co-authors have seen and agree with the manuscript's contents, and there is no financial interest to report. We certify that the submission is original work and is not under review at any other publication.

References

1. Kumar, B.; Manuja, A.; Gulati, B.; Virmani, N.; Tripathi, B.N. Zoonotic Viral Diseases of Equines and Their Impact on Human and Animal Health. *Open Virol. J.* **2018**, *12*, 80–98. [CrossRef]
2. Huang, C.; Wang, Y.; Li, X.; Ren, L.; Zhao, J.; Hu, Y.; Zhang, L.; Fan, G.; Xu, J.; Gu, X.; et al. Clinical Features of Patients Infected with 2019 Novel Coronavirus in Wuhan, China. *Lancet* **2020**, *395*, 497–506. [CrossRef] [PubMed]
3. Li, Q.; Guan, X.; Wu, P.; Wang, X.; Zhou, L.; Tong, Y.; Ren, R.; Leung, K.S.M.; Lau, E.H.Y.; Wong, J.Y.; et al. Early Transmission Dynamics in Wuhan, China, of Novel Coronavirus–Infected Pneumonia. *N. Eng. J. Med.* **2020**, *382*, 1199–1207. [CrossRef]
4. Paules, C.I.; Marston, H.D.; Fauci, A.S. Coronavirus Infections—More Than Just the Common Cold. *JAMA* **2020**, *323*, 707. [CrossRef] [PubMed]
5. Qu, J.; Yang, W.; Yang, Y.; Qin, L.; Yan, F. Infection Control for CT Equipment and Radiographers' Personal Protection During the Coronavirus Disease (COVID-19) Outbreak in China. *Am. J. Roentgenol.* **2020**, *215*, 940–944. [CrossRef] [PubMed]
6. van Doremalen, N.; Bushmaker, T.; Morris, D.H.; Holbrook, M.G.; Gamble, A.; Williamson, B.N.; Tamin, A.; Harcourt, J.L.; Thornburg, N.J.; Gerber, S.I.; et al. Aerosol and Surface Stability of SARS-CoV-2 as Compared with SARS-CoV-1. *N. Engl. J. Med.* **2020**, *382*, 1564–1567. [CrossRef]
7. Hietala, S.K.; Hullinger, P.J.; Crossley, B.M.; Kinde, H.; Ardans, A.A. Environmental Air Sampling to Detect Exotic Newcastle Disease Virus in Two California Commercial Poultry Flocks. *J. Vet. Diagn. Investig.* **2005**, *17*, 198–200. [CrossRef]
8. Li, Y.; Huang, X.; Yu, I.T.S.; Wong, T.W.; Qian, H. Role of Air Distribution in SARS Transmission during the Largest Nosocomial Outbreak in Hong Kong. *Indoor Air* **2005**, *15*, 83–95. [CrossRef]
9. Hefzy, E.M.; Wegdan, A.A.; Abdel Wahed, W.Y. Hospital Outpatient Clinics as a Potential Hazard for Healthcare Associated Infections. *J. Infect. Public Health* **2016**, *9*, 88–97. [CrossRef]
10. Marcel, J.-P.; Alfa, M.; Baquero, F.; Etienne, J.; Goossens, H.; Harbarth, S.; Hryniewicz, W.; Jarvis, W.; Kaku, M.; Leclercq, R.; et al. Healthcare-Associated Infections: Think Globally, Act Locally. *Clin. Microbiol. Infect.* **2008**, *14*, 895–907. [CrossRef]
11. Ilyas, F.; Burbridge, B.; Babyn, P. Health Care-Associated Infections and the Radiology Department. *J. Med. Imaging Radiat. Sci.* **2019**, *50*, 596–606.e1. [CrossRef] [PubMed]
12. Levin, P.D.; Shatz, O.; Sviri, S.; Moriah, D.; Or-Barbash, A.; Sprung, C.L.; Moses, A.E.; Block, C. Contamination of Portable Radiograph Equipment with Resistant Bacteria in the ICU. *Chest* **2009**, *136*, 426–432. [CrossRef] [PubMed]
13. Üstünsöz, B. Hospital Infections in Radiology Clinics. *Diagn. Interv. Radiol.* **2005**, *11*, 5–9. [PubMed]
14. Lawson, S.R.; Sauer, R.; Loritsch, M.B. Bacterial Survival on Radiographic Cassettes. *Radiol. Technol.* **2002**, *73*, 507–510.
15. Busi Rizzi, E.; Puro, V.; Schinina', V.; Nicastri, E.; Petrosillo, N.; Ippolito, G. Radiographic Imaging in Ebola Virus Disease: Protocol to Acquire Chest Radiographs. *Eur. Radiol.* **2015**, *25*, 3368–3371. [CrossRef]
16. Buerke, B.; Mellmann, A.; Stehling, C.; Wessling, J.; Heindel, W.; Juergens, K.U. Microbiologic Contamination of Automatic Injectors at MDCT: Experimental and Clinical Investigations. *AJR Am. J. Roentgenol.* **2008**, *191*, W283–W287. [CrossRef]
17. Wooltorton, E. Medical Gels and the Risk of Serious Infection. *CMAJ* **2004**, *171*, 1348. [CrossRef]
18. Buerke, B.; Puesken, M.; Mellmann, A.; Schuelke, C.; Knauer, A.; Heindel, W.; Wessling, J. Automatic MDCT Injectors: Hygiene and Efficiency of Disposable, Prefilled, and Multidosing Roller Pump Systems in Clinical Routine. *AJR Am. J. Roentgenol.* **2011**, *197*, W226–W232. [CrossRef]
19. Epidemiology Working Group for NCIP Epidemic Response, C.C. for D.C. and P. [The Epidemiological Characteristics of an Outbreak of 2019 Novel Coronavirus Diseases (COVID-19) in China]. *Zhonghua Liu Xing Bing Xue Za Zhi* **2020**, *41*, 145–151. [CrossRef]
20. Nienhaus, A.; Kesavachandran, C.; Wendeler, D.; Haamann, F.; Dulon, M. Infectious Diseases in Healthcare Workers-an Analysis of the Standardised Data Set of a German Compensation Board. *J. Occup. Med. Toxicol.* **2012**, *7*, 8. [CrossRef]
21. Schmidt, J.M. Stopping the Chain of Infection in the Radiology Suite. *Radiol. Technol.* **2012**, *84*, 31–48; qiuz 49–51. Available online: https://pubmed.ncbi.nlm.nih.gov/22988261/ (accessed on 11 January 2023). [PubMed]
22. Schmidt, J.M. Stopping the Chain of Infection in the Radiology Suite. *Radiol. Technol.* **2020**, *91*, 489–493. Available online: https://pubmed.ncbi.nlm.nih.gov/32381669/ (accessed on 11 January 2023).
23. Moher, D.; Liberati, A.; Tetzlaff, J.; Altman, D.G. Preferred Reporting Items for Systematic Reviews and Meta-Analyses: The PRISMA Statement. *PLoS Med.* **2009**, *6*, e1000097. [CrossRef] [PubMed]
24. El-Gilany, A.H.; Badawy, K.; Sarraf, B. Knowledge of Health Care Providers Os Standard Precautions and Infection Controla t Studentshospital, Mansoura University, Egypt. *TAF Prev. Med. Bull.* **2012**, *11*, 23–28. [CrossRef]

5. Abdelrahman, M.A.; Alhasan, M.; Alewaidat, H.; Rawashdeh, M.A.; al Mousa, D.S.; Almhdawi, K.A. Knowledge of Nosocomial Infection Control Practices among Radiographers in Jordan. *Radiography* **2017**, *23*, 298–304. [CrossRef]
6. Baird, M.; Zito, N.; Howden, L. The Awareness and Implementation of Infection Control Procedures among Radiographers. *Radiogr. Off. J. Aust. Inst. Radiogr.* **2002**, *49*, 61–65.
7. Cobb, A.; Lazar, B. Mobile Device Usage Contributes to Nosocomial Infections. *Radiol. Technol.* **2020**, *91*, 303–307.
8. Crofton, C.C.; Foley, S.J. An Investigation of Radiographers' Mobile Phone Use and the Success of an Awareness Campaign at Reducing the Nosocomial Infection Risks. *Radiography* **2018**, *24*, 57–63. [CrossRef]
9. Jayasinghe, R.D.; Weerakoon, B.S. Prevention of Nosocomial Infections and Standard Precautions: Knowledge and Practice among Radiographers in Sri Lanka -. *J. Med. Allied Sci.* **2014**, *4*, 9–16.
10. Nyirenda, D.; ten Ham-Baloyi, W.; Williams, R.; Venter, D. Knowledge and Practices of Radiographers Regarding Infection Control in Radiology Departments in Malawi. *Radiography* **2018**, *24*, e56–e60. [CrossRef]
11. Smith, A.; Lodge, T.D. Can Radiographic Equipment Be Contaminated by Micro-Organisms to Become a Reservoir for Cross Infection? *Synergy* **2004**, 12–17. Available online: https://www.proquest.com/docview/212420127?pq-origsite=gscholar&fromopenview=true (accessed on 11 January 2023).
12. Tavolacci, M.-P.; Ladner, J.; Bailly, L.; Merle, V.; Pitrou, I.; Czernichow, P. Prevention of Nosocomial Infection and Standard Precautions: Knowledge and Source of Information among Healthcare Students. *Infect. Control Hosp. Epidemiol.* **2008**, *29*, 642–647. [CrossRef] [PubMed]
13. Temesgen, C.; Demissie, M. Knowledge and Practice of Tuberculosis Infection Control among Health Professionals in Northwest Ethiopia; 2011. *BMC Health Serv. Res.* **2014**, *14*, 593. [CrossRef] [PubMed]
14. Tvedt, C.; Bukholm, G. Healthcare Workers' Self-Reported Effect of an Interventional Programme on Knowledge and Behaviour Related to Infection Control. *Qual. Saf. Health Care* **2010**, *19*, e7. [CrossRef] [PubMed]
15. Aso, M.; Kato, K.; Yasuda, M.; Takahashi, T.; Say, S.; Fujimura, K.; Kuroki, K.; Nakazawa, Y. [Hand Hygiene during Mobile X-Ray Imaging in the Emergency Room]. *Nihon Hoshasen Gijutsu Gakkai Zasshi* **2011**, *67*, 793–799. [CrossRef] [PubMed]
16. Giacometti, M.; Gualano, M.R.; Bert, F.; Minniti, D.; Bistrot, F.; Grosso, M.; Siliquini, R. Microbiological Contamination of Radiological Equipment. *Acta Radiol.* **2014**, *55*, 1099–1103. [CrossRef] [PubMed]
17. Olu, O.; Kargbo, B.; Kamara, S.; Wurie, A.H.; Amone, J.; Ganda, L.; Ntsama, B.; Poy, A.; Kuti-George, F.; Engedashet, E.; et al. Epidemiology of Ebola Virus Disease Transmission among Health Care Workers in Sierra Leone, May to December 2014: A Retrospective Descriptive Study. *BMC Infect. Dis.* **2015**, *15*, 416. [CrossRef] [PubMed]
18. Picton-Barnes, D.; Pillay, M.; Lyall, D. A Systematic Review of Healthcare-Associated Infectious Organisms in Medical Radiation Science Departments. *Healthcare* **2020**, *8*, 80. [CrossRef]
19. Carling, P.C.; Parry, M.F.; von Beheren, S.M. Healthcare Environmental Hygiene Study Group Identifying Opportunities to Enhance Environmental Cleaning in 23 Acute Care Hospitals. *Infect. Control Hosp. Epidemiol.* **2008**, *29*, 1–7. [CrossRef]
20. Kim, J.-S.; Kim, H.-S.; Park, J.-Y.; Koo, H.-S.; Choi, C.-S.; Song, W.; Cho, H.C.; Lee, K.M. Contamination of X-Ray Cassettes with Methicillin-Resistant Staphylococcus Aureus and Methicillin-Resistant Staphylococcus Haemolyticus in a Radiology Department. *Ann. Lab. Med.* **2012**, *32*, 206–209. [CrossRef]
21. Shelly, M.J.; Scanlon, T.G.; Ruddy, R.; Hannan, M.M.; Murray, J.G. Meticillin-Resistant Staphylococcus Aureus (MRSA) Environmental Contamination in a Radiology Department. *Clin. Radiol.* **2011**, *66*, 861–864. [CrossRef]
22. Tugwell, J.; Maddison, A. Radiographic Markers—A Reservoir for Bacteria? *Radiography* **2011**, *17*, 115–120. [CrossRef]
23. Bello, A.I.; Asiedu, E.N.; Adegoke, B.O.A.; Quartey, J.N.A.; Appiah-Kubi, K.O.; Owusu-Ansah, B. Nosocomial Infections: Knowledge and Source of Information among Clinical Health Care Students in Ghana. *Int. J. Gen. Med.* **2011**, *4*, 571–574. [CrossRef] [PubMed]
24. Huang, S.Y.; Philip, A.; Richter, M.D.; Gupta, S.; Lessne, M.L.; Kim, C.Y. Prevention and Management of Infectious Complications of Percutaneous Interventions. *Semin. Intervent. Radiol.* **2015**, *32*, 78–88. [CrossRef] [PubMed]
25. Boyle, H.; Strudwick, R.M. Do Lead Rubber Aprons Pose an Infection Risk? *Radiography* **2010**, *16*, 297–303. [CrossRef]
26. Khan, W.; Sullivan, K.L.; McCann, J.W.; Gonsalves, C.F.; Sato, T.; Eschelman, D.J.; Brown, D.B. Moxifloxacin Prophylaxis for Chemoembolization or Embolization in Patients with Previous Biliary Interventions: A Pilot Study. *AJR Am. J. Roentgenol.* **2011**, *197*, W343–W345. [CrossRef]
27. Paul, M.; Leibovici, L. Observational Studies Examining Patient Management in Infectious Diseases. *Clin. Microbiol. Infect.* **2017**, *23*, 127–128. [CrossRef]
28. Concato, J. Observational versus Experimental Studies: What's the Evidence for a Hierarchy? *NeuroRx* **2004**, *1*, 341–347. [CrossRef]

Disclaimer/Publisher's Note: The statements, opinions and data contained in all publications are solely those of the individual author(s) and contributor(s) and not of MDPI and/or the editor(s). MDPI and/or the editor(s) disclaim responsibility for any injury to people or property resulting from any ideas, methods, instructions or products referred to in the content.

MDPI
St. Alban-Anlage 66
4052 Basel
Switzerland
www.mdpi.com

International Journal of Environmental Research and Public Health Editorial Office
E-mail: ijerph@mdpi.com
www.mdpi.com/journal/ijerph

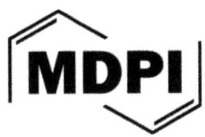

Disclaimer/Publisher's Note: The statements, opinions and data contained in all publications are solely those of the individual author(s) and contributor(s) and not of MDPI and/or the editor(s). MDPI and/or the editor(s) disclaim responsibility for any injury to people or property resulting from any ideas, methods, instructions or products referred to in the content.

www.ingramcontent.com/pod-product-compliance
Lightning Source LLC
LaVergne TN
LVHW070713100526
838202LV00013B/1084